Victory Over Disease

Resolving the Medical Crisis in the Crimean War, 1854–1856

Michael Hinton

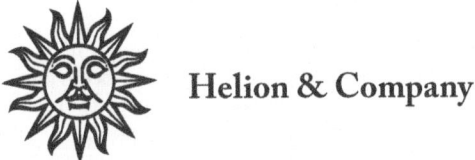 Helion & Company

Helion & Company Limited
Unit 8 Amherst Business Centre
Budbrooke Road
Warwick
CV34 5WE
England
Tel. 01926 499 619
Email: info@helion.co.uk
Website: www.helion.co.uk
Twitter: @helionbooks
Visit our blog http://blog.helion.co.uk/

Published by Helion & Company 2019
Designed and typeset by Mach 3 Solutions Ltd (www.mach3solutions.co.uk)
Cover designed by Paul Hewitt, Battlefield Design (www.battlefield-design.co.uk)

Text and figures © Michael Hinton 2019
Illustrations © as individually credited
Maps © Colin Robins 2019

Front cover: The coloured lithograph on the front cover is of the 93rd Highlanders of thin red line fame encamped on the Western Heights, Dover shortly after their return from the Crimea. It is by a well known local artist, William Burgess (1805–1861), and was one of three comparable lithographs published in *c.*1857. The other two depict the camps of the 41st Regiment, also on the Western Heights, and that of the 44th and 49th Regiments which was located near the Archcliffe Fort.
   The lithograph is preserved in the Dover Museum and Bronze Age Boat Gallery and it is pleasure to acknowledge the permission granted to reproduce it as it provides a suitably graphic demonstration of the Victory over Disease. The camp is clearly neat and tidy and the men look fit and well and this reflects what obtained during last six months of the regiment's time in the Crimea when there was not a single death among the NCOs and men treated for disease in the regimental hospital.

Every reasonable effort has been made to trace copyright holders and to obtain their permission for the use of copyright material. The author and publisher apologize for any errors or omissions in this work, and would be grateful if notified of any corrections that should be incorporated in future reprints or editions of this book.

ISBN 978-1-911628-31-6

British Library Cataloguing-in-Publication Data.
A catalogue record for this book is available from the British Library.

All rights reserved. No part of this publication may be reproduced, stored in a retrieval system, or transmitted, in any form, or by any means, electronic, mechanical, photocopying, recording or otherwise, without the express written consent of Helion & Company Limited.

For details of other military history titles published by Helion & Company Limited contact the above address, or visit our website: http://www.helion.co.uk.

We always welcome receiving book proposals from prospective authors.

Contents

List of Tables		vii
List of Figures		x
List of Maps		xiii
List of Abbreviations		xiv
Acknowledgements		xv
Author's note		xvii

1	Introduction		21
	1.1	Military campaigns, 1808–1852, and the prelude to the Crimean campaign	21
	1.2	The War with Russia 1853–1856	24
	1.3	Military medical knowledge in the mid-19th century	27
	1.4	Army Medical Department	29
		1.4.1 Drs Andrew Smith and John Hall, and Miss Nightingale	30
	1.5	Overview of the disease problems encountered in Bulgaria and the Crimea	31
	1.6	Misleading statistics	32
	1.7	Principal sources consulted	34

2	British Army of the East		41
	2.1	Organization and strength of the Army	41
		2.1.1 Recruitment	44
		2.1.2 Casualties relative to the length of time spent on active service	47
		2.1.3 Reception in the Crimea	49
		2.1.4 Stoicism of the troops	51
		2.1.5 Land Transport Corps	53
		2.1.6 Camp followers	54
		2.1.7 Concluding remarks	55
	2.2	Army Medical Department	55
		2.2.1 Medical officers and principal support staff	55
		2.2.2 Mortality among medical officers	60
		2.2.3 Hospital orderlies	60
		2.2.4 Staffing levels in general and regimental hospitals	62
		2.2.5 Medical Staff Corps	64
		2.2.6 Ambulance Corps	66
		2.2.7 Problems of communication	67
		2.2.8 Discontentment among the military surgeons	68

		2.2.9	Civilian surgeons	72
		2.2.10	Female nurses	75
		2.2.11	Medical supplies sent to the East	77
		2.2.12	Concluding remarks	77
	2.3	Commissariat		78
		2.3.1	Land transport	80
		2.3.2	Harbour facilities	86
		2.3.3	Provisioning the Army	87
		2.3.4	Royal Navy	95
		2.3.5	Concluding remarks	95
3	Provision of hospital facilities			97
	3.1	Turkey		100
		3.1.1	Scutari and Kuleli	101
		3.1.2	Abydos	104
		3.1.3	Smyrna	105
		3.1.4	Renkioi	111
		3.1.5	French hospitals	113
	3.2	Bulgaria		113
	3.3	Crimea		115
		3.3.1	General hospitals	116
		3.3.2	Regimental and divisional hospitals	121
		3.3.3	Provision for battlefield casualties	122
		3.3.4	Preparations for the second winter	124
	3.4	Mediterranean ports		124
	3.5	Other locations considered		128
	3.6	Comparison of hospitals		129
	3.7	Concluding remarks		131
4	Transportation and evacuation of invalids			132
	4.1	Initial planning and further developments		132
	4.2	The Black Sea theatre		137
		4.2.1	Evacuation from Bulgaria	137
		4.2.2	Invasion of the Crimea	137
		4.2.3	Transfer of patients from camp to Balaklava	140
		4.2.4	Preparation of vessels as hospital transports	150
		4.2.5	Embarkation of patients at Balaklava	153
		4.2.6	Employment of hospital transports	155
		4.2.7	Mortality among evacuees	157
		4.2.8	Disembarkation of patients at Scutari	159
		4.2.9	Causes célèbre	160
		4.2.10	Return to duty	162
		4.2.11	Concluding remarks	163
	4.3	Repatriation to England		164
		4.3.1	Provision of hospital transports	165
		4.3.2	Voyage to England	168

		4.3.3	Arrival in England	172
		4.3.4	Transportation from the port to other destinations	178
		4.3.5	Hospital facilities in England	179
		4.3.6	Onward journeys from hospital	189
		4.3.7	Number of invalids transported	190
		4.3.8	Post-war developments	191
	4.4	Concluding remarks		191
5	Diseases			194
	5.1	Diarrhoea and dysentery		195
	5.2	Cholera		202
		5.2.1	Clinical features	202
		5.2.2	Contemporary views on the cause, treatments and prevention	203
		5.2.3	Observations in camp	206
		5.2.4	Cholera in the Army, 1854–1856	207
		5.2.5	Concluding remarks	210
	5.3	Fevers		213
	5.4	Scurvy and Frostbite		215
	5.5	Other diseases		218
		5.5.1	Nosocomial (hospital acquired) infections	218
		5.5.2	Other infectious diseases	220
		5.5.3	Conditions typically associated with low mortality	223
	5.6	Non-medical hospital admissions and miscellaneous topics		223
	5.7	Intervals between admission and death		226
	5.8	Accidental deaths		227
	5.9	Concluding remarks		228
6	Casualties consequent upon action with the enemy			231
	6.1	General hospitals in the Crimea and Turkey		235
	6.2	Fatalities due to wounds or injuries		237
	6.3	Adjutant General's ledger		238
	6.4	Captain Sayer's analyses		242
	6.5	Outcome for wounded personnel		243
	6.6	Concluding remarks		246
7	Hospitals on the Bosphorus			247
	7.1	Mortality from disease in the Crimea and at Scutari		247
	7.2	Cholera		249
	7.3	Gunshot wounds (*Vulnus sclopitorum*)		249
	7.4	Conditions typically associated with low mortality		250
	7.5	Concluding remarks		250
8	Repatriation and discharge from the Army			255
	8.1	Repatriation for disease		256
	8.2	Repatriation for wounds and injuries		258
	8.3	Mortality among repatriated patients		259

	8.4	Reasons for discharge	259
	8.5	Potential future employment	260
	8.6	Concluding remarks	260
9	Commissions and committees of enquiry	261
	9.1	Hospital Commission	261
	9.2	Select Committee of the House of Commons	263
	9.3	Supplies Commission	267
	9.4	Sanitary Commission	269
		9.4.1 Scutari	270
		9.4.2 Crimea	274
		9.4.3 Responses to the report	283
	9.5	Select Committee on the Army Medical Department	285
	9.6	Royal Commission	286
	9.7	Concluding remarks	287
10	Reflections on the War	292
	10.1	Technology and medicine	292
	10.2	Victoria Cross, orders and medals	297
	10.3	Administrative reform	299
	10.4	Royal Patriotic Fund and other charities	300
	10.5	The British and the French	301
	10.6	Civilian disasters	303
	10.7	Power of the press and official publications	303
	10.8	Visual arts	304
	10.9	Memorials to the fallen	308
	10.10	A lasting legacy?	314
11	Afterword	315
Appendix: Principal personalities	322
Bibliography	326
Index	340

List of Tables

1.1	Summary of three amphibious invasions with limited objectives involving British forces, 1808, 1854, and 1915	21
1.2	The number of NCOs and men who suffered from wounds, sickness or injury during the campaigns in the Crimea and Gallipoli, and the South African War	23
1.3	The strength and losses in the principal corps of the Army of the East	26
1.4	Mortality from disease in the cavalry and infantry divisions which landed with the Expeditionary Army in the Crimea	31
1.5	Mortality rate for the whole campaign calculated using Colonel Tulloch's method, April 1854–June 1856	33
1.6	Mortality in the hospitals in England, Scutari, and Kuleli	34
1.7	Losses sustained by the British and French armies during the Crimean campaign	38
2.1	Deaths in the infantry regiments in relation to the time spent on active service in Bulgaria and the Crimea	48
2.2	Deaths in the infantry regiments in relation to the time spent on active service in Bulgaria and the Crimea together with those who were invalided	48
2.3	Number (%) medical staff employed in the Army of the East	77
3.1	The months during which the hospitals of the Army of the East were in operation, April 1854–June 1856	98
3.2	Admissions to and death from wounds and injuries in the general hospitals in the Crimea	130
4.1	Correspondence concerning the transfer of invalids from camp to Balaklava, December 1854–August 1855	140
4.2	Number of hospital ships departing from the Crimea during different phases of the campaign, September 1854–June 1856	158
4.3	The number of NCO and men in fifty-two infantry regiments who died in general hospitals and on board ship, and who were invalided home according to the month of arrival in the East	159
4.4	Press reports published following the arrival in British waters of ships conveying invalids	174
4.5	Generosity extended to invalids following their arrival in England	177
4.6	Number of passengers, including invalids, landed at Portsmouth during January and February 1855	184
5.1	Principal reasons for primary admissions into the hospitals of the Army of the East and also the deaths which occurred in the regimental and general hospitals and hospital ships with the exception of those killed in action, April 1854–June 1856	196

5.2	Twenty most common reasons for the admission of NCOs and men into hospital for disease, April 1854–June 1856	197
5.3	Ratio percent to strength during each month of admissions and deaths in General Return B	198
5.4	Gastrointestinal diseases, excepting cholera, diagnosed in NCOs and men, April 1854–June 1856	200
5.5	Conditions typically associated with low mortality listed in the *Medical and Surgical History*, 2, General Return A, April 1854–June 1856	224
5.6	Number of patients in cavalry, Guards and infantry regiments dying each week during the weeks following admission to hospital	227
5.7	Chronicles of contagion, AD 165–1918	230
6.1	Management of men suffering battlefield injuries	233
6.2	The wounds and injuries sustained by NCOs and men during the Eastern campaign, April 1854–June 1856	235
6.3	Numbers of NCOs and men admitted to hospitals in the Crimea and Turkey with gunshot wounds (*Vulnus sclopitorum*), September 1854–September 1855 and October–December 1855	236
6.4	The number of deaths among NCOs and men who sustained wounds and injuries, April 1854–June 1856	237
6.5	Time to death from fatal wounds and mechanical injuries	238
6.6	Casualties according to rank, 18 September 1854–8 September 1855	239
6.7	Number of casualties resulting from action with the enemy, 18 September 1854–8 September 1855	239
6.8	The proportion of officers and men killed during battles, siege operations, and assaults on Sevastopol, 18 September 1854–8 September 1855	240
6.9	Minimum, maximum, and median number of casualties sustained each day during siege operations, exclusive of the three principal assaults on Sevastopol, October 1854–September 1855	241
6.10	Distribution of casualties among officers and men according the number that were recorded on each day of the siege	241
6.11	Number of officers, sergeants and men who served in the cavalry, infantry, Royal Artillery, and RS&M during the Crimean campaign, together with the numbers who were killed and wounded	242
6.12	Number of officers, sergeants and men who served in the cavalry, infantry, Royal Artillery, and RS&M during the Crimean campaign, together with the numbers who were killed and wounded	243
6.13	The outcome for NCOs and men with gunshot wounds	244
6.14	Length of time taken for 4,015 NCOs and men to return to duty after treatment for wounds	245
6.15	NCOs and men disabled and discharged the service for wounds and other injuries	245
7.1	Conditions typically associated with low mortality listed in the *Medical and Surgical History*, 2, General Return A, April 1854–June 1856	251
7.2	Conditions typically associated with low mortality listed in the *Medical and Surgical History*, 2, General Hospital Returns I, April 1854–June 1856	252
7.3	Examples of misinformation on the state of the hospitals on the Bosphorus	253

8.1	The seven most common disease conditions recorded for the primary admission of NCOs and men into the hospitals of the Army and for their selection for evacuation to Turkey and England, and discharge from the Army	257
8.2	The number of NCOs and men with wounds and injuries who were admitted to hospital, repatriated to England, and discharged from the Army	258
8.3	The number of NCOs and men who died of disease during the voyage to England or after arrival	259
9.1	Responses of senior officers to questions posed by the Roebuck Committee during March 1855 on the health of the troops under their command	264

List of Figures

1.1	Hospital in Sebastopol. – Dr Duigan attending the wounded. (From a sketch by E.A. Goodall, *Illustrated London News*, 6 October 1855, p.404)	40
2.1	The number of cavalry and infantry regiments serving in the Army of the East, April 1854–June 1856.	42
2.2	The estimated strength of the cavalry and infantry regiments and the ordnance, April 1854–June 1856.	43
2.3	The age distribution of 70,425 NCOs and men in the cavalry and infantry 'who were sent to the East'.	44
2.4	Relationship between the numbers of NCOs and men in each year group and the mortality rate.	51
2.5	Mortality from disease in the Land Transport Corps and the Army, June 1855–March 1856.	54
2.6	Number, and the trend, of regimental and staff surgeons each month, April 1854–April 1856.	56
2.7	Embarkation of cattle, at Trieste for the Auxiliary Army in the East. (*Illustrated London News*, 15 July 1854, p.33)	80
2.8	Commencement of the railway works at Balaclava. (*Illustrated London News*, 10 March 1855, p.224)	83
2.9	Shipment of wooden barracks, on board "The White Falcon", at Southampton, for the French Army in the Crimea. (*Illustrated London News*, 3 February 1855, p.105)	93
3.1	The British hospital, Scutari (From a sketch by Julian Portch. *Illustrated Times*, 8 December 1855)	102
3.2	The Kukeieh (*sic*) Barracks, Constantinople – The Royal Artillery disembarking. (From 'The Jason'. *Illustrated London News*, 16 September 1854, p.260)	102
3.3	The English Hospital at Abydos. (*Illustrated London News*, 6 January 1854, p.244)	105
3.4	The hospital at Smyrna (From a sketch by Julian Portch. *Illustrated Times*, 24 November 1854, p.396)	106
3.5	The British hospital at Renkioi. (*Illustrated Times*, 1 December 1855, p.412)	112
3.6	Hospital and the quarters of the medical staff, Balaclava harbour. (From a sketch by Julian Portch, *Illustrated Times*, 11 August 1855, p.149)	117
3.7	New ambulance transport service. (*Illustrated London News*, 4 August 1855, p.156)	118

3.8	The new sanatorium, or Castle Hospital, at Balaclava. (From a sketch by Julian Portch, *Illustrated Times*, 11 August 1855)	118
3.9	The new Castle Hospital at Balaclava. (*Illustrated London News*, 28 July 1855)	119
3.10	Therapia, sketched from the Asiatic bank of the Bosphorus. (*Illustrated London News*, 6 August 1853, p.97)	121
3.11	Brigade hospital of the Light Division. (From a sketch by Julian Portch, *Illustrated Times*, 12 July 1856, p.4)	122
4.1	The Guards carrying a wounded officer from Inkerman. (*Illustrated London News*, 3 February 1855, p.116)	134
4.2	Morning: returning from the trenches. (*Illustrated Times*, 14 July 1855, p.89)	134
4.3	The sick-deck 'The Bellisle' hospital ship, in Faro sound. (*Illustrated London News*, 18 August 1855, p.220)	136
4.4	Siege of Sebastopol – Dr Smith's new hospital waggon. (*Illustrated London News*, 4 November 1854, p.448)	143
4.5	Ambulance for the wounded. (*Illustrated London News*, 30 December 1854, p.693)	144
4.6	French ambulances, before Sebastopol. (*Illustrated London News*, 16 December 1854, p.625)	146
4.7	Carrying the frost bitten to Balaclava. (*Illustrated London News*, 3 March 1855, p.213)	146
4.8	French cacolets carrying wounded before Sebastopol. (*Illustrated London News*, 27 January 1855, p.80)	147
4.9	"The Himalaya" steamship. (*Illustrated London News*, 21 January 1854, p.48)	169
4.10	Landing the wounded from 'HMS Retribution', at Portsmouth. (*Illustrated London News*, 17 February 1855, p.153)	175
4.11	Her Majesty inspecting the wounded troops, at Fort Pitt hospital, Chatham. (*Illustrated London News*, 10 March 1855, p.236)	181
4.12	Invalided soldiers before the hospital barracks, at Brompton. (*Illustrated London News*, 21 July 1855, p.69)	181
4.13	The Military hospital, Portsea. (*Illustrated London News*, 10 February 1855, p.128)	185
5.1	Primary admissions of NCOs and men to hospitals in Turkey, Bulgaria, and the Crimea, April 1854–June 1856.	199
5.2	Deaths of NCOs and men in regimental and general hospitals and on board ship, April 1854–June 1856.	199
5.3	Admissions for, and deaths from diarrhoea and dysentery, fevers, and cholera among NCOs and men, April 1854–June 1856.	201
5.4	Cumulative proportion (%) of deaths from diarrhoea and dysentery, fevers, and cholera among NCOs and men, April 1854–June 1856.	201
5.5	Admissions for, and deaths from cholera among NCOs and men, April 1854–June 1856.	208
5.6	Deaths among NCOs and men from cholera in the Army as a whole and the hospitals at Scutari, April 1854–June 1856.	209
5.7	Admissions, for, and deaths from fevers among NCOs and men, April 1854–June 1856.	214
5.8	Admissions, for, and deaths from scurvy among NCOs and men, April 1854–June 1856.	216

5.9	Admissions, for, and deaths from frostbite among NCOs and men, April 1854–June 1856.	216
5.10	Admissions of NCOs and men to hospital with gangrene or erysipelas, June 1854–June 1856.	221
5.11	Deaths of NCOs and men from gangrene or erysipelas, June 1854–June 1856.	221
6.1	Near Sebastopol – Ambulance waiting for the wounded. (*Illustrated London News*, 2 June 1855, p.540.	232
6.2	The Redan at sunset, September 8 – removing the wounded. (Sketched by E.A. Goodhall. *Illustrated London News*, 6 November 185, p.416)	232
6.3	The number of NCOs and men admitted to hospital with, or died from, gunshot wounds, April 1854–June 1856.	234
7.1	Deaths from diarrhoea and dysentery in regimental hospitals and the hospitals on the Bosphorus, September 1854–July 1855.	248
7.2	Deaths from continued fever in regimental hospitals and the hospitals on the Bosphorus, September 1854–July 1855.	248
7.3	Deaths from scurvy in regimental hospitals and the hospitals on the Bosphorus, September 1854–July 1855.	248
7.4	Deaths from frostbite in regimental hospitals and the hospitals on the Bosphorus, September 1854–July 1855.	249
8.1	The average daily number of vacant beds in the hospitals at Chatham, Chichester, Plymouth, and Portsmouth for each week from 21 February until 25 July 1856.	257
9.1	Winter clothing for the British troops in the Crimea. (*Illustrated London News*, 23 December 1854, p.649)	269
9.1	Mortality in British troops in the United Kingdom, 1840–1913.	288
10.1	A Sergeant Dawson and his daughter at Chatham by J.J.E. Mayall. (Royal Collection Trust/© Her Majesty Queen Elizabeth II, 2019) B A convalescent from Inkerman. (*Illustrated Times*, 9 June 1855, p.5)	308
10.2	The siege of Sebastopol – Burial of the dead in front of the Malakoff Tower. (*Illustrated London News*, 21 April 1855, p.384)	309
10.3	The battle-field of the Tchernaya – Burying the dead. (Sketched by Julian Portch, *Illustrated Times*, 15 September 1855, p.237)	309
10.4	Afternoon: The valley of the shadow of death. (*Illustrated Times*, 14 July 1855, p.89)	310
10.5	Graves at Scutari. (*Illustrated London News*, 24 March 1855, p.288)	310
10.6	Inkerman Mill – The scene or the recent explosion. (*Illustrated London News*, 8 December 1855, p.673)	312
10.7	Burial ground on Cathcart's Hill in the Crimea. (*Illustrated London News*, 2 February 1856, p.129)	312

List of Maps

3.1 Location of the general hospitals in Turkey and Bulgaria. (Map by Colin Robins, used with permission) 99
3.2 Location of the general hospitals in the Crimea. (Map by Colin Robins, used with permission) 99

List of Abbreviations

Add Ms:	Additional manuscripts
ADM:	Admiralty documents on the The National Archives
AG:	Adjutant General, also A(Assistant)AG
AoT:	Agent of Transports
AC:	Ambulance Corps
AMD:	Army and Ordnance Medical Department
AWC:	Army Works Corps
CEC:	Civil Engineering Corps
Deputy Secretary:	Deputy Secretary for War (Benjamin Hawes)
DG:	Director General
DIGH:	Deputy Inspector General of Hospitals
GOC:	General Officer Commanding
FO:	Foreign Office documents on the The National Archives
HCPP:	House of Commons Parliamentary Papers
HMS:	Her Majesty's Ship
IGH:	Inspector General of Hospitals, also D (Deputy)IGH
LTC:	Land Transport Corps
MOH:	Medical Officers of Health
MSC:	Medical Staff Corps
NCO:	Non-commissioned officer
PMO:	Principal Medical Officer
QMG:	Quartermaster General, also A(Assistant)QMG and D(Deputy) AQMG
RA:	Royal Artillery
RAMC:	Royal Army Medical Corps
RE:	Royal Engineers
RS&M:	Royal Sappers and Miners
TNA:	The National Archives
Undersecretary:	Undersecretary at War (Frederick Peel, MP)
VC:	Victoria Cross
WO:	War Office documents in The National Archives

Acknowledgements

This monograph has its origins in the research undertaken for a PhD thesis that was carried out at King's College London under the tutelage of Andrew Lambert, and to him I owe my thanks for his patience and wise council. Similarly, I wish to thank my commissioning editor at Helion & Co Ltd, Christopher Brice. Over the years I have written plenty of papers and essays for journals, as well as review articles and book chapters; but I nave never attempted a book before. His assistance in steering me through this tortuous process has been very much appreciated.

In addition, I am also particularly grateful to my friends Douglas Austin, Glenn Fisher, and Tony Margrave for the considerable help they have given while pursuing our common interest in the Crimean War; and for fun we had visiting various archives. I would like to thank additionally Douglas Austin for commentating on presentational matters, Tony Margrave for generously sharing his knowledge of the contents of The National Archives, and in particular the WO series, and Colin Robins for help in a multitude of ways. It is also a pleasure to acknowledge the assistance I have received over the years from the following; listed in alphabetical order: James Austin, John Barham, Michael Trevor-Barnston, Ann Bates, Jeff Bennett, Louise Berridge, Brian Best, Walter Bonnici, John Clewlow, Dave Cliff, Janet Corry, Larry Crider, Bill Curtis, Mark Davidson, Marianne Gilchrist, Alan Hedges, Tony and Jo James, Aled Jones, David Jones, David Kelsey, Norman Kirby, Peter Knox, Jérôme Lantz, René Maussion, Mike Hargreave Mawson, Tom Muir, Iffet Ozgonul, David Pick, Tim Pickles, Matt Pizzo, Helen Rappaport, Rod Robinson, John Rumsby, Hugh Small, Colin Smith, Keith Smith, Pete Starling, Megan Stevens, David Thurlow, Lee and Ken Tough, Paul Watkins, Bryan Williams, David Williams, Abigail Woods, and Gill Woods; and those no longer with us: Brian Abbott, Geoffrey Copus, Ken Horton, Bob Glover, Tony Lucking, James Mackie, and Michael Springman; and last, but certainly not least, to my wife Sheila for her considerable forbearance during the whole enterprise.

Over the years I have spent many happy hours in libraries and museums, for example, the Army Medical Services Museum, Bristol University Library, British Library, Brunel Institute, Caird Library, Florence Nightingale Museum, Kings College Library, London Guildhall Library, London Metropolitan Archive, London School of Hygiene and Tropical Medicine Library, National Army Museum Archive, National Archives of Scotland, National Library of Scotland, Nottingham University

Library, Royal College of Surgeons' Library, Royal College of Veterinary Surgeons' Library, Royal Society of Medicine's Library, Society of Apothecaries Archive, Society of Genealogists' Library, The National Archives, Tunbridge Wells Library, and Wellcome Trust Library, as well as a number of county record offices, particularly those in Gloucestershire and Wiltshire, and regimental museums, several of which have artefacts on medical interest. I have always been welcomed with unfailing courtesy, and I am obliged to the staff of all these institutions.

Author's note

My interest in the Crimean campaign was kindled during the 1990s when studying the history of my family. One of my 2x great grandfathers, James William Dewar, served in the 49th Regiment as a company commander, and as one of the town majors of Sevastopol following its occupation by the allies.

When I turned to the topic I was a Reader in Veterinary Public Health in the University of Bristol, and my principal research interest was infectious diseases. I was immediately attracted by just how much these shaped the course of the Crimean campaign. After my retirement in 2006 I was fortunate to register at King's College London to study for a PhD degree under Professor Andrew Lambert. My thesis finally emerged after a long gestation. This book, based in large measure on its contents, represents a further development.

I have concentrated as far as possible on primary sources, specifically because my aim was to produce an evidence-based account. There are many footnotes and I make no apology for them. When I started the project I had no preconceptions, because I knew little of the subject. It came as something of a surprise when I found it necessary to question seriously the contributions made by the talented and well-connected Florence Nightingale and the suitably-qualified Sanitary Commissioners – who were sent by the government to investigate matters on the spot in the spring of 1855. This may prove an unexpected and possibly unsympathetic conclusion for some of Nightingale's many admirers. However, I would ask them to heed the words of Fern Liddell who concluded her commentary on her book on the terrorist activities of some suffragettes:[1] 'A half history or a sanitised history, *or one that is based on inadequate research or a misinterpretation of the facts, either through ignorance of by design*, (author's italics), serves no one – it's a corruption. History should not be comfortable and it should not be safe. It should always challenge and it should always be challenged.'[2] On the other hand, to make use of the words of Major John Bennett, RAMC, my

---

1 F. Riddell, *Death in Ten Minutes: Kitty Marion: Activist, Arsonist. Suffragette* (London: Hodder & Stoughton, 2018).
2 *BBC History Magazine*, May 2018, pp. 66–7.

conclusions should not be seen to 'detract from [Nightingale]', rather they should 'remind us that other people were contributing to reform.'[3]

Having 'calmly weighed' the evidence, to use P.B. Maxwell's aphorism – quoted in its original context in Section 10.1[4] – it became clear to me that there is little tangible proof that Nightingale and the Sanitary Commissioners significantly influenced the improvement in the health of the Army in the Crimea. The principal problems were at the front, not in Turkey, and it was there that matters were gradually rectified, and the health of the troops began to improve during the early weeks of 1855.

And what about Mrs Mary Seacole? She arrived in the Crimea during March 1855 when the worst of the horrors of the winter were over. Her principal objective was to set up a catering establishment with her business partner Thomas Day. She never had a hospital and did not have formal access to any of the military hospitals. The so called 'British Hotel' proved a successful venture, at least until the Army began to evacuate the Crimea. Its management would have taken up most of her time and her opportunities for 'nursing' would have been limited – and carried out on an informal basis. She was obviously a much-liked and popular personality, but, in the final analysis her contribution to the overall 'Victory over Disease' would have been minimal. The absence of any medical records means that what ever she achieved cannot now be determined.

The most significant outcome of my investigations is summed up in Figures 7.1–7.4. These provide astonishingly clear-cut evidence that the problems in the hospitals on the Bosphorus merely reflected the situation in the Crimea. Therefore, improvements in survival at Scutari can be largely explained by an improved prognosis for the men selected for evacuation. Surprisingly, the conditions in the hospitals, though at times considerably less than satisfactory, seemed to have had relatively little influence on these events.

The historiography of the campaign has tended to concentrate on the disasters of the first winter and the perceived incompetence of the heads of department, while the contributions made by Nightingale and the Sanitary Commissioners have been over-emphasised. Inevitably this has established an unbalanced view of what actually took place. That view has been distorted further by commentators who to have failed to consider events in the strict order of their occurrence, and who have confused matters further by applying the direful knowledge of hindsight. As a consequence this aspect of the war has been inaccurately portrayed in both academic works and popular culture.[5]

---

3   J. Bennett, 'The Medical Service in the Crimea' In: *Redressing the Balance* (London: Florence Nightingale Museum Trust, 1991), pp.3–10.
4   Maxwell was one of the hospital commissioners, and author of an anonymous commentary of the Roebuck Committee Report; Anon [Peter Benson Maxwell], *Whom Shall We Hang? The Sebastopol Enquiry* (London: James Ridgeway, 1855).
5   For further thoughts on the peddling of misinformation see M. Hinton 'Reporting the Crimean War', *19: Interdisciplinary Studies in the Long Nineteenth Century*, 20 (2015), DOI: http://doi.org/10.16995/ntn.711.

Contemporary correspondence from Nightingale herself provides support for my conclusions. She informed Lord Panmure that: 'The men sent down to Scutari in the winter died because they were not sent down till half dead,'[6] and 'told Sidney Herbert unequivocally, Scutari was only a symptom of the army's malady, not a cause, and once things began to improve at Balaclava, things improved at Scutari. Once the men [...] began to get better food and the weather became warmer, their strength increased, they became more resistant to disease, the number arriving at Scutari went down, the wards became less crowded, and the medical personnel were under less pressure.'[7]

Similarly, the initial findings of the Sanitary Commissioners in the camps confirm that the Army was getting matters under control. They were: 'much surprised and gratified with the appearance of the camp and of the hospitals [...] as no sanitary recommendations were required from them for the upper camp.' and that there were 'no sanitary measure we could recommend [that they had] not seen carried out today in some phase or other.'[8]

There is thus little evidence to support the assertion that Nightingale made later to Lord Shaftsbury, that the Sanitary Commission 'Saved the British Army'[9] or indeed that their efforts were other than subsidiary. Rather, the progressive enhancement in the standard of living of the troops by providing adequate food, clothing, fuel and shelter, coupled with improvements in health care in the camps and general hospitals in the Crimea, from early in 1855. Those improvements resulted in the 'Victory over Disease' in 1856 – which Panmure acknowledged when proposing a vote of thanks to the armed forces in the House of Lords after the ratification of the Peace Treaty.[10]

It may well be too much to hope that my analyses will alter existing preconceptions, or prejudices about what happened in Crimea and Turkey during those fateful years. Perhaps the best I can expect is that some future commentators will take my conclusions into account and thereby provide a more balanced explanation of what actually took place. The 'Victory over Disease' was not due to the contributions of any one person, or even a group of individuals. Rather it represented the involvement of many people in many walks of life who worked, possibly unwittingly, for a common purpose and with such a gratifying result.

The last British troops sailed from the Crimea on 12 July 1856 and Scutari was finally evacuated a few weeks later. The Crimean campaign thereby became history

---

6   H. Small, *Florence Nightingale. Avenging Angel* (2nd edition) (London: Knowledge Leak, 2013), p.76.
7   G. Gill, *Nightingales: The Story of Florence Nightingale and her Remarkable Family* (London: Hodder and Stoughton, 2004), p.393–4.
8   The sanitary commissioners inspected the camps before Sevastopol on 26 April 1855 and this is an extract from a report of their visit prepared by Lieutenant Colonel Gordon, AQMG, for Major General Airey; TNA: WO 33/1/49/55, Inclosure 12 and WO 28/192.
9   E. Hodder, *The Life and Work of the Seventh Earl of Shaftsbury, KG* (London: Cassell, 1887), 2, p.195.
10 *Hansard*, 8 May 1856.

and nothing could be changed. Nightingale's greatest achievements, together with the germ theory which contributed to the elucidation of the infectious diseases that caused so such havoc amongst the troops, were yet to come.

Mike Hinton
Tunbridge Wells, 2019

1

Introduction

1.1 Military campaigns, 1808–1852, and the prelude to the Crimean campaign

Mark Harrison observed: 'Each theatre of operation [is] ecologically distinct and [presents] unique problems.'[1] It is inappropriate, therefore, to compare the medical aspects of different campaigns; except possibly in a superficial manner. Of the campaigns involving British troops during the first half of the 19th century it is only the Walcheren expedition that has certain similarities with the Crimean War. For example, both involved a sea-borne invasion, were of relatively short duration, had only a limited objective, were fought in a temperate rather than a tropical region, and were characterized by a high incidence of infectious diseases. However, the absence of detailed medical records from 1809 makes it impossible to make more than the simple comparisons set out in Table 1.1. The table includes reference to the Gallipoli campaign of 1915 as this has features similar to the other two.

Table 1.1 Summary of three amphibious invasions with limited objectives involving British forces, 1808, 1854, and 1915

Topic	Walcheren	Crimean campaign	Gallipoli
Dates	July–December 1809.	September 1854–July 1856, with the fall of Sevastopol on 8 September 1855.	March 1915–January 1916.
Invasion	Limited opposition.	Unopposed.	Opposed.
Principal strategic objective	Destruction of Flushing's port facilities: *Achieved*.	Destruction of Sevastopol's port facilities and prevention of Russian control of the Bosphorus: *Achieved*.	Control of the Bosphorus and access of the Black Sea: *Failed*.

1   M. Harrison, *The Medical War: British Military Medicine in the First World War* (Oxford: University Press, 2010), p.291.

Topic	Walcheren	Crimean campaign	Gallipoli
Principal forces	Army with essential naval support.	Army with essential naval support.	Army with essential naval support.
Principal belligerents	British v. French and Dutch.	British, French, Turks, and Sardinians v. Russians.	British, Empire forces, and French v. Turks.
Lines of communication	Short.	Long.	Long.
Military actions	Occupation and siege.	Pitched battles and trench warfare.	Principally trench warfare.
Naval losses	Minimal.	Minimal.	Considerable.
Disease problems	Serious epidemic of malarial fever that remained unresolved.	Serious epidemics of cholera and enteric disease which were resolved during the campaign.	Serious losses particularly from enteric disease and PUOs; problems that remained largely unresolved.
Mortality from disease	High.	High during the winter of 1854/55 for the diseases other than cholera.	Relatively low.
Casualties	No large scale evacuation of casualties.	Many casualties evacuated by sea to base hospitals.	Many casualties evacuated by sea to base hospitals.
Supplies	Some supplies obtained locally, except munitions.	All supplies brought by sea.	All supplies brought by sea.
Evacuation	Unopposed.	Unopposed.	Largely unopposed.

One attribute that distinguished the Crimean campaign from the two others was that the occupation continued after hostilities ceased and this allowed time to demonstrate that the medical problems had been overcome to provide a 'Victory over Disease'. By contrast, the 'Sanitary Disaster' was not resolved in the other campaigns, and it is this aspect of the Walcheren expedition which is particularly remembered.[2] The mortality rate from disease, but not wounds, was lower in the South African War and Gallipoli campaign (Table 1.2). A commission of enquiry convened after the Walcheren expedition exonerated the doctors but blamed the Medical Board. The members were dismissed, for 'poor planning and a failure to cope urgently with the disaster.'[3]

---

[2] See M.R. Howard, *Walcheren 1809: The Scandalous Destruction of a British Army* (Barnsley: Pen & Sword Military, 2012).
[3] J. Shepherd, *The Crimean Doctors: A History of the Medical Services in the Crimean War* (Liverpool: University Press, 1991), 1, pp.4–5.

Table 1.2 The number of NCOs and men who suffered from wounds, sickness or injury during the campaigns in the Crimea and Gallipoli, and the South African War

Location	Period	Force	Wounds			Sickness or injury		
			Number of cases	Deaths	Mortality (%)	Number of cases	Deaths	Mortality (%)
Crimean campaign*	1854–56	British	18,253†	1,761	9.5	144,390	16,297	11.5‡
South African War (p.271, Table 9a)§	1899–1902	British	21,292	1,835	8.5	404,126	13,682	3.5
Dardanelles (p.201, Table 5)§	1915–16	British	48,358	5,135	10.5	139,140	2,043	1.5

* *Medical and Surgical History*, 2, General Return A.
† This total included 10,691 and 1,270 cases of *Vulnus sclopitorum* (Gunshot wounds) and *Vulnus incisum* (Incised wounds) respectively; of whom 1,706 (16%) and 18 (1.5%) died.
‡ 8.5% if cholera is excluded.
§ The page and table number in the facsimile edition of T.J. Mitchell and G.M. Smith, *Medical Services: Casualties and Medical Statistics of the Great War*, (London: HMSO, 1931) published by the Naval and Military Press, Uckfield, and the Imperial War Museum.

When war with Russia appeared inevitable the Director General (DG) of the Army Medical Department (AMD), Dr, later Sir Andrew, Smith, had the foresight to send Drs D. Dumbreck, W. Linton, and J. Mitchell to make a reconnaissance in the Balkans and Turkey. Dumbreck visited the Danubian Provinces and made a number of sensible suggestions in his report.[4] For example, the need for more appropriate summer and winter clothing, prophylaxis against malaria, the adoption of strict hygiene measures, and the filtration of water. Smith requested the military authorities to implement Dumbreck's recommendations but in the most part no action was taken.

Smith had 'to create a wartime organization from scratch,' and, as only a short war in the principalities of Moldovia and Wallachia was envisaged there would have been little incentive for 'the Army Medical Department [and by the same token the Army as a whole] to have laid contingency plans for a prolonged campaign in the Crimea.'[5] The potential for a Sanitary Disaster was therefore present from the start, and this will be expanded upon later.

4 HCPP 1857–58 [2434] XXXVIII.Pt.I.1, Appendix 1 and summarized by N. Cantlie, *A History of the Army Medical Department* (Edinburgh: Churchill Livingston, 1974), 2, pp.18–9; Shepherd, *Crimean Doctors*, 1, p.39; and T. Scotland and S. Heys, *Wars, Pestilence and the Surgeon's Blade* (Solihull: Helion, 2013), pp.212–3.
5 T. Royle, *Crimea: The Great Crimean War 1854–1856* (London: Little Brown and Company, 1999), p.205–6.

1.2 The War with Russia 1853–1856

It is a well recognized fact that the British Army had been 'run down' since the Napoleonic War and it was hence under strength and relatively poorly equipped when war was declared, while the military infrastructure was more suited to defending the British Empire than fighting a European war.[6] The War with Russia was the only one in Europe between 1815 and 1914 that involved British troops and the conduct of the campaign tended to follow 18th and early 19th century military principles in several respects: 'Authority [was] concentrated in the commander and his small staff; [a system which proved] wholly unsuited to […] operations [requiring] co-ordination between the different branches of the Army, as well as between the Army and Navy.'[7] On the other hand, it involved the employment of modern technology including rifled muskets, steam-powered ships, an electric telegraph, a railway network, and vulcanized rubber products, steam-powered saw mills, and a floating bakery and factory ship.

Turkey declared war on Russia on 5 October 1853 following its occupation of the Danubian principalities of Moldavia and Wallachia (modern day Romania) on the pretext of preventing internal disorder.[8] The prospect of an escalation in hostilities increased following the Russian's destruction of a Turkish flotilla moored at Sinope (now Sinop) on 30 November 1853.[9] The British government responded by ordering the Mediterranean fleet to enter the Black Sea during January 1854; several regiments to embark for Malta on 22 February; and for a fleet to sail for the Baltic early in March. Relations with Russia continued to deteriorate and the British and French governments declared war on 28 March 1854.

The first allied troops arrived in Turkey during April 1854 and after some two months the British and French Armies moved to Bulgaria to support the Ottoman Army engaged with the Russians along the River Danube. The Turks put up a stout resistance and following the raising of the siege of Silistria on the 22 June 1854 the Russians withdrew across the River Pruth thus bringing the initial phase of hostilities to an end. Austria, which remained neutral, then occupied the principalities thus separating the combatants and confining hostilities to the Baltic and Black Sea theatres.

The allied armies remained in Bulgaria until shortly before landing in the Crimea on 14 September 1854. The main battles took place in the weeks that followed: at

---

6 See M.H. Kaufman, *Surgeons at War: Medical Arrangements for the Treatment of the Sick and Wounded in the British Army during the Late 18th and 19th Centuries* (London: Greenwood Press, 2000). p.131.
7 M. Harrison, *Medicine and Victory* (Oxford: University Press, 2004), p.11.
8 For details of the Bulgarian campaign involving the Ottoman and Russian armies see İ. Köremezli, *Ottoman War on the Danube: State, Subject, and Soldier, 1853–1856* (Unpublished PhD thesis, 2013: İhsan Doğramaci Bilkent University, Ankara).
9 For a Turkish account see M. Hinton, 'The Infamous Massacre at Sinope: a Turkish Perspective', *The War Correspondent*, 30:3 (2012), pp.19–22.

the Alma (21 September), Balaklava (25 October), and Inkerman (26 October and 5 November). Thereafter the conflict continued as static trench warfare. In July 1855 General Simpson, who succeeded Raglan, foresaw the likelihood of the allies spending a second winter in the Crimea when he informed Panmure that: 'Whether Sevastopol falls or not we are likely to remain on this ground for the protection of Balaklava and it becomes necessary to look to our supplies. Huts, stable huts, storehouses in camp. Clothing, boots, sabots, are matters of immediate consideration.' He then continued: 'I wish to record my conviction that our man cannot stand another winter in the trenches. Both officers and men are worn out. Their endurance and pluck are beyond all description, but this state of things cannot last, and human strength must yield to a continuance of the severe duty of the trenches.'[10] Fortunately this did not come to pass.

There was a further battle at the river Tchernaya on 16 August 1855, which involved the French and Sardinians, and two major assaults on Sevastopol on 18 June and 8 September. The French captured the Malakov tower on the second occasion and this resulted in the Russians evacuating the south of the city. This was then occupied by the British and French. There was little serious fighting following this and hostilities ceased officially on 27 April 1856 with the ratification of the Treaty of Paris signed on 30 March 1856. The bulk of the allied armies had left the Crimea by the end of June with the last British troops leaving Balaklava on the 12 July 1856.

After the war Captain Frederic Sayer, who served in the Crimea, published a book based on official documents available at Horse Guards.[11] An analysis showed that 3,905 officers and 93,959 sergeants and men served in the Army of the East with the infantry comprising 78 percent of the total force with the cavalry, artillery and the engineers accounting for 8.5, 11.5, and two percent respectively (Table 1.3). A summary of losses in the same table indicate that the losses in officers from all causes in each corps was approximately proportional to their total strength while for other ranks the losses in the cavalry and RS&M were relatively lower than those sustained by the infantry and to a less extent the artillery.

Within the Black Sea theatre, the principal focus of this monograph, the forcing of the river Alma was seen as a heroic military success and earned Lord Raglan a field marshal's baton while the battles of Balaklava and Inkerman were perceived as impressive feats of arms. These engagements proved indecisive and a stalemate ensued. This, coupled with the progressive deterioration of conditions at the front in the Crimea during the winter of 1854–55 had a destabilizing effect on the political situation and the Earl of Aberdeen and his coalition resigned at the end of January 1855.

10 Simpson to Panmure, 7 July 1855; TNA: WO 1/376. Panmure agreed on 28 July that it was necessary to plan for a winter in the Crimea, and the first point to be considered was housing the troops.
11 Captain Sayer, *Despatches and Papers Relative to the Campaign in Turkey, Asia Minor, and the Crimea during the War with Russia in 1854, 1855, 1856* (London: Harrison, 1857).

Table 1.3 The strength and losses in the principal corps of the Army of the East

Rank	Corps	Strength			Losses*			
		Embarked	Drafts	Total (% of total in row 5 or 10)	Deaths	Invalided	Deserters† & POW	Total (% of total on column 5)
Officers	Cavalry	287	140	427 (11)	37	144	2	183 (43)
	Infantry‡	1,497	1,498	2,995 (76.5)	306	1,072	8	1,386 (46)
	RA	120	268	388 (10)	23	145	0	168 (43)
	RE	3	92	95 (2.5)	20	31	0	51 (53.5)
	Total	1,907	1,998	3,905 (100)	386	1,392	10	1,788 (46)
Sergeants and men	Cavalry	4,868	3,425	8,293 (9)	1,172	920	96	2,188 (26.5)
	Infantry‡	43,639	29,660	73,399 (78)	17,302	11,464	494	29,260 (40)
	RA	3,095	7,628	10,723 (11.5)	1,483	2,117	0	3,600 (33.5)
	RS&M	403	1,241	1,644 (1.5)	241	157	4	402 (24.5)
	Total	52,005	41,954	93,959 (100)	20,198	14,658	594	35,450 (37.5)

* The total includes those killed in action and dying of wounds and disease.
† No officer deserted.
‡ The three Guards and 49 line regiments were itemized separately in the original table.

(Summarized from Sayer, *Despatches*, endpaper)

The Chancellor of the Exchequer in the new Government, Sir George Lewis, did not consider that the 'substitution of Lord Panmure for the Duke of Newcastle' would 'change the course of the campaign, or to convert failure into success.'[12] The news from the Crimea continued to cause concern for Viscount Palmerston's government, as confirmed by Lewis shortly before the fall of Sevastopol: 'As long as our Army remains in the trenches before Sebastopol, no Government can have any stability, our domestic politics are dependent on the events of the siege as they occur from day to day.'[13] This view was echoed by a remark made by the Earl of Clarendon, the Foreign Secretary, before the invasion to Lord Stratford de Redcliffe, the British ambassador in Constantinople: 'Until Sebastopol is taken there is no chance of [...] a binding peace. [...] the command of the Black Sea and the fate of Constantinople are in the hands of Russia and England and France are disgraced.'[14]

The War with Russia has been considered an inappropriate and pointless adventure by some commentators because it proved inconclusive since 'we had only driven the

---

12   Sir George C. Lewis to Sir Edmund Head, 2 February 1855; G.F. Lewis (ed.) *Letters of Sir George Cornewall Lewis, Bart.* (London: Longman, Green & Co., 1870), p.292.
13   Lewis to Head, 17 August 1855; Lewis, *Letters*, pp.297–8.
14   Clarendon to Stratford, 23 August 1854; quoted by Royle, *Crimea*, p.193.

robber from the gates of Turkey but we have refused to take him into custody' and that it was a peace that 'France insisted upon, and which the British people sulkily acquiesced in',[15] and in consequence the Black Sea only remained demilitarized for fourteen years. On the other hand, Hugh Small concluded that the conflict was not a 'historically irrelevant mistake' but suggested that (1) the Allies had fought a 'just' war, and that they had the moral support of all Europe in going to war in defence of the principle that nations, despite their differing ideologies, should coexist and not seek to expand their territory at their neighbours' expense; (2) the war was winnable given that Britain, the world's only superpower, with a relatively powerful France 'had a mighty ascendancy over unindustrialized Russia'; and (3) the objectives were limited and achievable, i.e. the liberation of the Russian peripheral vassal states and the prevention of Russian advances into British and French spheres of influence.[16]

1.3 Military medical knowledge in the mid-19th century

The health of the general public, particularly the urban poor, obtained an increasingly high profile during the 1840s[17] with the Health of Towns Commissioners concluding that: 'defective drainage, neglect of house and street cleansing, ventilation, and imperfect supplies of water, contribute to produce atmospheric impurities, which affect the general health and the physical condition of the population.'[18] Legislation was subsequently enacted, and it resulted in progress being made,[19] albeit not universally, with the appointment of qualified surveyors and inspectors of nuisances. Medical practitioners were originally employed on an ad hoc basis. The editor of the *Association Medical Journal* considered this policy unsatisfactory as preventive medicine was a legitimate new branch of medicine that was equally important as that of healing, being 'but sister branches of the same tree.'[20] However, despite this positive opinion preventive and community medicine, as we now know them, did not exist as disciplines in their own right. In this respect military surgeons were probably no more or less ineffectual than the majority of their civilian counterparts, whether they were

---

15 *Illustrated London News* 10 May 1856, p.798.
16 H. Small, *The Crimean War: Queen Victoria's War with the Russian Tsars* (Stroud: Tempus, 2007).
17 For an assessment of urban sanitary issues see H. Gavin, *Sanitary Ramblings* (London: John Churchill, 1848). Gavin, a Sanitary Commissioner, died following a shooting accident shortly after he arrived in the Crimea.
18 1st and 2nd Reports of the Health of Towns Commissioners dated June 1844 and February 1845, and quoted in the *Association Medical Journal*, 11 May 1855, p.434.
19 The Nuisances Removal and Diseases Prevention Act 1855 defined 'nuisances' as any 'filthy, unwholesome, or dilapidated house, building, or premises; any foul or offensive pool, ditch, gutter, watercourse, privy, urinal, cesspool, drain, or ash pit; any animal so kept as to be injurious to health; any decaying or offensive accumulation or deposit.'
20 *Association Medical Journal*, 4 May 1855, pp.411–2.

'miasmatist' or 'contagionists'.[21] In consequence, 'many of the subsequent criticisms of the medical services in the Crimea are unfair because they ignore the state of medical knowledge and treatment available at the time.'[22]

Before 1854 the army doctor received little specialised instruction in the medical or surgical problems encountered on service, and 'there was a near total neglect of teaching of the principles of hygiene and preventive medicine.'[23] Nevertheless, despite these shortcomings, the concepts of proverbs, such as 'Prevention is better than cure'[24] and 'Prevention is so much better than healing, because it saves the labour of being sicke,'[25] would have been appreciated by most medical men. However, at that time there were only two diseases for which specific methods of prevention were available, viz. vaccination against small pox and the issuing of lime juice to prevent scurvy, although the control of cholera would have been feasible, if Dr John Snow's explanation for the mode of transmission by contaminated water had been more widely known and generally accepted.[26]

An important principle of hygiene for an army on campaign was enunciated in Deuteronomy 23:12–13: 'Thou shall have a place also without the camp, whither thou shalt go forth abroad: and thou shalt have a paddle upon thy weapon; and it shall be, when thou wilt ease thyself abroad, thou shalt dig therewith, and shalt turn back and will cover that which cometh from thee.' The Medical Officers would have known of these verses as well as the writings of 18th century military surgeons such as Pringle[27] and Monro[28] who championed the importance of basic hygiene, and of the need to supply troops with an adequate diet and a supply of pure water, as well as keeping them well clothed and protected by adequate accommodation. Luscombe, writing after the Napoleonic wars, also made several sensible proposals about the care and effective management of soldiers which were equally as good as any of those recommended in 1858 by the Royal Commission chaired by Sidney Herbert.[29]

---

21 For further comment see A.E.W. Miles, *The Accidental Birth of Military Medicine* (London: Civic Books, 2009), pp.112–3.
22 C. Ponting, *The Crimean War: The Truth Behind the Myth* (London: Chatto and Windus, 2004), p.192.
23 Shepherd, *Crimean Doctors*, 1, p.14.
24 Latin proverb in D.C. Browning, *Dictionary of Quotations and Proverbs* (London: Chancellor Press, 1988), p.406.
25 T. Adams (1618) quoted by J. Simpson, *The Concise Oxford Dictionary of Proverbs* (Oxford: OUP, 1981), p.146.
26 These issues persist in the 21st century since it has been suggested that priority should have been given to sanitation and the provision of a clean water supply when tackling the cholera epidemic in Haiti, rather than the introducing a vaccination programme; P. Wampler, 'Pick Sanitation Over Vaccination in Haiti', *Nature*, 470 (2011), pp.175.
27 J. Pringle, *Observations on the Diseases of the Army in Camp and Garrison* (London: Miller and Wilson, 1752), and later editions.
28 D. Monro, *Observations on the Means of Preserving the Health of Soldiers, and of Conducting Military Hospitals* (2nd edition) (London: J. Murray, 1780), 1, pp.1–159.
29 E.T. Luscombe, *Practical Observations on the Means of Preserving the Health of Soldiers in Camp and in Quarters* (2nd edition) (Edinburgh: Archibald Constable, 1821), pp.108–15.

Pringle, who is considered the 'father of modern military hygiene', was well ahead of his time since 'even in the twentieth century' his ideas 'are thought by many doctors to be a comparatively recent discovery.'[30] This view echoes that of the editor of the *Association Medical Journal* who noted on 4 May 1855 that: 'Preventive medicine has within a few years been called into active existence, or [rather] revived; for many facts and opinions which seem to us novelties were well understood by older physicians.' However, when evaluating the seemingly unsatisfactory reports about the hospitals in Turkey and Crimea today it should be kept in mind that in the 1850s standards were different as even 'newly built mansions of Belgravia reeked of drains' and that the 'sanitation of Buckingham Palace' had 'so many defects the government suppressed [Playfair's] report.[31]

1.4 Army Medical Department

Surgeons were ranked 'above washerwomen and below tailors' during the reign of Henry V while by the time of Elizabeth I they were 'coupled with drummers and paid accordingly.'[32] Matters had improved by the beginning of the 19th century although Medical Officers remained in 'one of the lowest positions on the military hierarchy [and were] often regarded as neither a soldier nor a gentleman;' This situation prompted Jackson to recommend in 1803 that they should have military rank and powers equivalent to those of military officers and that a sanitary officer should be appointed to provide advice on the location for camps and hospitals; and to ensure compliance with regulations introduced to control epidemics.[33] Needless to say these suggestions went unheeded. Sir James McGrigor endeavoured to enhance the status of the army doctor when Director General of the AMD,[34] though in 1854 they still 'occupied a hybridized and inequitable position. Occupationally and geographically removed from civilian counterparts […] they were not fully integrated into the mainstream of the medical profession, neither were they equals, in terms of rank, pay, status, or conditions of service, of their fellow officers in the services.'[35] As a consequence Medical Officers still had little or no executive authority in 1854 and hence Dr, later Sir John, Hall, whose rank was equivalent to a Brigadier, was not involved

---

30   P. Starling, 'Sir John Pringle, 1707–1782: the Father of Modern Military Hygiene', *The War Correspondent*, 19:4 (2002), pp.48–9.
31   J. Bennett, 'The Medical Service in the Crimea' in *Redressing the Balance* (London: Florence Nightingale Museum Trust, 1991), pp.3–10.
32   J. Sweetman, 'The Crimean War and the Formation of the Medical Staff Corps', *Journal of the Society of Army Historical Research*, 53 (1975), pp.113–9.
33   Jackson (1803), quoted by Shepherd, *Crimean Doctors*, 1, p.7.
34   R. Blanco, 'Sir James McGrigor and the Army Medical Corps', *History Today*, 21 (1971), pp.132–9.
35   P. Bartrip, *Themselves Writ Large: The British Medical Association 1832–1996* (London: BMJ Publishing Group, 1996), p.114.

with operational planning. Surprising perhaps given that Raglan had been the Duke of Wellington's military secretary during the Peninsular War, and would have seen first-hand the advantages of the beneficial relationship between him and McGrigor.[36] Hall was thus 'kept in total ignorance of the movements of the army [...] until the last moment,'[37] although when things went wrong he was 'held accountable, both by [the military authorities] and the public, for its medical arrangements' and as a result 'no small measure of abuse was heaped on him and the department for what they termed its shortcomings.'[38] This issue will be considered later in Section 2.2.8.

1.4.1 Drs Andrew Smith and John Hall, and Miss Nightingale
Smith was based in London for the whole war. Hall, who was considered 'a gentleman of known ability and high character'[39] was recalled from India and joined the Army of the East as the Principal Medical Officer on 17 June 1854. Both men remained in post throughout the campaign, despite being subjected to considerable criticism, often unwarranted. They must have discharged their duties satisfactorily, however, as they retained the confidence of Newcastle and then Panmure, both of whom could have readily replaced them if they so wished.

There is but one biography each for Smith and Hall.[40] In contrast there is an extensive literature on Miss Nightingale, both her writings and numerous biographies.[41] As a consequence some commentators have tended to overemphasize events in Scutari

---

36 Cantlie, *A History*, 1, pp.338–9, 357 & 368.
37 Hall made this point to the Royal Commission on 22 June 1857; HCPP 1857–58 (2318) XVIII.1: *Report of the Commissioners Appointed to Inquire into the Regulations Affecting the Sanitary Condition of the Army, the Organization of Military Hospitals, and the Treatment of the Sick and Wounded*. (Hereafter: Royal Commission Report) and S.M. Mitra, *The Life and Letters of Sir John Hall M.D., K.C.B., F.R.C.S.* (London: Longmans, Green, 1911).
38 Hall to Smith; Smith, *Précis*, 2, Appendix 42. A 'rough copy' entitled 'Report of the Medical Arrangements for and Army in the Field rendered by Inspector General of Hospitals Sir John Hall, KCB, formerly Principal Medical Officer, British Army, Crimea, 20th January 1857' is preserved as RAMC: 527. There are minor textual differences between the two versions.
39 Special Correspondent, Scutari, 18 May 1855; *The Times*, 1 June 1854.
40 P.R. Kirby, *Sir Andrew Smith, M.D., K.C.B. His Life Letters and Works* (Cape Town: Balkena, 1965) and Mitra, *Life and Letters*, plus two essays on Hall by Major General Barnsley, RAMC, viz. R.E. Barnsley, 'Teeth and Tails in the Crimea', *Medical History*, 7 (1963), pp.75–9 and R.E. Barnsley, 'Sir John Hall', *Transactions of the Cumberland and Westmorland Antiquarian Society*, 64, (1966), pp.402–8. For a copy of the second essay see: RAMC: 524/15/10 and National Army Museum: 1967-10-14.
41 For example, Sir E. Cook, *The Life of Florence Nightingale* (London: Macmillan, 1913); Cecil Woodham-Smith, *Florence Nightingale 1820–1910* (London: John Constable, 1950); S.M. Goldie, *Florence Nightingale: Letters from the Crimea 1854–1856* (Manchester: Mandolin, 1997); H. Small, *Florence Nightingale: Avenging Angel* (2nd edition) (London: Knowledge Leak, 2013): G. Gill, *Nightingales: The Story of Florence Nightingale and her Remarkable Family* (London: Hodder and Stoughton, 2004); M. Bostridge, *Florence Nightingale: The Woman and Her Legend* (London: Viking, 2008); L. McDonald (ed.),

and to overlook what took place in the Crimea where the main Army was located; and, as will be explained, where the causes of the serious health problems experienced during the first winter were largely overcome. While Nightingale soon became immersed in dealing with the consequences of what was occurring at the front her terms of engagement did not extend to the Crimea, until the spring of 1856, and hence reports of her achievements in the Barrack Hospital are inevitably of limited relevance to the objectives of this monograph.

1.5 Overview of the disease problems encountered in Bulgaria and the Crimea

Disease will be considered in more detail in Chapter 5 but the topic is mentioned here merely to stress that only three categories of disease was responsible for the great majority of deaths as evinced by reference to the deaths in the regiments forming the one cavalry and five infantry divisions that landed in the Crimea in September 1854 (Table 1.4). The campaign was notable in that it took place during a European-wide cholera pandemic and this disease was responsible for nearly a quarter of all the deaths (24 percent). Bowel diseases and fevers were also prevalent and accounted for nearly two thirds (63 percent) while other conditions which were potentially fatal, such as respiratory disease, scurvy and frostbite, accounted for most of the remaining fatalities.

Table 1.4 Mortality from disease in the cavalry and infantry divisions which landed with the Expeditionary Army in the Crimea

Division (No. of regiments)	Total deaths*	Deaths (%) from:			
		Cholera	Bowel diseases	Fevers	Respiratory diseases
Cavalry (12)	935	353 (38)	267 (28.5)	204 (22)	42 (4.5)
Light (7)	2,532	633 (25)	984 (39)	448 (17.5)	66 (2.5)
1st (6)	2,511	641 (25.5)	911 (36.5)	608 (24)	96 (4)
2nd (6)	1,687	306 (18)	609 (36)	472 (28)	63 (3.5)
3rd (6)	2,347	527 (22.5)	780 (33)	668 (28.5)	94 (4)
4th (6)	1,779	349 (19.5)	861 (48.5)	292 (16.5)	76 (4.5)
Total	11,791	2,809 (24)	4,412 (37.5)	2,692 (23)	437 (3.5)

* These totals exclude deaths from wounds and mechanical accidents.

(*Medical and Surgical History*, 2, pp.217 & 220)

Florence Nightingale: The Crimean War (Waterloo, Ontario: Wilfred Laurier UP, 2010), 14; and L. McDonald, *Florence Nightingale at First Hand* (London: Continuum UK, 2010).

32 Victory Over Disease

1.6 Misleading statistics

The science of statistics was in its infancy during the mid-19th Century and some of the methods of data-handling appear unusual by today's standards. Nevertheless, the debate that followed the publication of the 3rd edition of Nightingale's '*Notes on Hospitals*' during 1863 illustrated some of the muddled thinking current at the time. The topic was re-evaluated in a paper entitled '*100 apples divided by 15 red herrings: a cautionary tale from mid-19th century on comparing hospital mortality rates.*'[42] It is not intended to enter into this debate in detail, but the two examples of misrepresentation described below illustrate the importance of analyzing data from first principles, as has been done in this monograph, and not to accept what has been previously published, and from which it may be possible to draw the wrong conclusions.

Colonel Tulloch's denominator: It is nonsensical to calculate the average weight of a growing child by adding the weights on each birthday and dividing the sum by the age in years. It is inappropriate, therefore, to adopt a similar approach for estimating the numbers at risk in the Army as this is influenced by gains from reinforcements and returning convalescents and losses from enemy action, disease, and redeployment. It is for this reason that the method adopted by Tulloch is questioned, viz. the totalling of the number of deaths during 'n' months and dividing the total by the average monthly strength during that period. However, this approach produces an exaggerated approximation as the denominator is bound to be less than the total number at risk. This is illustrated clearly when the whole campaign is considered (Table 1.5). Tulloch's denominator of 37,324 men was far too low given that the number sent to the East was about 2½-times greater at about 94,000.[43] His method gives a mortality rate of 44 percent when in reality it was under half of this value.

Miss Nightingale's mortality rates: Death is a once in a lifetime experience and so quoting a mortality rate in excess of 100 percent is illogical. Yet, Nightingale did so; as illustrated in Table 1.6. The cause of this distortion is the scaling up the rate to percent per annum. She justified doing this by suggesting that giving a percentage figure 'is simply misleading to the authorities, unless indeed, which is hardly likely, they are thoroughly *au fait* at statistical inquiries' because the 'standard comparison all over

---

42   I.E. Iezzoni, '100 Apples Divided by 15 Red Herrings: a Cautionary Tale from the Mid-19th Century on Comparing Hospital Mortality Rates', *Annals of Internal Medicine*, 124 (1996), pp.1079–85 and reproduced in D. Neuhauser and C.E. Blanchard (eds), *Florence Nightingale: Measuring Hospital Care Outcomes* (Joint Commission on Accreditation of Healthcare Organizations, 1999), pp.229–46.
43   Return provided by the AG, Horse Guards on 29 April 1856, and summarized in Sayer, *Despatches*, p.415

Table 1.5 Mortality rate for the whole campaign calculated using Colonel Tulloch's method, April 1854–June 1856

Year	Month	Estimated monthly strength*	No. of deaths†	Cumulative average monthly strength‡	Cumulative deaths	Tulloch's mortality rate (c6/c5)*100
1854	Apr.	8,265	3	8265	3	<0.1
	May	21,789	21	15,027	24	0.2
	June	25,122	17	18,392	41	0.2
	July	28,722	379	20,975	420	2
	Aug.	30,226	852	22,825	1,272	6
	Sep.	30,329	858	24,076	2,130	9
	Oct.	30,607	624	25,009	2,754	11
	Nov.	29,791	937	25,606	3,691	14
	Dec.	32,799	1,847	26,406	5,538	21
1855	Jan.	32,469	3,076	27,012	8,614	32
	Feb.	31,027	2,478	27,377	11,092	41
	Mar.	30,082	1,377	27,602	12,469	45
	Apr.	31,328	531	27,889	13,000	47
	May	35,063	543	28,401	13,543	47.5
	June	39,226	830	29,123	14,373	49.5
	July	42,919	414	29,985	14,787	49
	Aug.	44,414	507	30,834	15,294	50
	Sep.	48,243	208	31,801	15,502	49
	Oct.	48,812	145	32,696	15,647	48
	Nov.	49,942	206	33,559	15,853	47
	Dec.	50,089	116	34,346	15,969	46
1856	Jan.	50,881	87	35,098	16,056	46
	Feb.	50,319	39	35,759	16,095	45
	Mar.	55,000	49	36,561	16,144	44
	Apr.	54,452	37	37,277	16,181	43
	May	47,472	24	37,669	16,205	43
	June	25,935	6	37,234	16,211	44
General total		37,234	16,211	Not relevant		

*   Calculated from the *Medical and Surgical History*, 2, p.43, column 2 & 6.
†   Transcribed from the *Medical and Surgical History*, 2, pp.43 & 44, column 2, respectively, being the sum of those numbers recorded for the cavalry, ordnance (RA and RS&M), foot guards and infantry.
‡   The average strength calculated on the basis that the campaign had finished during the month in question, i.e. the sum of the strength for 'n' months in column 3 divided by 'n'.

34   Victory Over Disease

the civilized word would be in percentages *per annum*.⁴⁴ This approach may be useful for persuading policy makers to introduce change but it was not necessary because the valid statistic presented in the third column makes the point equally forcibly.

Table 1.6 Mortality in the hospitals in England, Scutari, and Kuleli

Location	Mortality	
	Rate percent per annum of sick population	Percent of cases treated
Eleven London General Hospitals	82	7.6
Fever Hospital	110.5	11.3
Military and Naval Hospitals in London	39	2.4
Scutari and Kuleli General Hospitals during four months*	203	19.8
During four weeks	319	32.1
During four week	415	42.7
Kuleli during four week	608	52
Scutari and Kuleli, summer 1855	34	2.2

* The dates are not stated but the context indicates that these losses occurred during the first winter.

(Adapted from *A Contribution to the Sanitary History of the British Army during the Late War with Russia* [Published anonymously], (London: Harrison, 1859), p.6.)

1.7 Principal sources consulted

Primary sources consulted include letters, despatches, and reports in the War Office (WO) and Foreign Office (FO) series in The National Archives (TNA) at Kew; the Royal Army Medical Corps (RAMC) archive; and the official and personal papers of key individuals preserved in various archives including the National Army Museum (NAM) and county record offices, as well as published and unpublished diaries and letters of other participants, both medical and military.

The digitization of published documents has facilitated the acquisition of relevant information. These include the *London Gazette*; the proceedings of both of Houses of Parliament in *Hansard*; and Parliamentary Papers (Blue Books) which provide statistical and documentary evidence, albeit usually with little or no analysis. Newspapers including *The Times*, *Daily News*, *Illustrated London News*, and other national and regional journals provided reports on the progress of the campaign as well as affording unbiased and sometimes commonplace factual information on daily life in the camps and elsewhere.

44   Royal Commission Report, p.367.

General Orders were issued by Headquarters on a daily basis and they provide information on the way that Army was administered as well as listing the arrival and deployment of personnel, including those who left the Crimea with a medical certificate.[45]

The Director General of the AMD kept copies of the letters he sent and received from the time he was told to prepare for service in the East until the end of war. A synopsis of these documents entitled *Précis of Letters Written and Received by the Director-General of the Army Medical Department in Reference to the Medical Arrangements Required at the Commencement and during the War with Russia 1854–55–56* (Hereafter: *Précis of Letters*) was printed in two volumes after the war, but not officially published. In addition to abstracts of numerous letters there are a number of appendices comprising tables of statistical data and listings of personnel, and drugs and equipment issued.[46]

The Crimean campaign was the first conflict for which a detailed account of the surgical and medical history of the infantry and cavalry regiments, and to a lesser extent the Royal Artillery and Royal Engineers, was published after the war, viz. the *Medical and Surgical History of the British Army which Served in Turkey and the Crimea during the War Against Russia in the Years 1854–55–56*.[47] The first volume provides, inter alia, details of the medical problems encountered by the 14 cavalry and 52 infantry regiments during each month, and for each there is a comprehensive table that lists the number of 'admissions into hospital and deaths' each month together with a separate column for the those who 'died in general hospitals during the war', but not those killed in action. The second volume comprises two principal parts that cover disease (pp.234–252), and wounds and injuries (pp.253–396). The section on disease concludes with five comprehensive tables, designated General Returns A–E, of which A will be the most commonly quoted in this monograph.[48] The second volume also

---

45 Copies of General Orders have been preserved in The National Archives, e.g. TNA: WO 28/50, WO 28/51, WO 28/130, and WO 28/131. Longhand transcriptions can also found in divisional order books in WO 28. After the war a compilation was published as: *General Orders Issued to the Army of the East, from April 30, 1854 to December 31, 1855 Selected by the Hon Sir Alex H Gordon*, (London: J.W. Parker, 1856).

46 The original documents or copies in out-letter books can frequently be found in the Royal Army Medical Corps archive, The National Archive, and other archives.

47 HCPP 1857-58 [2434] XXXVIII.Pt.I.1 & XXXVIII.Pt.II.1: *Medical and Surgical History of the British Army which Served in Turkey and the Crimea during the War Against Russia in the Years 1854–55–56* (Hereinafter: *Medical and Surgical History*, 1 & 2).

48 The rubrics for the General Returns A–E are: (A), Return showing primary admissions, by each month, into the hospitals of the Army of the East, from 10th April 1854, to 30th June 1856; also all the deaths which, during the same period, occurred in regimental and general hospitals, in hospital ships, or suddenly, of from violence, with the exception of those which occurred in action with the enemy; (B), Table showing the ratio percent, during each month, of the admissions and deaths in General Return A; (C), Return of deaths in the regiments of the Expeditionary Army, showing the duration of the diseases, wounds, and injuries, which proved fatal; (D), Return showing, by regiments, the ages of men, who were sent to the East and the ages of those who died there from disease and

includes tables, which have a similar format to General Return A, for the General Hospitals located on the Bosphorus (I) and at Abydos (VII), Smyrna (VIII), and Renkioi (IX) in Turkey; at Varna in Bulgaria (II); and in Balaklava (III), near the Castle (IV) and Monastery (VI), and in the Camp (V) in the Crimea; together with details of 187 voyages in which the sick and wounded were evacuated from the Crimea to Turkey (pp.465–77).

The government mindful of mounting disquiet among the British public engendered by the newspaper reports sent three commissions of enquiry to investigate matters on the spot, viz, the Hospital, Supplies, and Sanitary Commissions.[49] After the resignation of Aberdeen's administration the House of Commons convened a Select Committee chaired by Mr J. Roebuck, MP, to ascertain what had been going wrong, and who was to blame.[50] The reports of these initiatives provide an incomparable source of information of what transpired during the critical months after the invasion.

Three years after the war Harriet Martineau, a prominent sociologist and commentator, published her assessment of the reports of the various commissions, and Florence Nightingale's *A Contribution to the Sanitary History of the British Army*, which had been published anonymously.[51] The preface opened with the following sentence: 'This book is not a work of invention. It is no fancy-piece, but "an ower [Scots: over] true tale," as it would be easy to show.' Martineau then stressed that 'it is a grave work' and that she had attempted to; 'repress all weakening emotions' and thus 'avoid both censure and praise, and to be as impersonal as possible.' And in this she succeeded, and thus enhanced her book's value as a contribution on how the health of the Army might be improved and safeguarded in the future.[52]

Two more recent texts provide detailed and well balanced factual information on the medical problems were published in 1973 and 1991 respectively by Lieutenant

---

wounds; (E), Return showing, by centesimal ration, classes of diseases as they occurred in the Army, and in each regiment, namely, No. 1, of admissions of men into hospital; No. 2, of deaths in the East; No. 3, of invalids; and No. 4, of soldiers finally discharged after their return to England on account of disability contracted on service with the War with Russia.

49 HCPP 1854–55 [1920] XXXIII.1: *Report upon the State of the Hospitals on the British Army in the Crimea and Scutari*, (Hereafter: Hospital Commission Report); HCPP 1856 [2007, 2007–I] XX.1.497: *Report of the Commission of Inquiry into the Supplies of the British Army in the Crimea*, (Hereafter: Supplies Commission Report); and HCPP 1857 Session 1 [2196] LX.241: *Report to the Right Hon. Lord Panmure, G.C.B., etc. Minister at War, of the Proceedings of the Sanitary Commission Dispatched to the Seat of War in the East, 1855–56*, (Hereafter: Sanitary Commission Report).

50 HCPP 1854–55 (156) IX.Pt.I.7, (218) IX.Pt.II.1, (247) IX.Pt.III.1, & (318, 318–I) IX.Pt. III.365, 431, *Second, Third, Fourth and Fifth Reports of the Select Committee on the Army before Sebastopol*. (Hereafter: Select Committee, 2nd, 3rd, 4th, & 5th Reports respectively.) For further details see Shepherd, *Crimean Doctors*, 2, pp.373–411.

51 F. Nightingale, *A Contribution to the Sanitary History of the British Army during the Late War with Russia* (London: Harrison, 1859). [Published anonymously]

52 H. Martineau, *England and Her Soldiers* (London: Smith, Elder, & Co., 1859), p.v.

General Sir Neil Cantlie, RAMC, and John Shepherd, a retired surgeon.[53] In addition, Matthew Kaufman, sometime Professor of Anatomy at the University of Edinburgh, and two surgeons, Thomas Scotland and Steven Heys, considered the development of military medicine and surgery during the 19th century. Both books include chapters on the Crimean campaign;[54] and though the contents are of relevance to this monograph the reliance on non-archival sources has limited their value as a source of reference.

Cantlie considered the Crimean War in the context of developments which took place 'from the creation of the Standing Army in 1660 until the formation of the RAMC in 1898' and his account of the medical and surgical aspects of the campaign is set within the framework of ongoing military operations. References were made to the *Medical and Surgical History* and Smith's *Précis of Letters* as well as the reports of the Roebuck Committee, and the Hospitals, Sanitary and Royal Commissions, but not the Supplies Commission. Cantlie had access to the RAMC archive but there only two references to Hall's papers, and no references to medical journals or newspapers, the *London Gazette*, *Hansard*, or documents in The National Archives, National Army Museum, and other archives.

Shepherd's account is more comprehensive as it included two chapters on the Royal Navy, a topic beyond the scope of this monograph,[55] three on Miss Nightingale and the Scutari hospitals, and one each on commissions and committees, civilian surgeons, and the Turkish contingent. He made extensive use of reports in the medical press and scientific journals, personnel letters and diaries, *The Times* and *Illustrated London News*. He quoted secondary sources of a general nature and considered the *Medical and Surgical History* an 'indispensable text'. He had access to the RAMC archives but there are no references to Smith's *Précis of Letters*, Hall's papers, or to documents in The National Archives and National Army Museum.

The focus of this monograph is on events which influenced the health and wellbeing of the British Army while in Black Sea theatre, including particularly Bulgaria and the Crimea, and how these affected what occurred in the camps, on the hospital transport ships and in the general hospitals in the Crimea and elsewhere.

General accounts of the Crimean War have tended to concentrate on the causes and the conduct of the conflict, and one published in 1935 by General Sir G. MacMunn, RA. is particularly thought provoking.[56] Many of the books published during the last 25 years have touched on medical matters though the references were made *en passant*

---

53   Cantlie, *A History* and Shepherd, *Crimean Doctors*.
54   Kaufman, *Surgeons at War*, pp.129–79 and Scotland and Heys, *Wars, Pestilence*, pp.204–7.
55   For information on this topic see HCPP 1857 Session 1 (71) IX.797: *Medical Statistical Returns of the Baltic and Black Sea Fleets, during the Years 1854 and 1855*.
56   G. MacMunn, *The Crimea in Perspective* (London: G. Bell & Son, 1935).

as part of a general narrative and contain little or no detailed clinical or epidemiological information which might inform the analyses presented hereafter.[57]

It would be desirable to include a comparative element but there are no equivalent bodies of literature on the French, Turkish, and Sardinian armies, thus making it impossible to make detailed comparisons.[58] Suffice it to state that Bodart's summary suggests that despite initial praise for the French medical services it would appear that overall the French Army fared worse than the British during the campaign; and particularly during the final months, (Table 1.7).[59]

Table 1.7 Losses sustained by the British and French armies during the Crimean campaign

Nationality	Effective strength put into the field	Killed or died of wounds (%) = (c3/c2)*100	Died of disease (%) = (c4/c2)*100	Total fatalities (%) = (c5/c2)*100
British	98,000	4,602 (4.5)	17,580 (18)	22,182 (22.5)
French	310,000	20,240 (6.5)	75,375 (24.5)	95,615 (31)

[57] For example: C. Hibbert, *The Destruction of Lord Raglan* (Ware: Wordsworth Editions, 1999; originally published by Longmans, 1961); J.C. Curtiss, *Russia's Crimean War* (Durham, N.C.: Duke University Press, 1979); M.P. Lalumia (1984) *Realism and Politics in Victorian Art of the Crimean War* (Ann Arbour, Michigan: UMI Research Press, 1984); N. Rich, *Why the Crimean War?* (Hanover & London: University Press of New England, 1985); J.B. Conache, *Britain and the Crimea, 1855–56. Problems of War and Peace* (London: Macmillan, 1987); J. Sweetman, *Raglan from the Peninsula to the Crimea* (London; Arms and Armour Press, 1993); D.M. Goldfrank, *The Origins of the Crimean War* (London: Longman, 1994); R.B. Edgerton, *Death and Glory: The Legacy of the Crimean War* (Oxford: Westview Press, 1999); Royle, *Crimea*; U. Keller, *The Ultimate Spectacle: A Visual History of the Crimean War* (Australia: Gordon and Breach, 2001); I. Fletcher and N. Ishchenko, *The Crimean War: A Clash of Empires* (Staplehurst: Spellmount, 2004); Ponting, *Crimean War*; R.L.V. French Blake, *The Crimean War* (Barnsley: Pen & Sword Military, 2006); A. Troubetzkoy, *The Crimean War*, (London: Robinson, 2006); H. Rappaport, *No Place for Ladies* (London: Arum Press, 2005); Small, *Crimean War*; C. Badem, *The Ottoman Crimean War (1853–1856)* (Leiden: Brill, 2010); O. Figes, *Crimea: The Last Crusade* (London: Allen Lane, 2010); A.D. Lambert, *The Crimean War: British Grand Strategy, 1853–1856* (2nd edition) (Farnham: Ashford, 2011); and M. Melvin, *Sevastopol's Wars: Crimea from Potemkin to Putin* (Oxford: Osprey Publishing, 2017), with N. Ascherson, *Black Sea: Coast and Conquests: from Pericles to Putin* (London: Vintage Books, 2007) and N. Kent, *Crimea. A History* (London: C. Hurst & Co., 2016) providing accounts of the complex history of the Black Sea and Crimea from the classical times to the present day.

[58] For a review of the Turkish Medical Service see Shepherd, *Crimean Doctors*, 2, pp.562–8.

[59] G. Bodart, *Losses of Life in Modern Wars. Austria-Hungary: France* (Oxford: Clarendon Press, 1916), p.141. See also C. Bryce, *England and France before Sebastopol* (London: John Churchill, 1857); G. Milroy, 'On the Sickness and Mortality in the French Army in the East from 1854 to 1856', *British Medical Journal*, 17 April 1858 and *Medical Times and Gazette*, 1 May 1858; Royle, *Crimea*, p.441; and J. Barham, 'A Tragic Second Winter for the French Army', *The War Correspondent*, 24:1 (2006), pp.23–6.

Dr Bryce, a civilian surgeon concluded: 'France, on the contrary, in camp and country alike, enforced silence of speech and disuse of pens, other than official, concerning the real state of the Army [...] the sanitary state of [the French] troops soon became the reverse of what was then represented of it. [and the] frightful mortality from diseases was [not] exclusively the lot of the British Army,' as 'the French Army did not escape scathless from the first winter, so calamitous to the English.'[60] A report submitted to the Emperor Napoleon after the war contains a considerable amount of statistical information but no details on medical matters. In all 309,268 men were sent to the East of whom 67,058 (22 percent) died.

Following the cessation of hostilities Hall commissioned an assessment of the Russian Medical Department and the state of their hospitals in the Crimea, and a brief nine page report was published officially in 1857.[61] The Russians clearly faced immense difficulties during the war and many of these were due to a slow rate of mobilization on the part of the Russian government, rather than serious shortcoming in the Medical Service itself.[62] This conclusion resonates to an extent with the situation in the British Army, and like the British experience, matters improved as the campaign progressed. Nevertheless, the Russian losses were immense. There were 134,542 (16.4%) deaths among 822,025 sick patients while the comparable figures for these who were wounded were 15,971 (19%) and 83,777. Other commentators have suggested that number of Russians who died in the conflict probably exceeded 450,000 but 'the records are so poor it is impossible to analyse the causes of death.'[63]

A sketch of a Russian hospital made after the fall of Sevastopol, which has been mistakenly identified as being Scutari by some commentators, reveals that it had been abandoned with the patients in a very unsatisfactory condition after the hurried evacuation of the city (Figure 1.1).

Nikolai Pirogov is perhaps the best known of the many participating Russian surgeons. He is remembered for employing the system of triage to manage massed casualties in Sevastopol. However, it was not a new concept – it was employed in the 1790s by D.J. Larry, Surgeon-in-Chief to Napoleon's Imperial Guard.[64] An account of

---

60   Bryce, *England and France before Sebastopol*, pp.6–7 & 32.
61   HCPP 1857, Session 1 (135) IX.211: *Report on the Organisation of the Russian Medical Department and the Sanitary State of their Crimean Hospitals.*
62   For a review see Y. Naumova, 'Russian Medical Service during the Crimean War: New Perspectives', *19: Interdisciplinary Studies in Long Nineteenth Century,* 20 (2015).
63   Ponting, *Crimean War*, p.334.
64   I. Robertson-Steel, 'Evolution of Triage Systems', *Emergency Medicine Journal,* 23:2 (2006), pp.154–8. Incidentally, no specific reference to the term triage has so far been found in contemporary British documents, though it is likely the surgeons would have automatically categorized their patients in a similar manner, given it was a matter of common sense so to do.

Pirogov's career has been published,[65] while other summaries of his achievements are in general terms and none can be validated numerically for comparative purposes.[66]

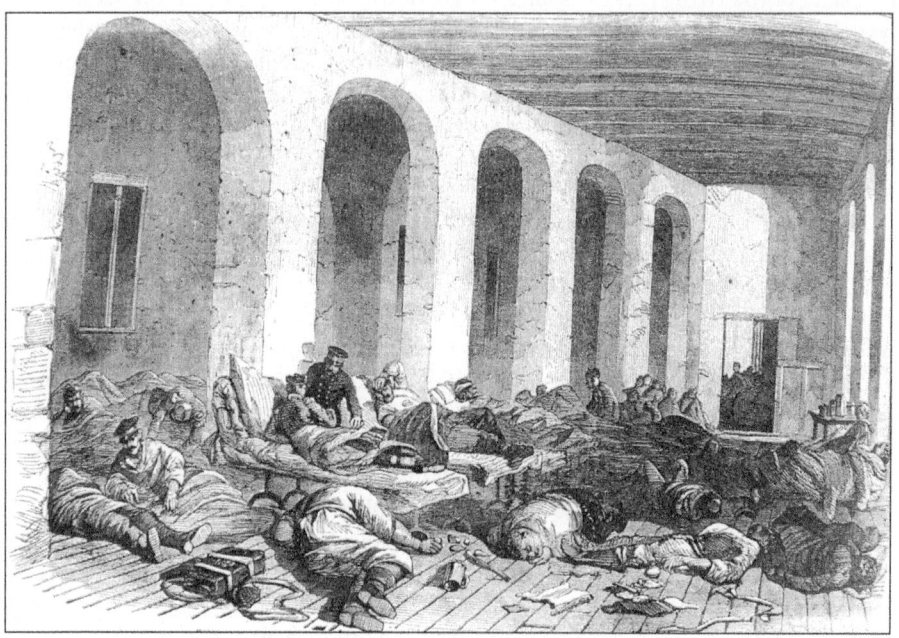

Figure 1.1 Hospital in Sebastopol. – Dr Duigan attending the wounded. (From a sketch by E.A. Goodall, *Illustrated London News*, 6 October 1855, p.404)

65 I.F. Hendriks, J.G. Bovill, P.A. van Luijt, and P.C.W. Hogendoorn, 'Nikolay Ivanovich Pirogov (1810–1881): a Pioneering Russian Surgeon and Medical Scientist', *Journal of Medical Biography* (2016) DOI: 10.1177/0967772016633399.
66 For example, Curtiss, *Russia's War*; V. Porundominsky, *Pirogov in Sevastopol* (Moscow: Young Guard, 1965) Translated by A. Kennaway; Royal Society of Medicine Library, WZ 100 (Pir); Royle, *Crimea*; Fletcher & Ishchenko, *Crimean War*; Figes, *Crimea*; and Melvin, *Sevastopol's Wars*.

2

British Army of the East

Three aspects of the organization of the Army of the East will be considered in this chapter, viz. a general overview and more detailed considerations of two non-military components of the force, namely the Army Medical Department (AMD) and the Commissariat.

2.1 Organization and strength of the Army

Combat units: Preparation for the Eastern campaign commenced early in 1854 when several cavalry and infantry regiments, together with elements of the Royal Artillery (RA), and a small number of Engineers, were mobilised for service overseas. When fully constituted, the Army comprised 14 cavalry and 52 infantry regiments, which included two battalions of the 1st Regiment and Rifle Brigade (Figure 2.1),[1] together with the RA, Royal Engineers (RE), and Royal Sappers and Miners (RS&M).[2]

The last infantry regiment arrived after the fall of Sevastopol and hence all the regiments were present in the Crimea for only about two months before 13 cavalry regiments were withdrawn to Turkey for the winter of 1855/56.[3]

The initial six divisions of the Army were reorganised in August 1855 into seven each with two brigades, except the cavalry that had three. A further reorganisation to form two *corps d'armée* was planned after the fall of Sevastopol but this was not put into effect.

The infantry regiments sent to the East early in the campaign were between 900 and 1,000 strong; thereafter the new regiments usually numbered between 500 and 850. The cavalry regiments were smaller; the first ten to arrive numbered a little over 300.[4]

---

1   The two battalions of the 1st Regiment and the Rifle Brigade were treated as separate units in the Order of Battle.
2   The RE (officers) and RS&M (other ranks) were amalgamated during 1856 to form the Corps of Royal Engineers.
3   Collated from the regimental returns in the *Medical and Surgical History*, 1.
4   Summarized from the endpaper in Sayer, *Despatches*.

42 Victory Over Disease

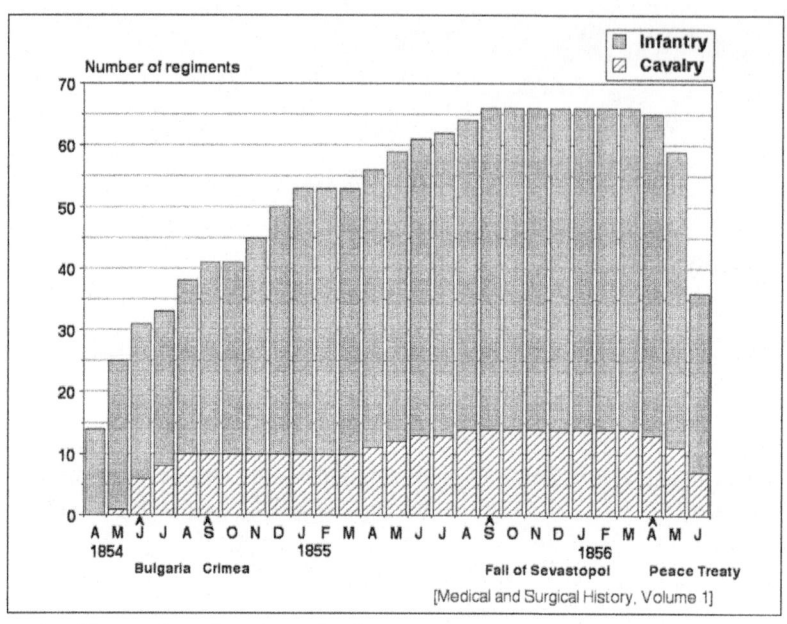

Figure 2.1 The number of cavalry and infantry regiments serving in the Army of the East, April 1854–June 1856.

The Army increased in size during the summer of 1854; the numbers remained relatively stable during the winter of 1854–55 indicating that losses from enemy action and the effects of disease were balanced by the arrival of reinforcements. The buildup recommenced in May 1855 and continued until the fall of Sevastopol when the numbers stabilized once again. A final augmentation occurred early in 1856, presumably in anticipation of a campaign that never materialized. (Figure 2.2)[5]

The Army numbered about 26,000 at the beginning of the campaign[6] while a return dated 1 April 1856 indicated that despite the losses, it had increased to about 60,500 excluding the Land Transport Corps (LTC).[7] The proportional strength of the principal corps being: infantry including the guards (75.5 percent), RA (12), cavalry (10.5), and RS&M (2).[8] In all it was calculated that the total number of NCOs and men sent to the East up to the end on March 1856 was about 94,000.[9]

5 The figures were calculated from *Medical and Surgical History*, 2, p.43. The Ordnance included the Royal Artillery and Royal Sappers and Miners.
6 Adapted from Sayer, *Despatches*, p.416.
7 For details of the order of battle during the campaign see R. McGuigan, *Into Battle. British Orders of Battle for the Crimean War, 1854–56* (Bowdon: Withycut House, 2001).
8 Summarized from the endpaper Sayer, *Despatches*, but excluding the LTC and the British German and Swiss Legions.
9 Returns provided by the Adjutant General and summarized by Sayer, *Despatches*, p.415.

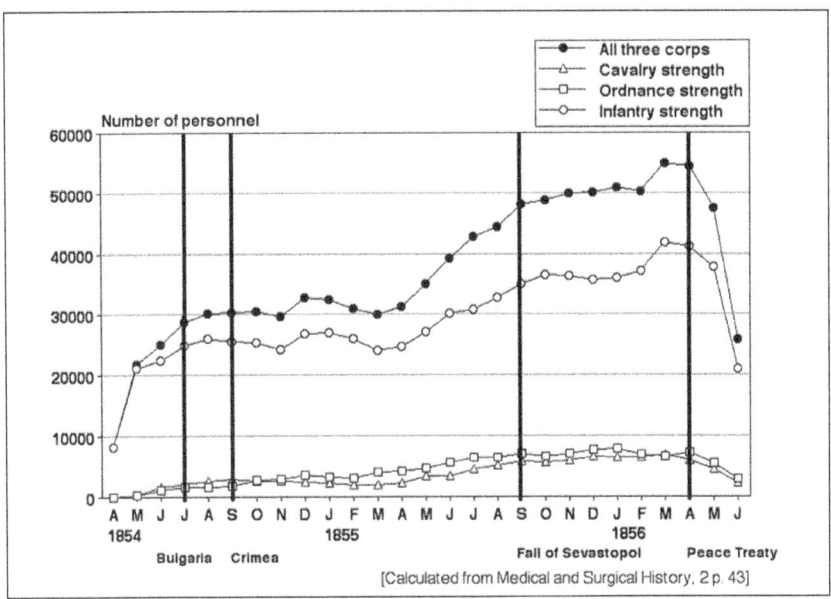

Figure 2.2 The estimated strength of the cavalry and infantry regiments and the ordnance, April 1854–June 1856.

Civilian departments: The three principal non-military departments included the AMD, Chaplains' Department,[10] and Commissariat. The Commissariat was initially under the control of the Treasury, but later the War Department, was responsible for supplying provisions, including food, clothing, and other necessities. During 1855 a LTC[11] was established with the aim of relieving military personnel from transporting stores and equipment.

Three 'ad hoc' corps, the Medical Staff Corps (MSC), Civil Engineer Corps (CEC), and Army Works Corps (AWC), were raised in response to the manpower crisis that became apparent soon after the invasion. The CEC constructed the railway and was probably the most effective although in Sweetman's opinion all were unsuccessful ill-conceived ministerial initiatives and 'that their collective experience supports the popular conclusion that Britain went into the Crimean War ill-prepared.'[12] Nevertheless, despite an unpromising start the MSC and also the LTC eventually evolved into permanent military organizations.

---

10 For a list of chaplains who served with the British Army see M.H. Mawson, 'Chaplains of the Crimean War', *The War Correspondent*, 20:1 (2002), pp.28–36 & 20:2 (2002), pp.34–41.
11 The LTC was the precursor of the Royal Corps of Transport.
12 J. Sweetman, '"Ad hoc" Support Services during the Crimean War, 1854–5', *Military Affairs*, 52 (1988), pp.135–40.

2.1.1 Recruitment

Luscombe, writing after the Napoleonic Wars, recommended that recruits should be over 19 years of age and that those employed in agriculture or by outdoor 'manufacturers' were preferable to the town dwellers working in sedentary occupations.[13] An analysis of the age structure of over 70,000 NCOs and men in the cavalry and infantry regiments revealed that the Army contained a high proportion of young men since two thirds were 25 years or under with nearly a quarter being teenagers, with about one eighth being below the minimum age recommended by Luscombe (Figure 2.3).[14]

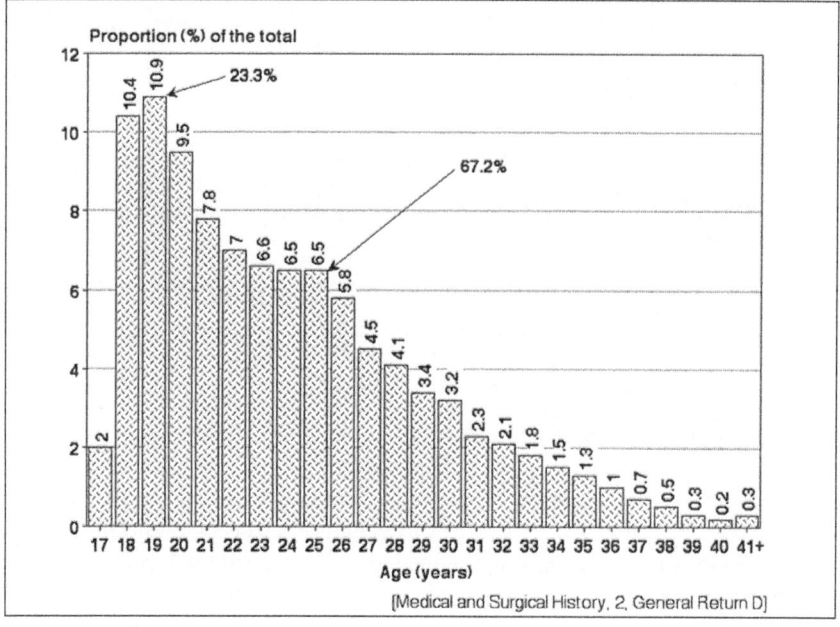

Figure 2.3 The age distribution of 70,425 NCOs and men in the cavalry and infantry 'who were sent to the East'.

The British Army was relatively small by comparison with those in continental Europe and the need to send a seemingly large proportion of its strength to the East prompted the Queen to express her concern to Newcastle on 3 July 1854:

> The Queen feels very uneasy at the very defenceless state in which the country will be left, not from any want of confidence arising from the present conjuncture

---

13 Luscombe, *Practical Observations*, pp.108–15. He was sometime a surgeon with the 2nd Dragoons and 34th Regiment.
14 *Medical and Surgical History*, 2, General Return D.

or affairs, but from a strong sense of the impolicy and danger of leaving this great country in such a state for we never can foresee what events may not suddenly spring up at any moment (like Greece for instance) which may require a force to be in readiness for any particular purpose.[15]

Fortunately her fear of possible insurrection or civil disorder proved unfounded.

Selection of recruits: Within a month of the invasion W.G. Romaine, the Deputy Judge Advocate General, a civilian barrister at Headquarters, was minded to write home: 'We do not have half enough artillery men, engineers, sappers or doctors;'[16] while after the hurricane of 14 November 1854 the Quartermaster General, Major General R. Airey privately informed Major General G.A. Wetherall, the Adjutant General, at Horse Guards that: 'If we don't get reinforced strongly [...] we shall go to the wall, and the English Army be lost! We can't re-embark before an offensive army [...] Our Govt always looks alive too late.'[17],

This state of affairs could not have been lost on the government but the reduction in the size of the army following 1815 meant the deficiency could not be corrected within weeks. The reasons for this were provided by Viscount Hardinge in his evidence to the Roebuck Committee on 10 May 1855. There had been little strategic need to maintain a permanent reserve of trained troops since the defeat of Napoleon, and since then existing regiments had been reduced in strength, and that the 'peace establishment [was] very low indeed; [and after] we made the first effort to send out 25,000, we could do nothing but send out young recruits.'[18]

In an attempt to rectify this deficit the selection criteria were modified.[19] The minimum height for the cavalry was reduced and the maximum age for enlistment into infantry of the line was raised from 25 to 30 years.[20] No minimum age was specified though a Memorandum of 5 January 1855 stipulated that no lad under 17 should be recruited into the infantry as it was 'desirable' that they 'should be of sufficient age and strength to immediately enter upon the duties of soldiers.'[21] Nevertheless,

---

15 J. Raymond (ed.), *Queen Victoria's Early Letters* (London: B.T. Batsford, 1963), p.202.
16 Romaine to C.J. Selwyn, 22 October 1855; C. Robins (ed.), *Romaine's Crimean War* (Stroud: Sutton Publishing, 2005), p.33.
17 Airey to AG, Horse Guards, 13 November 1854; National Army Museum: 1962–10–94–1. For additional comments on the problem of recruitment see I. Binnie, '"Lions led by Jackasses" or fourteen interesting facts about the Crimean War', *The War Correspondent*, 35:2 (2017), pp.27–31.
18 Circular Memorandum No. 912, 22 January 1855; TNA: WO 123/151 and Select Committee, 4th Report, p.234.
19 TNA: WO 123/141 and Select Committee, 4th Report, p.353.
20 For a discussion on the problems of recruitment into the cavalry after the first winter see A. Dawson, *Letters from the Light Brigade* (Barnsley: Pen & Sword Military, 2014), pp.193–5.
21 TNA: WO 123/151.

about two percent of men in the line regiments were 17 years of age or under (see Figure 2.3).[22]

The bounty paid to cavalry and infantry recruits at the beginning of the war was £5/15/6d and £4 respectively. This was increased to £7/15s and £6 on 30 October 1854 and then again to £10 and £8 on 22 January 1855.[23]

Sidney Herbert, the Minister at War, also contributed to the recruitment initiative by issuing a circular letter to officers commanding militia regiments on 20 November 1854. It was intended to limit the demand on these regiments to a quarter of their strength though the bounty payable was to be increased substantially from £1 to £7.[24]

Hardinge subsequently admitted to the Roebuck Committee that many of the recruits were 'too young' as they were 'almost gristle' rather than 'bone and muscle.' He conceded, but without admitting it directly, that this policy must have influenced the losses sustained during the first winter as 'it was impossible to expect [them to] stand the inclemency of the climate and the hard work in the trenches in the same manner as [...] soldiers would have done in 1808,' when a substantial reserve of trained troops aged between 25 and 35 years would have been available.[25]

Hall also noted on occasions that the recruits arriving in the Crimea were 'sickly young boys' or 'mere delicate boys, no stamina and physically unfit for the field [...], these useless boys should be detained at the depot.'[26] The inference from this is that the Queen's Regulations were being overlooked by the officers commanding regiments and depots at home as they were responsible for ensuring that 'no one is selected [...] who is not in every respect calculated for the performance of the duty required of him.'

Incidentally, Dr R. Battersby, a Medical Officer at Chatham, saw the problem from a different perspective. He tended soldiers repatriated from the East, and concluded that: 'In consequence of the pressing demand on soldiers, the relaxed criteria relative to the examination of recruits [...] was carried too far.' The 'physical force' of the Army was 'by no means augmented,' and the 'half-grown, sickly-looking men, who should never have been enlisted should be more 'pitied than condemned for having undertaken duties, the nature of which they were ignorant of, and physically unable to perform.'[27] A further cause of sympathy was enunciated by an unnamed correspondent writing after the action of 9 September 1855: 'There was a considerable number of men in draughts which came out last week [...] who had only enlisted a few days, and who had never fired a rifle in their lives!'[28]

The problem of recruitment continued to be vexatious and Palmerston found it necessary to instruct Panmure on 10 June 1855 not to 'let departmental or official

---

22 *Medical and Surgical History*, 2, General Return D.
23 Select Committee, 4th Report, p.352.
24 *The Times*, 21 November 1854.
25 Select Committee, 4th Report, p.234.
26 RAMC: 397/F/RT/1/2.
27 *Medical and Surgical History*, 2, pp.228–9.
28 *Berrow's Worcester Journal*, 29 September 1855.

or professional prejudices and habits to stand in our way; we must override all such obstacles and difficulties. The only answer [is] the thing *must* be done. We *must* have troops.'[29] It is fortunate perhaps that significant hostilities ceased some three months later, and there was no campaigning during 1856.

Enlistment of Foreign nationals: One of the consequences of the shortage of man power was the passing of the Enlistment of Foreigners Act in December 1854. It was a controversial policy as the mercenaries would be citizens of neutral countries and there would be complex implications as a consequence of the countries' domestic legislation and international law. The topic is outside the objectives of this monograph; suffice it to say mercenaries were recruited into the British German, Swiss, and Italian Legions and these were held in reserve at Kuleli, Smyrna, and in Malta respectively. None saw active service.[30]

The possibility of recruiting men from North America was also investigated. This proved impractical and the initiative increased diplomatic tension between Great Britain and the USA. This resulted in President Franklin Pierce dismissing 'the British minister to the United States, J.F.T. Crampton, and [revoking] the exequators of the British Consuls at New York, Philadelphia, and Cincinnati' on 28 May 1856.[31]

Turkish troops attached the British Army: The Turkish Contingent and Osmanli Irregular Cavalry, not to be confused with the Turkish Army commander by Omer Pasha, were in British pay. They were concentrated sometime at Kertch (now Kerch) and comprised eight cavalry and sixteen infantry regiments together with artillery.[32] The Osmanli Irregular Cavalry had seven regiments.[33] The absence of any worthwhile medical records precludes any further consideration of these units.

2.1.2 Casualties relative to the length of time spent on active service
The length of time an infantry regiment spent on active service influenced the proportion of men who died from disease and wounds and injuries or were invalided home. As expected, the rates were highest in regiments arriving prior to the invasion of the Crimea and these tended to become less with decreasing length of time on campaign, as evinced by data from two sources summarized in Tables 2.1 and 2.2.

---

29 G. Douglas and G.H. Ramsey (eds), *The Panmure Papers*, (London: Hodder and Stoughton, 1898), 1, p.232.
30 Sayer, *Despatches* gave the strength of the German and Swiss Legions as 3,738, and 2,036 respectively.
31 For details on the 'enlistment controversy' J.B. Brebner, 'Joseph Howe and the Crimean War Enlistment Controversy between Great Britain and the United States', *Canadian Historical Review*, (1938), pp.300–27.
32 McGuigan, *Into Battle*, pp.78–79.
33 R. Stevenson, 'The Osmanli Irregular Cavalry: Organising Britain's Bashi-Bazouks', *The War Correspondent*, 33:1 (2015), pp.35–42.

Table 2.1 Deaths in the infantry regiments in relation to the time spent on active service in Bulgaria and the Crimea

Month of arrival (1854–55)	Number of regiments	Median numbers with (range) and [Proportion (%) of median admissions]				
		Admissions to hospital	Total deaths [c4/c3*100]	W&I deaths* [c5/c3*100]	Cholera deaths [c6/c3*100]	Other deaths [c7/c3*100]
Apr.–June	25	2,925 (2,232–3,944)	399 (237–650) [13.5]	50 (9–86) [1.7]	83 (35–152) [2.8]	246 (147–467) [8.5]
July–Sep.	6	2,596 (1,737–2,857)	342 (200–497) [13]	25 (20–50) [1]	53 (36–82) [2]	250 (128–413) [9.5]
Oct.–Dec.	9	2,101 (1,725–2,840)	221 (124–550) [10.5]	17 (7–56) [0.8]	59 (10–195) [2.8]	159 (69–377) [7.5]
Jan.–Mar.	3	1,577 (1,332–2,690)	86 (71–104) [5.5]	7 (2–10) [0.5]	33 (20–41) [2]	56 (28–64) [3.5]
Apr.–June	6	1,652 (1,047–1,918)	84 (63–102) [5]	9 (1–21) [0.5]	43 (18–74) [2.5]	30 (15–41) [1.8]
July–Sep.	3	1,159 (335–1,176)	30 (10–33) [2.5]	1 (0–1) [<0.1]	12 (4–20) [1]	12 (5–18) [1]

* W&I = Wounds and injuries.

(Summarized from the tables in the regimental histories in the *Medical and Surgical History*, 1)

Table 2.2 Deaths in the infantry regiments in relation to the time spent on active service in Bulgaria and the Crimea together with those who were invalided

Month of arrival (1854–55)	Number of regiments	Median numbers with (range) and [median % of median strength]		
		Men sent to the East	Deaths [c4/c3*100]	Invalids [c5/3*100]
Apr.–June	25	1,570 (1237–2341)	460 (265–784) [29]	288 (133–444) [18.5]
July–Sep.	6	1,398 (1321–1783)	395 (257–458) [28]	205 (184–359) [14.5]
Oct.–Dec.	9	1,267 (1079–1477)	246 (137–570) [19.5]	202 (153–279) [16]
January–March	3	1,177 (1069–1187)	94 (77–109) [8]	129 (67–199) [11]
Apr.–June	6	998 (928–1092)	93 (73–146) [9.5]	120 (84–169) [12]
July–Sep.	3	918 (701–927)	30 (9–38) [3]	31 (11–32) [3]

(Summarized from Sayer, *Despatches*, end paper)

2.1.3 Reception in the Crimea

The Royal Navy was responsible for overseeing the transportation of troops to the East with the military authorities, particularly the QMG's department, taking charge once they landed. In theory this should take place only when 'tents and blankets were ready for them.'[34] These instructions were amplified a few weeks later: 'Officers in command of troops coming to join the Army [are] responsible that every article of equipage (blankets, camp kettles, water canteens, haversacks, tents, hospital marquees, intrenching tools, and hospital panniers) are disembarked and in a state of readiness to be carried on the march by the soldiers themselves, together with two days rations.'[35]

On occasions disembarkation was delayed by 'boisterous weather' and once ashore things did not go smoothly when the military authorities failed to make adequate provision for the new arrivals. Various reports confirmed that matters deteriorated noticeably from the beginning of November 1854. On 6 January 1855 Newcastle complained to Raglan that he had heard that a detachment of Guards had marched to camp without a guide, and, after getting lost found on arrival in camp that nothing had been prepared from them.[36]

In an attempt to ameliorate the situation the troops were given some time to acclimatize before moving to the plateau to do duty in the trenches, though the official histories of the Grenadier Guards and the 14th 18th, 34th, 39th, 71st, and 90th Regiments noted that this policy did not necessarily make it easier for the men as they did not escape exhausting fatigues, cholera or other enteric diseases.[37]

Illness following arrival: Many men landing during the first nine months after the invasion fell ill, often with a fatal result, particularly when cholera was present in the camps. At the beginning of January 1855 Hall pointed out, with good reason, that the poor health was due to several interrelated factors which if corrected should result in improvement:

> It is quite true that all newly arrived regts and [...] recruits [...] have suffered more than others from disease. Cholera [appeared] about the middle of November and proved very destructive. [...] The weather was wet, cold, and tempestuous, the duty necessarily severe, and the exposure of the men in the trenches necessarily very great. Supplies of all kinds were obtained with great difficulty for want of transport, and from the almost impassable state of the roads [...] Fuel was exceedingly scarce, and cooking consequently imperfectly performed. The shelter of bell tents, many of which were old, thin and torn, was inadequate to the climate and season of the year. There was no want of disposition on the part

---

34 QMG to Captain Hamilton, 28 November 1854; TNA: WO 28/137.
35 QMG, Memorandum, 22 December 1854; TNA: WO 28/196.
36 TNA: WO 6/70/111.
37 For details see the *Medical and Surgical History*, 1.

of any one to remedy the evils that existed, but at one time means were wanting, and the difficulties [...] almost insurmountable. Of late [...] the men are better clad, and fed, and the duty is lighter, and great efforts are made to get them more comfortably housed [...] At a distance it is not easy to comprehend all the difficulties [...] and a number of unforeseen accidents [...] have added to embarrassment perplexing enough in themselves.[38]

Dr R. Lyons, a pathologist who had been sent to the East by Panmure to investigate the disease afflicting the Army, also recognized these problems. He noted in his official report that: 'Amongst even well-matured constitutions the hardships and fatigues, trials, privations, and exposure of campaigns, such as those of the past year in the Crimea, [...] prove largely productive of disease, and induce much mortality. But in the undeveloped frames and the unripe strength of the ill-seasoned recruit, such causes operated with two-fold energy, and with more than doubly fatal effect.'[39]

Incidentally, this issue was revisited after the war by Kinglake, who candidly summarized the position after the storm of 14 November 1854, and thereby supported Hall's assessment:

[The] reinforcements [...] did not effect a [...] sustained augmentation of the number of men [...] for the new-comers [when] subjected to the hardships [...] fell sick with appalling rapidity [to become] a superadded assemblage of hospital sufferers than an actual accession to strength. [...] the 9th Regiment [...] sickened so fast, that [after a few days they had] only a small remnant left. The Guards had received some strong draughts of men [...]; yet [at the end of January] the three battalions could only muster [...] 312 men. [...] The 63rd Regiment may almost be said to have disappeared.[40]

As the living standards and the weather improved during the course of 1855 the health of the new arrivals became less of a concern and, after the fall of Sevastopol, Hall was able to write more optimistically: 'The newly arrived regiments are getting acclimatized and we may reasonably expect [...] improvements in the general health of the Army, as duty will be less severe, and the weather is becoming cool and pleasant.'[41]

Incidentally, the importance of training and leadership, and the provision of satisfactory living conditions, were illustrated by the experience of the LTC during the second winter. Many recruits were too young and callow to cope and they sickened

---

38 Hall to Military Secretary, 25 January 1855; RAMC: 397/F/CO/1/1/1333.
39 HCPP 1857 Session 2 (2229) XVIII.533: *Report of the Pathology of the Diseases of the Army of the East*, (Hereafter: Pathology Report), pp.vii–viii. For a review of the report see *Glasgow Medical Journal*, 4 (1857), pp.129–46.
40 A.W. Kinglake, *The Invasion of the Crimea* (Edinburgh: Blackwood, 1891), 7, pp.178–9.
41 Hall to Simpson, 19 September 1855; RAMC: 397/F/CO/1/2/3134.

and died in relatively large numbers in comparison with the regular soldiers working alongside them who generally remained fit and capable of work. However, the employment of sufficient officers and NCOs to enforce discipline and order, and the improvement in the weather and living conditions, benefited their health towards the end of the campaign.

Mortality in relation to age: Nearly a third of the men joining the Army during the campaign were 21 years of age or under, and hence it is understandable that Hall concluded that these youths had a higher rate of mortality than the older troops, as nearly a quarter of the deaths from disease occurred in the younger lads. However, when the mortality rate was calculated with respect to age the converse was true as a higher proportion of the older troops died although the fatalities among those aged 36 or more accounted for only about five percent of all the deaths from disease (Figure 2.4).[42]

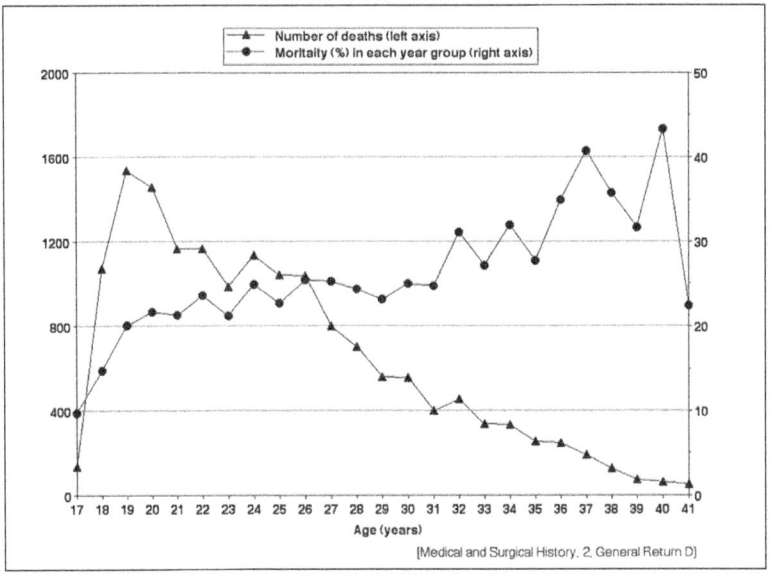

Figure 2.4 Relationship between the numbers of NCOs and men in each year group and the mortality rate.

2.1.4 Stoicism of the troops

The bad news received from the front did not seem to stem the flow of men volunteering to join up, perhaps a consequence of the considerable increase in the bounty offered to new recruits. The British Army was thus composed of volunteers, and this might account in part for their tenacity and forbearance in the face of adversity. For example,

---

42   The figures were calculated from the *Medical and Surgical History*, 2, General Return D.

letters written by two civilians, Charles Holte Bracebridge, one of Nightingale's companions, and Peter Benson Maxwell, one of the Hospital Commissioners, both refer to their stoicism.[43] This could explain why only twenty suicides were reported during the whole campaign.[44] Major General Estcourt, the Adjutant General also noted that: 'The regiments which fought their way here are the best; they bear their hardships wonderfully,'[45] while Assistant Surgeon Taylor wrote on 14 February 1855 that: 'The men never complain, and in this respect the officers [...] might take a creditable example from [them].'[46] Later, the future Viscount Wolesley, then Lieutenant G.J. Wolesley, 90th Foot, concluded:

> In the winter of 1854–55 I made frequent visits to Balaklava [...] All [the men] had a care-worn look that bespoke over work, insufficient food, and incipient disease. [...] In the midst of unavoidable misery, as also when struggling in danger, what an uncomplaining fellow is the British soldier! He was always energetic, either cursing his mule [...] or laughing at his comrade who had stumbled into some deep rut. [...] were I to live forever I should never forget the uncomplaining resignation of our soldiers throughout [the winters] appalling miseries.[47]

Further evidence of devotion to duty is provided by a report sent to the Ambassador in Constantinople on 3 February 1855:

> When the draft was mustered on deck [in Constantinople] some soldiers joined them from below, and requested [the medical officer] to let them go [back to the Crimea]. Several [were] so weak that they supported themselves on their muskets, but there they were equipped in heavy marching order [and begged] to be allowed, not to go home, but to return to the trenches. [...] If this is not real heroism, I know not what is, and, as such devoted gallantry is displayed in a manner which rarely attracts notice.[48]

Similarly, evacuees landing at Falmouth during February 1855 reported that 'they had undergone considerable hardships, but no more than troops were often exposed to by the contingencies of war; and that they firmly believed that their sufferings were unavoidable, and produced by causes over which their officers had no control.' In addition, Raglan had been 'universally kind and attentive to their condition and interests,

---

43 C.H. Bracebridge, letter, 13 November 1854; RAMC: 494 and P.B. Maxwell to Herbert, 8 January 1855; Wiltshire and Swindon History Centre: 3057/F8/II/B/363.
44 *Medical and Surgical History*, 2, General Return A.
45 Estcourt to AG, Horse Guards, 8 January 1855; National Army Museum: 1962-10-95.
46 Quoted by Cantlie, *History*, 2, pp.142–3.
47 Viscount Wolesley, *The Story of a Soldier's Life* (London: Archibald Constable, 1903), 1, pp.138–9.
48 J.H. Skene to Stratford, 3 February 1855; TNA: FO 352/41B.

and was continually to be seen in the lines,' while many of the men were 'so redolent of *esprit de corps* in the cause' that many declared they would be delighted to return and have 'another slap at the Russians.'[49] Likewise, many of those arriving on *Tynemouth* also expressed 'a desire to go out again.'[50]

In his despatch to Panmure dated 9 September 1855 reporting the fall of Sevastopol Simpson recorded that: 'The hardships and privations endured by many of the regiments [...] were endured by both officers and men with patience and unmurmuring endurance worthy of the highest praise and gained them the deserved applause and sympathy of their country.'[51] He also issued a General Order locally in which he availed 'himself of this opportunity to congratulate and convey his warmest thanks to the general officers, officers, and soldiers of the several Divisions, to the Royal Engineers and Artillery, for their cheerful endurance of almost unparalleled hardships and sufferings, and for the unflinching courage and determination which on so many trying occasions they have evinced.' This was later published in the British newspapers. Likewise, an unpublished draft of a history of the war prepared at Horse Guards echoed Simpson's sentiments: 'Great as the sufferings of the Army were it is gratifying to record the fortitude and cheerfulness with what the soldiers bore up against them, and continued to the last a strict performance of their duties and a regard to discipline which must now reflect great credit upon the British Army.'[52]

It is a testimony to the phlegmatic nature and good discipline of the British soldier that despite having lethal weapons within easy reach and living cheek by jowl in less than satisfactory conditions only three men were arraigned during the campaign for killing a fellow soldier, and only one was hanged.[53]

2.1.5 Land Transport Corps

The first draft of NCOs and artificers arrived from England on 22 April 1855 and the 'Turks in charge of the Commissariat' were then distributed among the infantry divisions and to a depot in Balaklava. Men, 'mainly Asiatics', were then recruited by agents 'at the Dardanelles, Constantinople, and various places in Asia' and sent to Crimea 'without medical inspection.' The headquarters and depot comprising two wings were moved to 'a knoll on the east of Kadikoi' in June 1855 and this site 'proved much more healthy than the huts at Balaklava.'

The living conditions and the provision of health care for the corps was generally unsatisfactory from the start and this was reflected in a relatively higher mortality from disease than that experienced in the main army during the period June 1855–March

---

49 *West Britain and Cornwall Advertiser*, 9 February 1855.
50 *Daily News*, 7 May 1855.
51 *London Gazette* and *The Times*, 22 & 24 September 1855 respectively.
52 TNA: WO 28/199/2. The paragraph was annotated 'omit' suggesting that it would not have appeared if a published version had been printed.
53 M. Hinton, 'Capital Punishment in the Crimea', *The War Correspondent*, 29:1 (2011), p.38 and TNA: WO 28/199/2.

1856 (Figure 2.5). Of 358 deaths recorded 147 (41 percent), 125 (35 percent), and 47 (13 percent) were caused by fevers, cholera, and dysentery or diarrhoea respectively. 'In short, the men [...] were little better in regard to exposure and hard work, hut and hospital accommodation in the winter of 1855–56 than the men of the line during the previous winter.'[54]

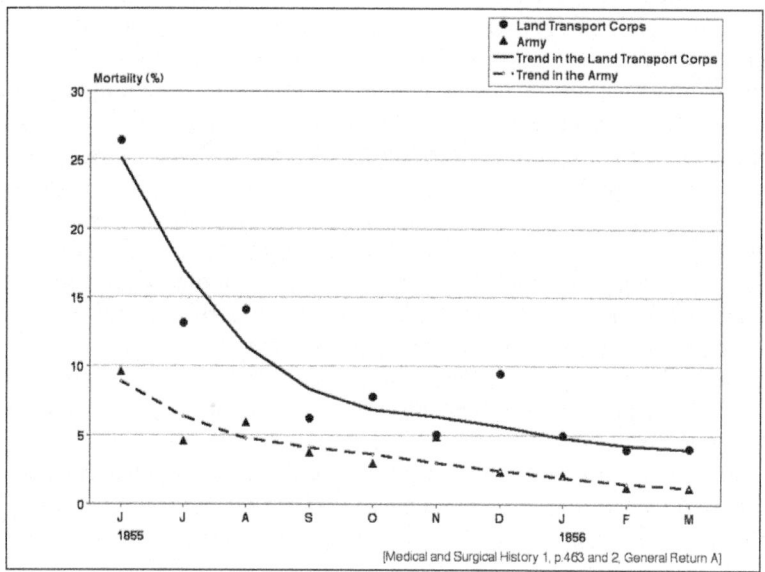

Figure 2.5 Mortality from disease in the Land Transport Corps and the Army, June 1855–March 1856.

2.1.6 Camp followers

A large population of civilians and camp followers congregated within the allied lines. The Army, including the AMD, had no responsibility for them and hence no details of their numbers or disease status were collected or published. Nevertheless, some individuals had to be provided for, although not necessarily at the public expense, given General J. Simpson's response to a letter from Hall dated 16 August 1855: 'There is hardly any person in Balaklava, who does not receive some pay [...] and I therefore recommend that no patient be treated free of expense, but be charged hospital stoppages.'[55]

---

54 For further details see *Medical and Surgical History*, 1, pp.460–5, on which this section is based.
55 Smith, *Précis of Letters*, 2, Appendix 7.

2.1.7 Concluding remarks

The British Army was composed of volunteers who, though they may have been tempted to join the colours for the bounty paid, nevertheless exhibited courage and stoicism in the face of danger and hardship.

Many of the men sent to the East were young and immature and they would have found it difficult enough to cope with the vicissitudes of camp life and the arduous duties in the trenches under normal circumstances, let alone during the first winter of the campaign when the environmental conditions on the plateau had deteriorated, particularly after the hurricane of 14 November 1854. In addition, some of the new arrivals were let down by the military authorities because of a failure to make adequate provision for their well-being following disembarkation. Inevitably this had a deleterious effect on their health and ultimately their chances of survival from cholera and other enteric diseases that were prevalent in the Army at the time. This topic that will be considered further in later chapters.

2.2 Army Medical Department

McGrigor retired as Director General in 1852 and his place was taken by Smith who was paid less than half of his salary, and whose status would inevitably have been diminished thereby. At the time of Smith's appointment there were 667 medical officers distributed between the staff (185) and regiments including the RA stationed in the UK, Colonies, and India (482). Smith had control over the staff medical officers, but little over the regimental medical officers who were under the orders of their commanding officers. There were also 80 regimental medical officers and a few others in India, paid for by the Honourable East India Company, and over whom Smith had no authority.[56]

2.2.1 Medical officers and principal support staff

Maxwell, a hospital commissioner, considered that under normal circumstances the number of surgeons employed at the beginning of the campaign should have been more than adequate; and thus the forward planning could not be faulted.[57] However, as it transpired, circumstances proved far from normal, and a considerable number of additional medical personnel and support staff served during the campaign. Several published and unpublished returns have survived but none appear complete, and there are inconsistencies between them.[58] In order to demonstrate how the medical services

---

56 Cantlie, *A History*, 2, pp.3–4.
57 Anon [Maxwell], *Whom Shall We Hang? The Sebastopol Enquiry* (London: James Ridgeway, 1855), p.186.
58 Unpublished sources: (1) A monthly return on the Army's strength prepared by the AG contained the names of these individuals in the grades; TNA: WO 3/1730–1731; (2) The medical staff serving in the Army of the East; TNA: WO 33/3B/68–56/11–2 (Cabinet

evolved during the campaign the foregoing analysis will be restricted to one unpublished summary table prepared by Hall from records available to him locally, and which listed the numbers of personnel employed on the medical staff, and in the regiments, from April 1854 until April 1856.[59]

Military surgeons: The number of regiments increased throughout the campaign until shortly after the fall of Sevastopol (Figure 2.1) and hence the number of regimental surgeons in post increased from April 1854 until the end of 1855 when the numbers stabilized at about 240 (Figure 2.6). When the staffing levels were related to the size of the Army the ratio of surgeons to men reduced from 1:320–335 while in Bulgaria to 1:170–155 in the spring of 1855, after which the ratio widened to 1:210–245.

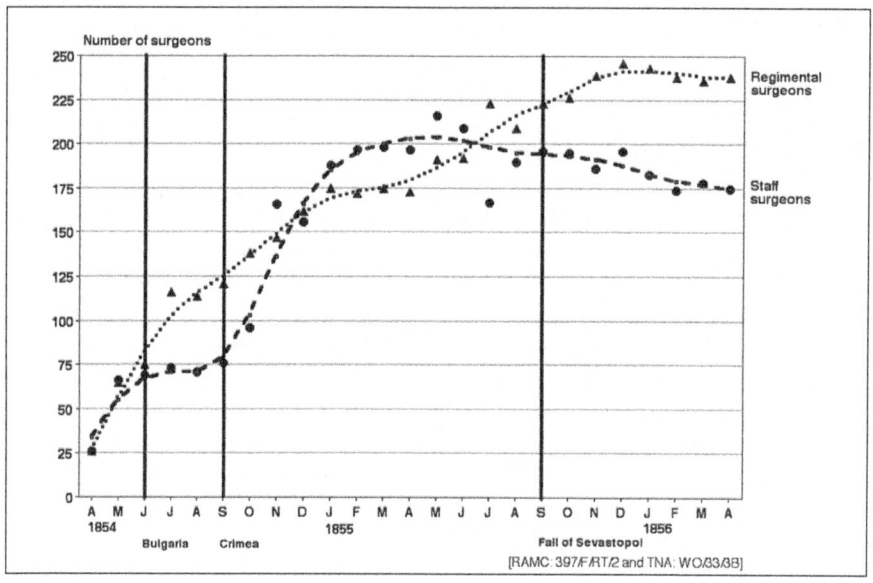

Figure 2.6 Number, and the trend, of regimental and staff surgeons each month, April 1854–April 1856.

paper) and RAMC: 397/F/RT/2 (Hall's longhand version); and (3) An incomplete collection of longhand monthly returns of the strength of the Army Medical Department in TNA: WO 28/193; and published sources: HCPP 1854–55 (126) XXXII.431: *(Turkey). Return of the Medical Officers Attached to the Forces Serving in Turkey*; HCPP 1854–55 (428) XXXII.421: *Medical Officers (Army and Navy)*; HCPP 1857 Session 1 (133) IX.11L: *Return of the Names of Officers [...] of the Army* etc.; the *Medical and Surgical History*; Smith, *Précis of Letters*, 1, Appendix 8; the *Army Lists* for the years of the campaign; and General Orders.

59 The Army's monthly numerical strength is included in a printed version (TNA: WO 33/3B/68–56/11–2) but not in a longhand draft (RAMC: 397/F/RT/2). It is not clear if this table included surgeons in the RA.

Relatively few staff surgeons were employed in Bulgaria. The numbers increased after the invasion to reach about 200 during the summer of 1855, after which time the strength decreased to about 175 by April 1856 (Figure 2.6). The ratio of staff surgeons to men widened during the build-up of the Army in Bulgaria to exceed 1:400. It then reduced to 1:150–160 during the first winter before gradually widening to just over 1:300 when peace was declared.

The need to provide sufficient medical officers on hospital ships and in the general hospitals prompted Hall to ask Raglan to permit the transfer of the third assistant regimental surgeon to the medical staff so they could be deployed on detached duty when required.[60] Newcastle indicated that he favoured an increase in the complement of both regimental and staff assistant surgeons and on 29 January 1855 informed Raglan that that the third assistant surgeon could be transferred to the medical staff, as the size of the regiments had been reduced and the numbers in hospital increased.[61] Hall also pointed out it was usual for regiments to be 'disembarrassed of their sick' by placing them 'under treatment in General Hospitals,' thus leaving the remaining surgeons 'free to meet contingencies as they arise.' Hall concluded that 'No injury can accrue for the proposed alteration as it is equally easy to attach a staff medical officer temporarily to regiments when required.'[62] This opinion, which was subsequently endorsed by the Hospital Commissioners who considered that under normal circumstances a surgeon, an assistant surgeon, and a apothecary (*sic*: ? a dispenser) should be sufficient for an infantry regiment.[63] It was forwarded by Raglan to the War Office with the following comment:

> I am not disposed to question [Hall's] opinion, but I attach so much importance to the maintenance of the regimental hospital system so long as circumstance[s] [...] allow, that I earnestly recommend that this diminished number may be kept as efficient as possible, and that [surgeons] should not be transferred from [their] Corps [...] on slight grounds, the advantage of them knowing the men [...] being incalculable.

In his reply to Raglan Panmure wrote: 'I [...] suppose that the varying requirements of the service will best be met by empowering your Lordship to make [...] such disposition of the medical strength [...] whither staff or regimental, as with the assistance and advice of the senior medical officer, you may judge expedient.'[64]

---

60 Hall, diary entry, 27 November 1854; RAMC: 524/15/6 and AG, Horse Guards to Raglan, 19 August 1854; TNA: WO 3/116.
61 *Hansard*, 12 December 1854 and TNA: WO 6/70.
62 Hall to Military Secretary, 13 February 1855; RAMC: 397/F/CO/1/1/1442 and TNA: WO 1/371/463–6.
63 Hospital Commission Report, p.49.
64 Panmure to Raglan, 16 February 1855; TNA: WO 6/70/232–3. The despatch was annotated by Lt. Col. Lefroy: 'Lord Panmure's despatch [...] seems to close this correspondence.'

The shortage of surgeons remained an issue, and later in the year Smith informed Hall efforts were being made to supply replacements for absent surgeons, and suggesting that staff officers should be attached to regiments during their absence.[65] In the latter part of 1855 the possibility of replacing the third assistant surgeon with a dispenser of medicines was discussed,[66] and Panmure approved of this policy, at least initially.[67] A few weeks later dispensers, many of whom had worked with chemists, were sent to the Crimea for regiments not having a third assistant surgeon,[68] an initiative that probably accounted for the increase in the number of dispensers recorded by Hall during early 1856. This policy did not find favour at Horse Guards, however, and it was 'withdrawn in consequence of the opinion of the Commander-in-Chief.' This decision was opposed by Smith who considered that the continued want of staff assistant surgeons 'would be more felt if the Army took to the field in the spring [of 1856].'[69]

Incidentally, the appointment of dispensers to regiments raised problems regarding their status as most had not completed a medical training and did not equate to surgeons of the lowest rank. This dilemma necessitated Hall to inform Smith of:

> The anomalous and unpleasant position, in which the dispensers attached to regiments are placed. The appointments being a new one and not defined by authority some Commanding Officers have objected to consider them as officers belonging to the mess of the regiments. It is probable this difficulty will be obviated by a new warrant, but if not, it would be well [...] to have the question defined and settled by authority.[70]

Smith replied to say that the 'Secretary for War has decided that dispensers attached to infantry regiments are to be regimental officers, and have been commissioned accordingly.'[71] Hall passed this information to the AG[72] who informed a divisional commander of the decision that dispensers should be 'received in every respect as such.'[73]

Dispensers of medicines: The number of dispensers increased following the invasion of the Crimea to 24–38 between February 1855 and April 1856 when the number

---

65 Smith to Hall, 7 August 1855; Smith, *Précis of Letters*.
66 Cantlie, *A History*, 2, p.176.
67 Smith to Undersecretary, 14 September 1855 and Smith to Hall, 5 October 1855, Smith, *Précis of Letters*.
68 Smith to Hall, 7 November 1855; Smith, *Précis of Letters*.
69 Smith to Undersecretary, 24 January 1856; Smith, *Précis of Letters*.
70 Hall to Smith, 29 February 1856; RAMC: 397/F/CO/1/2/4323.
71 Smith to Hall, 18 March 1856; Smith, *Précis of Letters*.
72 Hall to AG. 13 April 1856; RAMC: 397/F/CO/1/2/4617.
73 AG to GOC, 1st Division, 14 April 1856; TNA: WO/28/125.

increased to 54. This presumably reflected the attachment of dispensers to regiments in lieu of the third assistant surgeon as mentioned above.

Hospital dressers: The difficulty in obtaining sufficient qualified medical practitioners prompted Smith to send out twelve dressers and their arrival was recorded during the following month, December 1854.[74] The numbers increased to 36 in March to May 1855 before declining gradually to eleven by April 1856.

Apothecaries, purveyors, and support staff: A Royal Warrant delineating conditions of service for apothecaries was signed on 23 October 1854.[75] Only three were employed during the campaign, namely, G.H. Reade, who died at Scutari on 28 November 1854 and was succeeded by J. Mackintosh, and F. Fernandez who served in the Crimea from October 1854 until June 1856.

The duties of the Purveyor included the provision of hospital equipment, the rations for patients and staff, hospital extras and medical comforts, the cooking of meals and diets, washing of hospital and patients' clothes, cleanliness of all parts of the hospital except the wards, payment of staff, arrangement of funerals, and drawing up of wills.'

Smith and Hall made no reference to purveyors in their returns, possibly because they were not part of the AMD until the issuing of a Royal Warrant on 31 October 1855,[76] though the department was placed under Hall's orders in detailed instructions of his duties issued by the War Office on 14 November 1854.[77]

An analysis of the arrivals of purveyors and purveyor's clerks recorded in the General Orders revealed that the staff of this department did not increase significantly until the beginning of 1855 with new arrivals joining the Army throughout the rest of that year. Five clerks were promoted to Purveyor during February and March 1855 and their number was deducted from the number of clerks.

The provision of medical services during the campaign was a considerable undertaking but it appeared from Smith's return that despite this there were few store keepers employed and little clerical assistance.[78] Five of the fourteen medical clerks served only in the Crimea while one, who did two tours of duty, served in Scutari, Bulgaria and the Crimea. The number of clerks available for duty did not exceed three until July 1855. Thereafter, staffing increased regularly until April 1856. Some clerks were retained in Scutari until August 1856, presumably to assist with organizing the final departure from Turkey.

---

74   Smith to Hall, 9 November 1855; Smith, *Précis of Letters*.
75   *The Lancet*, 18 November 1854.
76   Cantlie, *A History*, 2, p.60.
77   Printed pamphlet in the Herbert papers; Wiltshire and Swindon History Centre: 2057/F8/III/B/299, and reproduced in Select Committee, 2nd Report, pp.701–3.
78   *Medical and Surgical History*, 1, Appendix VIII, p.525.

2.2.2 Mortality among medical officers

Of 752 medical officers employed during the campaign, 418 (56 percent) reported sick, 48 (six percent) died, and 186 (25 percent) were invalided home.[79] The loss of medical officers during the summer of 1854 and the first winter would have compounded the medical problems during this period, and from time to time: 'sickness amongst the orderlies and the medical officers [was] very considerable.'[80]

Of staff surgeons who died almost half served in the Crimea and half in Turkey, while the preponderance of regimental surgeons died near the front. Incidentally, a further list of surgeons and support staff stationed on the Dardanelles and Bosphorus and who died during the campaign was included in Smith's *Précis of Letters*.[81] The names of the medical officers who died were subsequently inscribed on a memorial at Military Hospital erected at Netley after the war. Sadly, the monument was destroyed when the hospital was demolished.[82]

The mortality rate among medical officers during the first year of the campaign was 13 percent and in the second, two percent. This figure was within the annual rate recorded during 1839–1854, viz. 2–6 percent (median 3.1).[83]

2.2.3 Hospital orderlies

Before war was declared Smith proposed the creation of a 'Hospital Corps of at least 600 men to serve as hospital orderlies and ambulance waggon drivers.'[84] The suggestion was accepted in principle by Newcastle and Hardinge, but nothing was decided in advance of the troops arrival in Turkey and consequently the PMO at Scutari had to 'recruit ward-masters, ward orderlies, stewards, storekeepers, and cooks, from men left behind at Scutari, many of whom would have had 'no formal training and in all probability would be the poorest soldiers in their respective units' being 'bad characters with long crime sheets.'[85, 86]

A General Order dated 4 July 1854 required the 3rd Division to provide orderlies and attendants at the General Hospital in Varna while the provision of hospital staff in the Crimea continued on an 'ad hoc' basis until a General Order of 11 May 1855 (see below), although 55 volunteers from the depots at Chatham were sent out to Scutari towards the end of 1854.[87]

---

79 Smith to Undersecretary at War, 3 March 1856; Smith, *Précis of Letters*.
80 Hall to Smith, 19 March 1855; Wellcome Library: MS 8520, ff.307–10.
81 Smith, *Précis of Letters*, 2, Appendix 35.
82 For a photograph see Shepherd, *Crimean Doctors*, 2, Plate XXXVI.
83 Royal Commission Report, Appendix VIII.
84 Smith to Military Secretary, 18 February 1854; Smith, *Précis of Letters* and TNA: WO 43/987.
85 Cantlie, *A History*, 2, pp.11 & 20.
86 Hall issued a printed document on 13 August 1854 outlining the duties of hospital stewards and ward-masters; RAMC: 397/F/CO/2/1.
87 AG, Horse Guards to Raglan, 15 December 1854; TNA: WO 3/116.

Maxwell, one of the Hospital Commissions, informed Herbert privately that that 'the hospital [at Scutari] is not sufficiently provided with orderlies' and that:

> evil arises from the practice of removing hospital orderlies [...] well enough to return to their regiments, so that surgeons have always to deal with wretched and unskilled convalescents [...] this might be attended with great advantage if the soldiers [taken] to do duty as orderlies, were left in that situation, [because, if they] shewed a capacity for learning their business, they would seem very efficient, and a smaller number would probably suffice than is now required.

He then pointed out that 'most of [the hospital's] bad points would disappear if an efficient body of orderlies could be organized,' but 'the system will not work well [if] such duties are entrusted to rude uneducated men of sickly health, miserable habits, and more miserable propensities [and] it is but natural to shrink in dismay from the consequences of entrusting such duties to such men.'[88]

Following receipt of this correspondence Herbert summarized his views to Smith: 'all authorities concur to the entire failure of the hospital orderlies [and] press for a permanent establishment devoted to this work, and to this only!'[89] The points made privately by Maxwell were reiterated officially by the Hospital Commissioners who regarded 'this branch of the hospital service as most unsatisfactory' and added that: 'The ward-masters and assistant ward-masters are generally intelligent and respectable non-commissioned officers but they do not possess that degree of experience [...] which ought [...] be an indispensable condition to their employment [...] in our military hospitals [and] the cooks are but indifferently acquainted with the peculiar style of cooking required in hospitals.'[90]

Later Maxwell gave evidence to the Roebuck Committee:

> The whole system of hospital orderlies was radically defective [...] The men were [...] not of a strong constitution, but very often convalescents [...] or not sufficiently strong to stand the hard work of the trenches. They did not volunteer, but were ordered [...] Their work was incessant [...] and they were very ignorant of their duties [and] upon being sufficiently recovered [were] ordered back to active service [...] and raw recruits [...] substituted in their place.[91]

One of the nurses at Scutari recognized that some men 'thought well of as patients' showed 'a negligence, hardness, and indifference' after becoming orderlies. She also indicated that no orderly 'comes back sober' after leave to go out, although she accepted

---

88 Maxwell to Herbert, 10 November and 5 & 10 December 1854; Wiltshire and Swindon History Centre: 2057/F8/III/B/356 & 359–60.
89 Herbert to Smith, 24 December 1854; Select Committee, 4th Report, pp.343–4.
90 Hospital Commission Report, p.32
91 Select Committee, 2nd Report, p.671.

that they had some excuse, given that they were 'confined day and night to the pestilential air of the sick wards' and 'had to perform offices for the dead and dying much more trying than any we had to do; they were expected in addition to their day's work sit up every third night.'[92]

Inevitably, despite the acceptance of the importance of this issue, it was not until June 1855 that the embodiment of the MSC was finally authorized (see Section 2.2.5).

2.2.4 Staffing levels in general and regimental hospitals

At the end of 1854 nearly 800 men were employed at Scutari 'as orderlies, ward-masters, charge of stores, etc.' which gave a ratio of 1:6–7 patients and that 'the regulation of 1:10 at home could not be carried out here' as 'attending the sick being very hard'. It was concluded, however, that 'most of the men are efficient and fit for service.'[93]

In April 1855 the ratio was still about 1:7 overall, the General Hospital had space for 905 patients and 129 orderlies, the Barrack Hospital, 1,683 and 240, and the Palace Hospital, 400 and 63,[94] while another return listed the deployment of 577 non-medical hospital staff as: 14 head ward-masters, 50 assistant ward-masters, 450 orderlies, eight head cooks, 35 assistant cooks, 11 surgery men, two bath men, four dead house men, and three barbers.[95] Similarly, the scale of the commitment in the Crimea can be gauged by a return made in July 1855 listing the names of 21 NCOs and 222 privates employed as orderlies in the 'Hospital establishments in Balaklava and on [...] sick ships.'[96]

The allowance of one orderly to ten patients could prove inadequate in General Hospitals with smaller wards, and particularly those in the Crimea, since one man in a ward could not carry out the routine duties in the day, attend to seriously ill patients, and then undertake night duty on a regular basis.[97] Hall, therefore, informed the AG that three orderlies for two wards was the minimum to ensure they were kept clean and the sick properly cared for. Nineteen orderlies for the 21 wards in the General Hospital at Balaklava were inadequate and an additional 13 were required.[98]

Information on the 'number of orderlies and other hospital attendants employed' in regimental hospitals, and their 'general fitness for their duties' was sought by a questionnaire circulated by the Hospital Commissioners on 3 December 1854. The answers suggest that most surgeons were relatively satisfied with their hospital staff,

---

92 S. Terrot, *Reminiscences of Scutari Hospitals in Winter 1854–55* (Edinburgh: Andrew Stevenson, 1898), p.38.
93 Paulet to AG, 30 December 1854; TNA: WO 28/186.
94 PMO, Scutari to Smith, 5 April 1855; Smith, *Précis of Letters*.
95 Deputy Secretary for War to Smith, 31 July 1855; Smith, *Précis of Letters*.
96 Commandant, Balaklava to AG, 27 July 1856; TNA: WO 28/194.
97 Dr Matthews to PMO, Balaklava, 30 April to 16 May 1855; Royal Commission Report, Appendix LXXIX, pp.191–2.
98 Hall to AG, 7 May 1855; RAMC: 397/F/CO/1/1/2031.

all of whom were soldiers of the regiment, although problems arose when the regular personnel became sick, and had to be replaced by inexperienced men, while on occasions the number allowed by regulation could prove inadequate, although there was scope to draft in fatigue men on occasions.

Early in 1855 Newcastle informed Brigadier the Hon. W. Paulet the commandant on the Bosphorus, that Smith was engaged in: 'the organization of a permanent hospital staff to supersede the use of orderlies taken from the ranks [as it was] obvious that the hospital duty cannot be well performed by a succession of fresh and inexperienced hands possessing no interest in the permanent well-being of the establishment.'[99] Dr A. Cumming, the PMO at Scutari, was informed privately that 'We are also sending out stewards and ward-masters, selected by Smith, and we hope gradually to give you a corps of permanent hospital orderlies to replace your ever changing body.'[100] Paulet also received similar advice from the Hospital Commissioners who noted that:

> One of the most obvious defects [...] is the utter absence of a trained body of orderlies [also hospital sergeants, ward-masters, and cooks. The task which devolve on these men requires [the employment] of persons of intelligence and respectable character, good constitution and active habits [and who have] undergone some training. [...] and those who prove themselves duly qualified should not be removed except for misconduct or incapacity.[101]

The shortage of manpower meant that men could not be spared from the Crimea and hence additional orderlies would have to be sent from England.[102] Despite the apparent interest of ministers, progress was slow and Smith continued to hear 'of inefficiency of the orderlies [and stressed] the necessity for some remedy being immediately adopted to remedy [this] evil.'[103]

The temporary assignment of convalescent and other soldiers detached from their regiments for hospital duties could cause problems following their recall for regimental duty at short notice. For example, Hall informed Raglan on 28 December 1854 that the absence of orderlies when the QMG [Airey] visited the General Hospital in Balaklava was because those from one regiment had be withdrawn by the military

---

99 Newcastle to Paulet, 5 January 1855; TNA: WO 33/1/8/55 & WO 6/70 and Wiltshire and Swindon History Centre: 2057/F8/III/C/65.
100 Herbert to Cumming, 5 January 1855; Wiltshire and Swindon History Centre: 2057/F8/III/C/15.
101 Commissioners to Paulet, 26 January 1855; Hospital Commission Report, p.346. Incidentally, on 12 February Paulet informed Raglan that he 'never withdrew or changed [orderlies] except for gross misconduct;' National Army Museum: 1968-07-393-8.
102 AG to Paulet, 13 January 1855; TNA: WO 28/186
103 Smith to Military Undersecretary, 26 March 1855; Select Committee, 2nd Report, p.704; Royal Commission Report, Appendix LXXIX, p.46; Smith, *Précis of Letters*; and *The Lancet*, 28 July 1855.

authorities before a new draft had arrived.[104] The issue was eventually clarified by a General Order of 11 May 1855 which obliged infantry regiments to select four 'efficient' men as permanent orderlies for the General Hospitals at Balaklava and the sick ships. The Order was amended on 7 June to require regiments to replace orderlies who became non-effective.

The work of the orderlies was arduous, and some requested to return to their regiments on that account,[105] while others succumbed to disease, and some died. This situation probably provided the stimulus for a further Order on 17 May authorizing hospital sergeants and orderlies to receive free rations and an extra 8d and 4d a day as an inducement.[106] This payment was backdated to 1 May and on 22 May the terms were extended to orderlies on hospital ships etc., while on 10 October 1855 the payment of a 6d field allowance, in addition to these allowances, was confirmed.[107]

Problems persisted however and the need for a Hospital Corps, which could cater for 1,500 sick, and the provision of an 'extensive' Purveyor's Department remained an imperative,[108] although the issue was not resolved until the arrival of members of the MSC a little before Christmas 1855.[109]

2.2.5 Medical Staff Corps

The embodiment of the MSC was authorized by an Order in Council on 30 June 1855 and confirmed by Royal Warrant on 20 September 1855.[110] The objective was to recruit literate men of 'intelligence and highest character'[111] with the recommendation from Panmure that the NCOs should be fit enough for hospital duty though 'not quite so robust' as required 'for active duty in the field'.[112] The bounty and levy money was the same as for line regiments at home; the term of enlistment, ten years; age, 25–35 years; minimum height, 5ft 2ins; and pay, 2/- per day.[113] The principal duties were: 'to attend upon and assist generally [...] patients, to apply [...] simple portions of their

---

104 RAMC: 397/F/CO/1/1/1204 and National Army Museum: 1968-07-293.
105 For correspondence on orderlies see Royal Commission Report, Appendix LXXIX, pp.191–5.
106 Hall informed Smith on 19 May that the increase in pay and free rations was to encourage recruiting; RAMC: 397/F/CO/1/1/1219 & 2127 and Smith, *Précis of Letters*. Smith replied on 8 June 1855 to say he hoped that this policy would ease matters until the Hospital Corps could be organized; Smith, *Précis of Letters*.
107 TNA: WO 1/369. The allowance of 6d a day was granted to NCOs and men by a Royal Warrant dated 16 August 1855. It was back-dated to 1 July and announced in a General Order on 21 September 1855.
108 Hall to Smith, 8 October & 5 November 1855; RAMC: 397/F/CO/1/2/3322 & 3524.
109 National Army Museum: 1968-07-380-8B.
110 For details see Sweetman, 'The Crimean War', pp.113–9 and Cantlie, *A History*, 2, pp.149–50 & 171.
111 Deputy Secretary for War to AG, Horse Guards, 11 May 1855; TNA: WO 123/14, RAMC: 397/F/GO/2/6, *The Lancet*, 7 July; and *Association Medical Journal*, 27 July 1855.
112 Deputy Secretary for War to AG, Horse Guards, 11 May 1855; TNA: WO 123/151.
113 Circular Memorandum, 25 June 1855; TNA: WO 123151.

treatment, to keep clean the portion of their ward under their charge, to collect the foul linen and distribute clean linen [...] and generally to attend to the wants of the patients.'[114]

The HQ was at Chatham and the full complement was to be 10 companies of 120 men. Each would cater for 500 patients and would comprise two sections of 102 and 18 NCOs and men in the Surgeon's and Purveyor's Department respectively.[115] Smith suggested that officers promoted from the ranks would be 'less likely to be sensitive, or apt to take umbrage at the light in which their position and duties might be received and perhaps remarked on by the officers of the more strictly combatant class.'[116]

On 15 September 1855 the AG at Horse Guards ordained the MSC should be 'under the general superintendence and control of the PMO of each hospital' but 'military discipline [will] be maintained and enforced by the officer commanding on the station.'[117] Smith, nevertheless, requested Hall to keep a 'defaulters book' and that the men should be informed that a record of their offences would thus be retained.[118] Smith also considered the Corps should remain under the control of the AMD and not be employed for military duties, and he informed Hall that he was endeavouring to 'place within his reach men whom no military authorities can affect.'[119]

Smith was informed in mid-June that 37 sergeants, 27 corporals and 178 privates had volunteered,[120] and by the next month recruiting ceased as there were sufficient men for eight companies.[121] The first contingent of 300 men, including hospital stewards and ward-masters arrived at Scutari during November 1855. Some replaced regimental orderlies,[122] while others were sent to the General and Castle Hospitals in Balaklava.[123] Incidentally, the AG [Colonel the Hon. W.L. Pakenham] made the point privately to the AG [Wetherall] at Horse Guards that the men had been 'enlisted under several warrants' and as a consequence they were 'in a fix' as the 'mode of dealing with them was very confused.'[124]

Several drafts of men 'perfected in their respective duties' were sent to the East from time to time[125] until the depot was broken up during May 1856, although last

---

114 See Wiltshire and Swindon History Centre: 2057/F8/III/B/237 for the proposed regulations for the Corps.
115 Cantlie, *A History*, 2, p.426.
116 Cantlie, *A History*, 2, p.149.
117 TNA: WO 123/151; RAMC: 397/F/CO/1/3; and RAMC: 397/F/GO/2/5.
118 Smith to Hall, 23 November 1855; RAMC: 397/F/CO/1/3.
119 Smith to Hall, 22 November 1855; Smith, *Précis of Letters*.
120 Smith, *Précis of Letters*.
121 *The Times*, 24 July 1855.
122 Cantlie, *A History*, 2, p.171.
123 Medical Department Memorandum, 18 December 1855; National Army Museum: 1968-07-380-8B.
124 Pakenham to AG, Horse Guards, 26 February 1856; National Army Museum: 1962-10-97-1.
125 *The Times*, 24 November 1855; 1 & 25 January, 19 February, 13 March & 10 May 1856.

detachment did not return to Chatham until 17 August, after leaving Scutari on 31 July.[126]

2.2.6 Ambulance Corps

Some 35 years before the war J. van Millingen made a proposal for a Hospital Ambulance Crops[127] but this advice went unheeded. The development of the corps had thus to be commenced from scratch. Of 341 volunteers sent to Bulgaria with the Hospital Ambulance Corps 27, 30, 141, and 121 were 34 or younger, 35–40, 40–45, and 45–50 years old respectively, and two were over 50.[128] The men had the reputation for drunkenness and bad behaviour although subsequent enquiries by Colonel A.M. Tulloch concluded this was unjust as all had 'received good characters from their corps' with sixty having between one and six good conduct badges, and seven the Good Conduct Medal. The aim was to have about 100 drivers selected from cavalry regiments with the remainder 'employed as hospital orderlies and servants for medical staff.' However, this came to nothing as sickness diminished their ranks drastically and hence by December 1854 it became necessary to:

> solicit the aid of the French ambulance to transport our sick down to Balaklava: artillery waggons were ordered to afford assistance, and finally the cavalry horses were employed for that purpose, by which means such men as were able to sit on horseback were got away, but a great number of sick, whom it was not desirable to remove, were left in the field hospitals by this arrangement.[129]

The AMD was let down by both the government and military authorities because they failed to provide adequate land transport for the sick and wounded, and it was essential that any unit employed for this purpose should comprise trained able-bodied men, be equipped with spring carriages and pack animals with pannier seats, and be supported by farriers, wheelwrights, and other tradesmen.[130]

Smith favoured having ambulances under the control of AMD, and not the QMG, because the divisional PMO was the best judge of the invalids' needs and should possess the 'power of independent action.' He also stated that the Army would never derive full advantage of its AMD if it was rendered ineffective by regulations that made it subservient to the judgement and interference of Military Officers.[131] His view

---

126 *The Times*, 18 August 1856.
127 Cantlie, *A History*, 1, p.375 and J. van Millingen, *The Army Officer's Manual upon Active Service* (London, 1819) quoted by Shepherd, *Crimean Doctors*, I, p.7.
128 Memorandum prepared by Colonel Tulloch; Supplies Commission Report, pp.194–6.
129 Hall's comments to Smith on the Supplies Commission Report; Mitra, *Life and Letters*, p.484.
130 G. Fisher, 'The Failure of the Ambulance Corps in the Crimean War', *Journal of the Society of Army Historical Research*, 91 (2013), pp.161–81.
131 Smith to Military Secretary, 17 July 1855; Smith, *Précis of Letters*.

did not prevail, however, and neither did it for 'the PMO of every campaign fought in the remainder of the 19th Century.'[132]

The integration of the Ambulance Corps into the LTC was under consideration during March 1855.[133] Raglan supported the recommendation made for this development on 24 May by Colonel W.M.S. McMurdo, the Director General of the LTC, and Panmure ordered this to be done in July 1855.[134] McMurdo noted in early September that the Ambulance Corps 'would fall to pieces if [he took] it up just now; it is so fragile,' and it would be 'better to leave it where it is in its present state.'[135] Integration was finally achieved during December 1855.[136]

2.2.7 Problems of communication

An army is run on a top down basis through a chain of command and hence Smith would have been expected to direct all communications on management matters to Hall. However, the distances between the Crimea and London meant that it could take a month or more for letters to pass between them. This resulted in Smith disregarding protocol and corresponding directly with the PMO at Scutari, and merely informing Hall that the exigencies of the Service demanded it.[137] By so doing he effectively assumed executive control of the Scutari hospitals and the PMO, who held the same rank as Hall, looked to London for instructions. Hall thus faded out of the picture, although there is no indication that he protested formally against this abrogation of his powers.[138] This practical solution meant that there was little justification for Hall to visit Scutari again following his visit in October 1854, and hence any criticism levelled against him for not doing so is unjustified.[139]

It would seem that the Minister of War also appreciated this problem, because, from early January 1855, he began to correspond directly with the military commandant on the Bosphorus. His first despatch contained detailed instructions and advice on what was required of him.[140]

2.2.8 Discontentment among the military surgeons

The Queen's Regulations provided basic instructions on the management of hospitals and duties of medical officers but there was no guidance on the expected relationship

---

132 Cantlie, *A History*, 2, p.147.
133 Commandant, Ambulance Corps to QMG, 12 March 1855; TNA: WO 28/197.
134 TNA: WO 1/374/313; and Military Secretary separately to Smith and Simpson, 17 July 1855; Smith, *Précis of Letters* and TNA: WO 28/175.
135 Memorandum prepared by the DG, Land Transport Corp on 4 September in response to a General Order to be issued on 6 September 1855; TNA: WO 28/110.
136 General Order, 28 December 1855.
137 Smith to Menzies and Smith to Hall, 2 November 1854; Smith, *Précis of Letters*.
138 Paraphrased from Cantlie, *A History*, 2, p.70.
139 For example, Shepherd, *Crimean Doctors*, 2, p.609.
140 Newcastle to Paulet, 6 January 1855; TNA: WO 6/70/112–33 (longhand copy) and TNA: WO 33/1/8/55 (Cabinet paper).

between them and their commanding officer.¹⁴¹ This lack of clarity proved a problem at times since some senior officers did not consult them on any matter, particularly those who thought that surgeons were there only 'to treat sickness, not to prevent it.'¹⁴² In essence medical officers had little or no executive powers, a problem summarized by an unnamed military officer in the Light Division:

> Attached to the Division is a Deputy Inspector General of Hospitals, who is said to be 'in medical charge;' and to each brigade a Staff Surgeon of the 1st class, having more direct charge in general matters of each regiment in his brigade. [...] in no one instance has the medical officer [...] been consulted as to the [camp] site occupied. Surely this demands an enquiry. [...] It is the duty of military medical men to acquaint themselves [...] with such sanitary subjects that prevent sickness, always more important than its cure. No such study is requisite before [military] officers in the British Army are placed upon the staff, whereas in France and Germany [they are instructed in] the particular duties they are called on to perform.¹⁴³

Not unexpectedly these sentiments were echoed in the medical press, since the problems encountered were exacerbated by 'the want of fuller power and authority in the heads of the Army Medical Department' and not 'from any absence of ability or deficiency of skill, is a sufficient proof of the necessity there is for entrusting all purely sanitary arrangements to properly qualified medical men.'¹⁴⁴

It would seem that some politicians and other commentators failed to appreciate the weak position of medical officers within the military hierarchy. For example, Charles Newdegate, MP, suggested to the House of Commons that the failings in the Crimea were not due to 'the regimental service of the army, which some hon. Members condemned as being aristocratic,' but to the Medical Department and Commissariat, which were 'not in the hands of the noblemen and gentlemen of the army,' and that he [Newdegate] 'trusted that hon. Members would speak with common fairness of the noblemen and gentlemen who, as officers of the army, had done their duty, and not attribute to them discredit for calamities for which they were in no way accountable.'¹⁴⁵ This defamatory slur was subsequently supported publicly by

---

141 *The Queen's Regulations and Orders for the Army 1844* (3rd edition), (London: Parker, Furnivall, and Parker), pp.285–90.
142 Cantlie, *A History*, 2, p.26. For example, General Brown's response to a reasonable request about the provision of medical stores on 10 June 1854, viz. 'Refer [...] to the PMO informing him that I by no means approve of the tone of this, and that in my judgement Dr Alexander had better defer such suggestions and strictures until they are asked for;' Royal Commission Report, Appendix LXXIX, pp.136 & 160.
143 Letter, 2 September 1854; *Daily News*, 21 September 1854.
144 Editorial, *Association Medical Journal*, 4 May 1855.
145 *Hansard*, 19 February 1855.

Palmerston, an intervention considered by W.H. Russell to be as a 'most extraordinary and uncalled-for insult.'[146] Not surprisingly it also provoked an angry editorial in the *Association Medical Journal*:

> If, then, as Lord Palmerston affirms, the army surgeons have shown a 'want of capacity, a want of energy, a want of intellect and vigour', it must be for some reasons peculiar to the army – the army system. The charge commonly made against army surgeons, is a want of moral courage in boldly making complaints, for fear of the injury to their promotion. And to what is this moral cowardice owing? Is it not to the practice of the higher military authorities to depress in every way the 'doctor', to consider him as belonging to an inferior class, and to treat him as such, until he believes it, and loses his spirit? And having done this, the authority who has depressed him and his branch of the service blames him for a want of energy, intellect, and vigour, when he sees the men rotting like sheep.[147]

The dissatisfaction of the medical officers at the front was aggravated by Raglan's tendency to follow the practice adopted by Wellington and Hardinge in earlier campaigns and to name only senior staff and regimental officers in official despatches, and thereby omitting to acknowledge other combatants. This prompted the editor of *The Lancet* to decry Raglan's failure to 'acknowledge the devoted services of the Army surgeons', while a couple of weeks later a trenchant editorial in the *Medical Times and Gazette* listed the injuries sustained by several medical officers during combat.[148] Hall also expressed his concerns privately to the PMO, Scutari: 'A thankless office we doctors have to perform. We work hard with no reward [...] Had we neglected or abused means placed at our disposal, then we might have been ashamed, but circumstanced as we have been I feel that we have all done our duty, not only done it but done it most conscientiously.'[149]

Hall was not a lone voice, however, as exemplified by a graphic account penned by a surgeon at the front:

> For a considerable period [I was] within twenty-five yards of the advancing Russian columns, and amid a perfect hailstorm of grape, canister, round shot, shell, and bullets [...] when three round shot passed close by me [...] each shot striking a man, killing two outright, [...] and mangling in a frightful manner the right arm of the third. The 'thud' with which the formidable missiles struck against the accoutrements and bodies of the men, was the strangest and most appalling sound I ever heard.[150]

146 Despatch dated 13 March; *The Times*, 29 March 1855.
147 *Association Medical Journal*, 18 May 1855.
148 *Medical Times and Gazette*, 11 November 1854. On 13 January 1855 the editor accused Raglan of 'cowardly and unjust' behaviour towards Medical Officers.
149 Hall to Menzies, 7 December 1854; RAMC: 397/F/CO/1/1/1042.
150 *Medical Times and Gazette*, 30 December 1854 and Shepherd, *Crimean Doctors*, 1, p.232.

This report prompted the journal's editor to comment: 'Surely, when medical men incur such dangers [...] it is too bad to deny them a share of the honours and rewards so ungrudgingly bestowed upon other classes of officers.' Smith was also anxious that medical officers should receive recognition and requested Hall to 'send him, periodically the names of all the officers he can recommend,' as he wished to show medical officers that 'laudable and successful exertions do not pass unnoticed.'[151] Smith's anxieties persisted, however, and a few weeks later he wrote to Horse Guards:

> It is generally admitted that highly valuable services have been rendered [by] Medical Officers [...] exposed to hardships and dangers from the enemy, as well as from disease, fully equal to any other class. Rewards for good service [have] been liberally granted, but not to [...] Medical Officers, which [...] has tended to produce discouragement likely to operate unfavourably to the interests of the service. [...] When the morbid excitement roused by misrepresentations against the Medical Department shall have subsided [...] the public will applaud [...] the services of the Medical Officers [...] the public generally [...] recognise the self-denying labours of the devoted men, who [...] did so much to mitigate the sufferings, and to console [...] those whom their professional skill could not preserve from the grave.[152]

The continued failure of the establishment to acknowledge the contribution made by the medical profession also elicited a degree of bitterness at the front: 'I cannot tell you how depressing the continued slight of the services of the Regimental Surgeons is to us all. The [*London*] *Gazette* [reports] honours and promotions to the regimental officers [...] But we have no friends, no parliamentary interest, and are not merely passed over unnoticed, but absolutely maltreated.'[153]

Clearly the medical profession remained unhappy and shortly after the conclusion of peace the editor of *The Lancet* returned to the issue:[154]

> The want of proper appreciation [...] of medical officers is shown in many ways, in none more so than the conferring of decorations. [...] medical officers are entitled to double distinction, first, as soldiers; and, secondly, as professional men. The surgeon of the 7th Hussars who rallied some of the Guards on the heights of Inkermann (*sic*), gallantly led them to [rout] the Russians, and [save] the Duke of Cambridge, was entitled to distinction as a soldier; but are not [...] the late Dr Jackson, Dr. Trotter, or Dr John Davy, entitled to distinction for their services in the army in a professional and scientific point of view?

---

151 Smith to Hall, 16 February 1855; RAMC: 397/F/CO/1/2/2892.
152 Smith to Military Undersecretary, 17 August 1855; Smith, *Précis of Letters*.
153 Undated letter from a regimental surgeon; *Medical Times and Gazette*, 2 June 1855.
154 *The Lancet*, 19 April 1856.

A number of the senior medical officers did receive recognition by the award of the Order of the Bath and other orders bestowed by Britain's French, Turkish and Sardinian allies. In addition, three regimental surgeons were awarded the Victoria Cross, namely, Assistant Surgeons T.E Hale, 7th Regiment, and H.T. Sylvester, 23rd Regiment, and Surgeon, later DIGH, J. Mouat, 6th Dragoons (see Section 10.2).

Growing discontent amongst the military surgeons about pay and conditions was exacerbated by the better employment conditions offered to civilian surgeons. This resulted in three memorials being sent to the War Office between July 1855 and April 1856.[155] The first from 49 assistant surgeons did not receive Smith's support and Panmure subsequently rejected it because it had been published in *The Lancet* before he had considered it.[156] The second was from more senior regimental surgeons who were aggrieved because they did not receive a share of the honours accorded to combatant officers, especially as they were also exposed to enemy fire, and this differentiated them from the other civilian departments.[157] This memorial was forwarded to Panmure by the Smith and it was anticipated that a new Royal Warrant would be issued, but this proposal was rejected by the Treasury. A third memorial, however, prompted the convening of a House of Commons Select Committee on the Medical Department chaired by Augustus Stafford, MP, and it was on their recommendation that a new Royal Warrant was promulgated.[158] It redefined the terms of service, remuneration, and the status of military surgeons and was signed by Her Majesty's command by the Minister of War on 1 October 1858.[159]

The AMD was a civilian department and medical officers, unlike their military counterparts, were not entitled to a soldier servant. The daily allowance for hiring a servant was increased from 1/6d to 3/- but this was insufficient to meet the high rates of pay demanded by civilians.[160] In consequence, some surgeons were forced 'to draw their own rations, cook their own food, and water their own horses,' and 'carry out these tasks under the eyes of their brother officers made an undignified spectacle which brought contempt upon the Department.'[161] Matters were exacerbated by senior medical staff needing three horses or more to fulfil their duties, and, as their care

---

155 For details see Cantlie, *A History*, 2, pp.181–3.
156 *The Lancet*, 8 September 1854. The editor strongly supported 'our military brethren [who] should be classed amongst the purely military branches of the service, and should reap its share of the honours accorded to them.'
157 *Medical Times and Gazette*, 13 October 1855.
158 HCPP 1856 (331) XIII.359: *Report from the Select Committee on the Medical Department [Army]*. (Hereafter: *Select Committee on the Medical Department*).
159 The text was reproduced in *The Lancet*, 28 October 1858 and Cantlie, *A History*, 2, pp.428–32.
160 General Order, 30 October 1854.
161 Cantlie, *History*, 2, p.132.

would take much of a servant's time, a second servant was sorely needed, especially as the medical officer would suffer considerable hardship if his only servant was sick.[162]

Raglan eventually took up the surgeons' case when he enquired of Horse Guards, through the AG, if a scheme could be devised for improving the medical officers circumstances with respect to servants. The shortage of military personnel made it impractical to provide the numbers required, and it was hoped that civilian servants could be procured from 'among the people who are constantly arriving from Constantinople or elsewhere.'[163] The matter was considered at the highest level because Smith was informed by the Deputy Secretary for War on 26 July 1855 that Panmure agreed that medical staff officers should not have to waste their time doing things that 'properly devolve on servants.' He suggested that men should be enlisted into the MSC for the purpose; presumable from among the 50 servants allocated to each company of the Corps.[164] After the war Smith recommended the servants allowed to medical officers should be determined according his rank relatively to military officers.[165]

2.2.9 Civilian surgeons

A few civilian surgeons accompanied the Army to Bulgaria and the Crimea. These appeared to have been employed informally, presumably on Raglan's authority, and as they were not part of the Army establishment Hall made no reference to them in his returns.

The shortage of medical officers after the invasion 'necessitated the filling of our hospitals *ex necessitate rei* with very young surgeons.' Herbert then suggested to Smith that there would be an advantage in employing more experience civilians whose services would be dispensed with once the war was over.[166]

Towards the end of 1854 Lord Blantyre took up this issue by suggesting to Aberdeen, the Prime Minister, that civilian surgeons should be recruited as additional medical officers. His letter was forwarded to Smith via Herbert who commented that 'Lord Blantyre suggests improvement in our military hospitals by employment of civilians with better pay and allowances.' Smith stated his reservations the next day:

> [Blantyre's proposition is] wild and [...] calculated to disorganize everything. If the Medical Department had power in itself to effect what it considers necessary we have no want of assistance from without. The Department has in itself men

---

162 PMO, 4th Division to Hall, 18 December 1854; Royal Commission Report, Appendix LXXIX, p.166.
163 AG to AG, Horse Guards, 26 May 1855 and AG to GOC, 3rd Division, 20 May 1855; TNA: WO 28/109.
164 Smith, *Précis of Letters*. This opinion was sent to the AG in the Crimea by AG, Horse Guards on 7 August 1855; TNA: WO 28/180; and Deputy Secretary to Smith, 7 August 1855; Smith, *Précis of Letters*.
165 Royal Commission Report, p.lxxii.
166 Herbert to Smith, 24 December 1854; Select Committee, 4th Report, pp.343–4.

competent to all and every duty and I do hope they will not be insulted by the adoption of such a measure [...] They [...] must either support the servants of the public or sacrifice them and permit a chaos to be established.[167]

Not surprisingly Hall was against mixing civilian and military medical officers in the same establishment,[168] while the Revd H.P. Wright, the principal chaplain, shared this reservation, when he suggested to Herbert that military surgeons were preferable to civilians as they would manage hospitals better under campaign conditions.[169] Conversely, in his assessment of the Scutari hospitals, the Hon. the Revd S.G. Osborne recommended that they should be 'placed under the management and control of civilians.'[170] This system of management was adopted at Smyrna and Renkioi, but not in the military hospitals.

Newcastle announced the employment of civilian doctors on 29 January 1855 because the 'present state of the Army and of the hospitals, [makes it] necessary [despite opposition] to introduce into the army hospitals the civilian element.'[171] Their employment was thus a political initiative taken when matters were pressing, although prompted to an extent by public opinion, and the fact that physicians were needed as the principal clinical problems were medical, not surgical.[172]

The policy proved controversial, not least because the 'civils' were paid better than their military counterparts and most were spared the dangers and privations of serving near the front.[173, 174] This caused resentment amongst the medical officers and Hall called Smith's attention 'to the [...] extravagantly high rate of remuneration they receive [...] This inequality of pay has occasioned much discontent'[175] although he conceded that he could not say this of 'the gentleman who have been doing duty in camp who have [...] exerted themselves with great zeal and [...] cordiality towards

---

167 Blantyre to Aberdeen, 19 December, Aberdeen to Herbert, 22 December, and Smith to Herbert, 23 December 1854; Wiltshire and Swindon History Centre: 2057/F8/III/B/241.
168 Raglan to Panmure, 11 March 1855; TNA: WO 1/272/202.
169 Wright to Herbert, undated; Wiltshire and Swindon History Centre: 2057/F8/III/B/246. Wright also stressed the need for adequate support staff and suggested that these could be provided from militia regiments.
170 S.G. Osborne, *Scutari and its Hospitals* (London: Dickinson Brothers, 1855).
171 *Hansard*, 29 January and *Medical Times and Gazette*, 3 February 1855. For a discussion on civilian surgeons see Shepherd, *Crimean Doctors*, 2, pp.412–51.
172 Mr Augustus Stafford, *Hansard*, 19 March 1855
173 The medical press was divided on the issue; the *Association Medical Journal* generally favoured employing civilians, while *The Lancet* supported for the military surgeons, and pressed for improvement in their status.
174 The civilian orderlies were paid better making it difficult to recruit Maltese; DAQMG, Malta to QMG, 25 May 1855; TNA: WO 28/197.
175 The civilian director at Smyrna was reportedly offered £2,000 p.a. while Smith was paid £1,300; *The Lancet*, 17 February 1855.

those whom they were associated [...] we have been fortunate in securing their assistance.'[176]

The hospital in Smyrna opened during February 1855 and was staffed by medical officers for a few weeks until replaced by civilians from mid-March. Its location far from the front meant that was inappropriate to send seriously ill or wounded soldiers there and it was under-utilized, receiving only 1,887 patients during the ten months it was open. The prefabricated hospital at Renkioi designed by I.K. Brunel received its first patients during October 1855 and it was from the start a civilian operation under the superintendence of Dr E.A. Parkes.[177] Apart from the publication of tables that listed admissions and deaths each month at Smyrna and Renkioi there was no analysis of their performance in the *Medical and Surgical History*, though Parkes published a report on the formation and management of the hospital in 1857.[178] Hall also expressed his view on civilian hospitals in his draft memoirs: 'Had the Medical Department [the same means and facilities] given to the civil establishments [...] they would have accomplished as much, or more [...] at considerably less cost to the public, and with equal efficiency, so far as the real wants of the sick were concerned [...] and their admission into military establishments was of questionable utility.'[179]

In like manner Hall pointed out to the Royal Commission during June 1857 that the civil hospitals proved expensive and, with the benefit of hindsight, unnecessary as sufficient beds were available in military hospitals.[180] This was not entirely an expression of bitterness, however, as Newcastle, a prime mover in the establishment of the hospital at Smyrna, entertained similar sentiments when he visited there some two months before the fall of Sevastopol:

> The present staff [...] is decidedly too large, it consists of Colonel Storks, Dr Meyer, 25 other doctors, 13 lady nurses, 23 paid nurses, 47 military orderlies, and 36 civil orderlies. Besides these Colonel Storks has under him Major Chads

---

176 RAMC: 397/F/CO/1/2/2884 and Smith, *Précis of Letters*. Incidentally, Hall's report to Raglan on the assault on the Redan included the names of the 'following gentlemen belonging to the civil establishment who did their duty zealously, viz. Dr Mcleod, Mr Wordsworth, Dr Frazer, and Dr Lyons;' RAMC: 397/F/CO/1/2/2412.
177 For details see D. Toppin, 'The British Hospital at Renkioi 1855', *The Arup Journal*, 16:2 (1981), pp.3–20 and C. Silver, *Renkioi Brunel's Forgotten Crimean War Hospital* (Sevenoaks: Valonia Press, 2007).
178 E.A. Parkes, *Report on the Formation and General Management of Renkioi Hospital on the Dardanelles, Turkey*, (War Department, April 1857). Incidentally, the death of 50 (four percent) of 1,330 patients admitted to the hospital at Renkioi might appear an endorsement for the undoubted brilliance of Brunel's design. However, this is not the case as the comparable figures for the Army as whole were better, viz. 740 (two percent) deaths from disease among 36,794 hospital patients; see *Medical and Surgical History*, 2, General Return A & General Hospital Returns IX.
179 RAMC: 397/F/RT/2 and Mitra, *Life and Letters*, p.378.
180 Evidence given on 19 June 1857; Royal Commission Report, p.180.

and six other officers making in all a number about equal to the patients at the present time. [...] That they are further from the seat of war than is desirable there can be no doubt, so indeed are those on the Bosphorus. [...] I doubt whether any so good a location can be found between it and Constantinople, and if this is the case, the political importance of retaining our hold upon this place until the close of war is manifest.[181]

In his account of the AMD Cantlie noted that the Select Committee on the Medical Department condemned making the hospitals at Smyrna and Renkioi independent of Smith. He considered that the establishment of a hospital at Smyrna was unjustified in retrospect, while the opening of the hospital at Renkioi, when others were closing, was 'a step of doubtful administrative value' taken by the Secretary of State alone as Smith played had no part in it. 'Both hospitals were, therefore, examples of the futility of a dual method of hospital planning directed on the one hand by the Medical Department and on the other by the Secretary of State.'[182]

In all thirty civilian surgeons were employed officially by the Army with three doing two tours of duties.[183] Between one and three were in post until February 1855 when the number increased to 15 by which time the troops' health was improving and mortality falling. The numbers employed remained between 15 and 22 until March 1855 when their services were dispensed with following the cessation of hostilities.

2.2.10 Female nurses

Nurses were employed in the Savoy military hospital in London during the English Civil War.[184] It was thus not a new phenomenon when, in 1803, Jackson referred to the employment of female nurses in medical, but not surgical wards;[185] while 'in the colonies coloured women were considered the best nurses in the world.'[186] Since then much has been written on the topic and opinions tend to be polarized, and frequently obscured by entrenched religious or chauvinistic attitudes. Suffice it to state, nurses were not deployed in the regimental hospitals where most men were treated. As it turned out relatively few were employed in the general hospitals and, as their contribution was necessarily limited, Shepherd opined that it is unlikely that improvements in the mortality rates at Scutari were due to better nursing.[187]

---

181 Diary entry, 13 July 1855; University of Nottingham: Ne/2F/10/1.
182 Cantlie, *A History*, 2, pp.170 & 199.
183 *Medical and Surgical History*, 1, Appendix VIII. This total does not include surgeons employed at Smyrna and Renkioi.
184 D. Flintham, *Civil War London* (Solihull: Helion, 2017), p.31.
185 R. Jackson, *Remarks on the Constitution of the Medical Department of the British Army* (London: Cadill & Davies, 1803), pp.82–3.
186 W. Fergusson, *Notes and Recollections of a Professional Life*, (London: Longman & Co., 1846), p.63.
187 Shepherd, *Crimean Doctors*, 2, p.520.

Some pro-nursing commentators have criticized the military authorities, including the AMD, for a lack of enthusiasm towards their employment. Not surprising, perhaps, as it was a political initiative introduced without discussion or advanced planning. The nurses were, thus, superimposed on a management structure unprepared for employing civilians of either gender and not bound by the Mutiny Act, and for whom no formal logistical provision had been made. Responsibility for their maintenance was assumed later by the military authorities although it has been inferred by some commentators that the AMD was remiss for not directly providing for their care. However, this is an unwarranted criticism, because there was no mandate for the AMD so to do without being authorized by the Commander of the Forces.

The services of the small number of nurses employed in the Crimea were seemingly appreciated. For example, following the resignation of Mrs Bridgeman and the Roman Catholic nurses, Codrington wrote the following appreciation to Hall on 4 April 1856:

> I request you to assure that lady of the high estimation in which her services and those of the nurses are held by us all; founded as that opinion is on the experience of yourself, the medical officers of the hospital and of the many patients, who during 14 or 15 months have benefited by their care. I am quite sure that their unfailing kindness will have the reward that Mrs Bridgman values, viz. the remembrance and gratitude of those who have been the subject of such disinterested attention.[188]

Several biographies of Nightingale deal *in extenso* with her relationship with Hall and the Purveyor in the Crimea, David Fitzgerald; particularly with respect to the management of the general hospitals in the Crimea and the employment of the nurses following the fall of Sevastopol. In the final analysis the debate was little more than a clash of personalities, and to some extent religious bigotry – Fitzgerald was a Catholic – than anything else. It had little obvious relevance to the general health of the troops who were principally cared for in regimental hospitals, and where no female nurses were employed. That the physical appearance of the general hospitals, and the way they were managed, could have been improved is not in question, but any upgrading would have been cosmetic rather than essential, and, by the end of 1855 there was little incentive for the authorities to invest in extensive infrastructural improvements in the camps or elsewhere.

Mrs Mary Seacole, a popular and well-liked personality from Jamaica, ran the so called British Hotel with her business partner Thomas Day. She practiced herbal medicine but her impact on the health of the Army as a single handed doctress who arrived after the worst of the first winter was over would have been limited. She did not have a hospital and was not employed officially in any of the military hospitals.[189]

---

188 National Army Museum: 1968–07–380–8B.
189 For a biography see J. Robinson, *Mary Seacole. The Charismatic Black Nurse who became a Heroine of the Crimea* (London: Constable, 2005).

2.2.11 Medical supplies sent to the East

Immense amounts of medical stores were forwarded for the use of the Army and details of these can be found in the *Medical and Surgical History*.[190] The items listed included medical comforts (e.g. alcoholic beverages, dried vegetables, preserved meats, sugar, and other food stuffs); hospital stores and equipment; and medical and surgical stores.

2.2.12 Concluding remarks

The provision of health care for the Army of the East proved a prodigious undertaking. The numbers of those who served on the medical staff, as opposed to those on the strength of the regiments, is given in Table 2.3. Inevitably it took time to increase the manpower in all branches of the medical services and for those employed to gain experience after a prolonged period of peace in Europe; and, although some would have seen service in India and at other foreign stations, that would not necessarily have equipped them for campaigning in Europe.

Table 2.3 Number (%) medical staff employed in the Army of the East

Country*	Staff medical officers	Apothecaries and dispensers	Dressers	Support staff†	Civilian surgeons‡
T	62 (15)	24 (45)	23 (55)	11 (61)	21 (70)
B	1 (0.2)	0	0	0	0
C	153 (37)	13 (24.5)	7 (16.5)	6 (33.5)	5 (16.5)
T & B	1 (0.2)	1 (2)	0	0	0
B & C	5 (1)	0	0	0	0
T & C	130 (31)	14 (26.5)	12 (28.5)	0	4 (13.5)
T, B & C	66 (16)	1 (2)	0	1 (5.5)	0
Total	418	53	42	18	30

* T, Turkey; B, Bulgaria; C, Crimea.
† Storekeepers, bookkeepers, and medical clerks.
‡ This return does not include civilian surgeons stationed at Smyrna and Renkioi as they were not part of the military establishment.

(Adapted from *Medical and Surgical History*, 1, Appendix VIII)

The development of the medical services was seriously compromised by the collapse of the health of the Army during the months following the invasion. The cause of this was not medical in nature, but, as will be explained in later chapters, it was the result of the combined effects of exposure, overwork, malnutrition and living in unhygienic conditions. The health of the troops did not improve until their living standards improved and the weather became milder.

190 See *Medical and Surgical History*, 1, pp.526–30, 531–54, & 555–60.

Another important issue facing Hall and his senior colleagues was that they had little or no executive authority as this was vested in the Commander of the Forces and implemented by the AG, QMG, and the officers commanding divisions, the RA and RE. This meant that their opportunity to influence events was limited as they were not involved routinely in the planning of the activities of the Army, both military and domestic. Inevitably this resulted in the AMD being ill-prepared on occasions for what was expected, and for which they got unreasonably criticised.

A further complication was the fact the military officers tended to regard surgeons as their social inferiors and this resulted in problems, both administrative and personal. Raglan was also criticised for failing to acknowledge the part played by the medical officers in the face of the enemy, though a degree of recognition was ultimately achieved with the award of a number of orders and medals, including three VCs (see Section 10.2).

The employment of civilian surgeons on an official basis was a political initiative, taken when matters were pressing. It proved controversial and caused resentment among medical officers because their conditions of service were better, particularly with respect to pay, and for those stationed in the hospitals in Smyrna and Renkioi life was much easier. Hall also expressed his displeasure at this situation although he paid tribute to those of whom he had first-hand experience. For example, after the war he wrote in his *Observations* that he had 'much satisfaction' in praising their conduct, but they were not 'superior to military surgeons.'[191]

Finally, the employment of both civilian doctors and female nurses was, in Shepherd's opinion, a failed 'experiment' [...] as it neither relieved 'the situation in the Crimea' nor promoted 'a closer liaison between the army medical services and the civilian doctors.' However, he concluded that overall 'much good came out of it' since the 'evolution, in time, of the territorial army medical officer and the RNVR medical officer who have supported the regular services in times of war may be thought to have stemmed from this Crimean interlude.'[192]

2.3 Commissariat

The supply of campaigning armies over the ages has been the subject of several monographs,[193] but in the final analysis this highly complex topic can be summarized

---

191 RAMC: 397/F/RT/2 and TNA: WO 33/3B.
192 Shepherd, *Crimean Doctors*, 2, pp.412–51.
193 For example, J. Sinclair, *Arteries of War* (Shrewsbury: Airlife Publishing, 1992); M. Christopher, *Logistics and Supply Chain Management* (2nd edition) (London: Financial Times Management, 1998); and M. van Creveld, *Supplying War. Logistics from Wallenstein to Patton*, (2nd edition) (Cambridge: University Press, 2004), though none make any specific reference to the Crimean campaign.

succinctly by the axiom 'an army marches on its stomach;'[194] or put another way the Commissariat is 'the stomach of the Army. Without it, or an inefficient one, the line and the artillery (the limbs) are worthless.'[195]

The benefits of an effective commissariat were appreciated by Wellington after the battle of Talavera in 1809; and 'by recognizing it [he] assured himself of ultimate success.'[196] However, this hard learnt lesson did not result in any worthwhile reforms at the time, or in the years before 1854. In consequence the administrative shortcomings in the Commissariat became apparent soon after active warfare commenced in 1854. These problems were exacerbated by the late start of the campaign and the absence of well-made roads and harbour and storage facilities in and around Balaklava.

Sweetman analysed the administration of the Army at the time and concluded that in the long term the 'real British success of 1855' was not attained in the operational theatres, but in London where the 'reorganisation of army administration' was achieved.[197] This topic will be considered further in Section 10.3. It is unlikely, however, that strategic changes in governmental organization, for example the transfer of the Commissariat from the Treasury to the War Department during December 1854, would have had an immediate impact at the front given that improvements in the troops' well-being commenced during early 1855; and well before any reforms introduced in London could have taken effect.

The supply of the Army during the first winter was investigated by the Supplies Commissioners, Sir John McNeill and Colonel Alexander Tulloch. Their findings were published in a 728 page report which identified several obvious shortcomings.[198] For example, it was impossible for the troops to obtain fuel and vegetables for themselves and until such that these items were supplied by the Commissariat the men suffered unnecessarily as they could not keep warm and cook their food, and the unbalanced diet led to the onset of the effects of malnutrition including scurvy. The Commissioners also criticised the delay in providing facilities for baking bread locally and obtaining sufficient cattle of good quality to provide fresh meat (see Figure 2.7). On the other hand, in defence of the department's performance, the Commissary General wrote to the QMG on 8 January 1855: 'The Commissariat did not foresee, any more than any other departments, that the army would not be in its present situation, otherwise precautionary measures might have been taken to mitigate some of the evils and inconveniences now experienced.'[199]

---

194 E. Knowles (ed.), *The Oxford Dictionary of Phase and Fable* (Oxford: University Press, 2004). It is not certain whether this phase should be attributed to Napoleon or Frederick the Great.
195 A. Sterling, *The Highland Brigade in the Crimea* (Minneapolis: Absinthe Press, 1995, but first published in 1895), pp.ix–x.
196 Fortescue, *History of the British Army*, quoted by Cantlie, *A History*, 1, p.319.
197 J. Sweetman, *War and Administration: The Significance of the Crimean War for the British Army* (Edinburgh: Scottish Academic Press, 1984).
198 Supplies Commission Report.
199 Filder to Airey, 16 January 1855; Select Committee, 3rd Report, p.409.

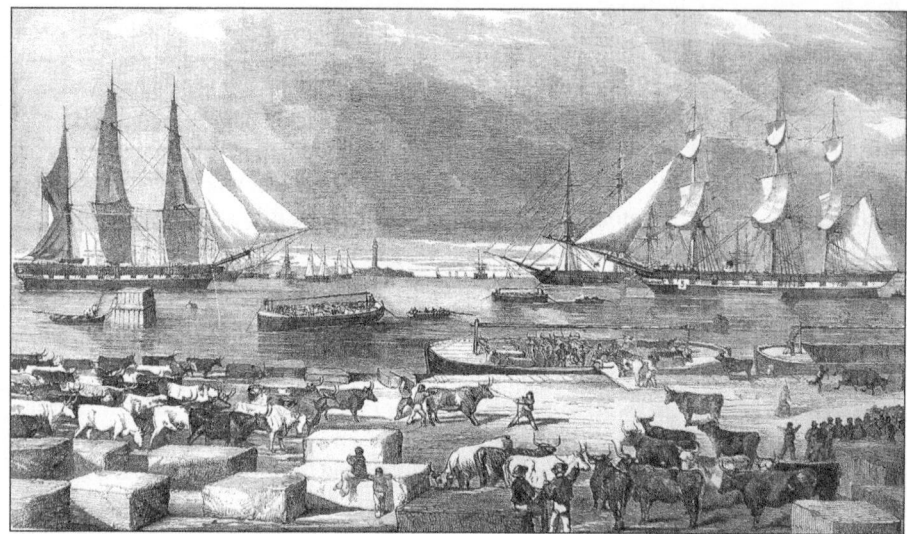

Figure 2.7 Embarkation of cattle, at Trieste for the Auxiliary Army in the East. (*Illustrated London News*, 15 July 1854, p.33)

The discussion hereunder focuses principally on some of the problems encountered in supplying the Army during the winter of 1854–55, and how matters were developed during the following months.

2.3.1 Land transport
Land transport in the Crimea proved the ultimate Achilles heel. Raglan considered that it was his 'principal want and a serious one,'[200] while the problem was expressed succinctly by Maxwell, one of the hospital commissioners, when he wrote privately to Herbert from the Crimea on 8 January 1855:

> Everybody says that the government and the public have met all the wants except one. They have sent plenty to Balaklava, but have taken no steps to bring that plenty to camp. In short, Sir, you have sent everything 3,000 miles, but the whole distance is 3,006, and the last six are more difficult to overcome than the 3,000.'[201]

This opinion should not have surprised Herbert, however, as the 'crux of the supply problem [...] the inadequate road' had been 'identified in London long before the winter weather arrived and made the road almost unusable.'[202] Newcastle, who was one

---

200 Quoted by Sweetman, *War and Administration*, p.55.
201 Wiltshire and Swindon History Centre: 2057/F8/III/B/363.
202 Ponting, *Crimean War*, pp.188–9.

of the 'political victims of the Crimean winter,' who was responsible for introducing 'the measures which improved the position by the spring' such as the 'railway, huts, sanitary officers and Land Transport Corps [...] thereby benefiting Palmerston.'[203] The railway proved crucial in keeping the Army 'operational and demonstrated how important modern supply systems would be in warfare' though the 'effective organization of the LTC was not achieved until the autumn of 1855.'[204]

The Commissariat was empowered to pay for provisions obtained locally, and for land and water transport. It could also enter into contracts for ordnance stores, building materials, etc., and was responsible for superintending the issue of provisions, forage, fuel and light, and these 'duties were blended with the Army, Ordnance, Navy, and many other branches of the public service.'[205] In the context of the Crimean campaign the Commissariat relied heavily on the Royal Navy for sea transport as without its 'zealous cooperation' it would prove 'impracticable to keep the Army properly provided; Constantinople being the principal depot from which we draw our supplies.'[206] Fortunately, the British merchant fleet was the largest in the world and the relatively high proportion of steam-powered vessels meant that they could operate in most weathers, and critically during the stormy winter months.[207] Overall there was no serious shortage of shipping though on occasions there were short-term problems associated with hold-ups in the harbours, the inability to charter ships locally at short notice, delays in obtaining coal for steamers, and adverse weather conditions hampering the progress of sailing vessels.

Correspondence and reports on land transport matters reveal that the roads deteriorated from early November 1854, while after the hurricane of the 14 November the Commissary General appreciated the long-term problem posed by this unforeseen setback when he informed Raglan the next day that the losses sustained had placed: 'the Army in a critical condition with respect to the supply of provisions and forage. More food may arrive but the loss of forage is irreparable as only pressed hay of which none can be obtained from Turkey can be conveyed in sufficient quantity to meet the consumption of the Army.'[208] A problem that may not have occurred if Filder's earlier request to the Treasury for large quantities of baled hay had been sent from England and a suitable equipped transport corps had been provided.[209]

---

203 See Anon [Maxwell], *Whom Shall We Hang?*, p.80 and Lambert, *Crimean War*, p.201.
204 Ponting, *Crimean War*, pp.335–6 & 190.
205 See H.G. Hart, *The New Annual Army List, and Militia List for 1856* (London: John Murray, 1856), p.386.
206 Filder to Military Secretary, 14 December 1854; TNA: WO 62/13.
207 Comprehensive lists of the merchant ships chartered by the government for transport purposes were published in three Blue Books, viz. HCPP 1854–55 (24) XXXIV.229; HCPP 1854–55 (283) XXXIV.235; and HCPP 1856 (345) XXXIV.341.
208 TNA: WO 62/13. Incidentally, Russell reported that twenty days supply of hay and corn were lost; *The Times*, 14 December 1854.
209 See comments by MacMunn, *The Crimea in Perspective*, pp.241 & 244.

Two days after the hurricane of 14 November an officer from the QMG's department was ordered to Constantinople with wide discretionary powers to obtain large quantities of clothing and other items.[210] The Ambassador in Vienna was also instructed by the Foreign Secretary to procure both clothing and huts for the Army,[211] while the GOC in Corfu took the initiative and forwarded 500 blankets, 1,500 flannel shirts, 1,115 pairs of trousers, and 200 gregos (cloaks) to Constantinople.[212] Supplies from England were also en route, for example, *Alster* called at Malta on 28 December with huts, tons of woollen clothing, and 30,000 articles of fur clothing.[213]

Roads: The poor condition of the roads limited the weight carried by carts and pack animals and when these became impassable for wheeled transport the effect of the losses of pack animals due to malnutrition and exposure became increasingly evident. It proved impracticable to replace them, however, because any new arrivals could not be fed for want of forage.[214] Incidentally, the Supplies Commissioners concluded that this factor had a greater effect on limiting the supply of the Army than the shortage of wheeled transport and animals.[215]

In order to keep the Army supplied during the winter of 1854–55 increasing reliance had to be placed on the resources available in divisions and regiments, and on the over-worked troops for whom the round trip to Balaklava frequently took 'twelve hours, during the whole of which time they were without food, shelter, or rest.'[216] There can be little doubt that this additional excessive labour contributed to the length of the sick list.

Questions were asked by Russell and others, including Panmure, as to why the roads had not been upgraded in advance of winter. This was probably a reflection of manpower shortages and the operational priorities of the siege rather than either an error of judgement or intentional negligence on the part of the QMG's department, given the colossal effort that was subsequently required for the construction of roads after the ending of the siege.[217] A point of view, which highlighted one of the fundamental problems facing Raglan and his successors, namely the shortage of manpower,

---

210 The list included 22,000 blankets or rugs, 4,000 Guernsey frocks, 7,600 woollen drawers, 36,000 socks, 26,000 stockings and mitts, 24,000 gregos (cloaks), 2,000 Turkish boots, stove, and tarpaulins for tent floors, and 4,700 camp kettles; TNA: WO 28/28/196.
211 Westmorland to Raglan, 10 December 1854; TNA: WO 28/155.
212 GOC, Corfu to Raglan, 18 December 1854; TNA: WO 28/197.
213 *Malta Times*, 2 January 1855.
214 Raglan to Newcastle, 30 January & 10 February 1855; TNA: WO 33/1/17/55 & WO 28/199/1.
215 Supplies Commission Report, p.18.
216 Supplies Commission Report, p.16.
217 On 2 October 1855 Major R. Barnston noted in a letter that 6,550 men were working on the public roads to Balaklava and made the comment 'I wonder where Lord Raglan would have got 6,550 men to have made the road this time last year!'; M. Trevor-Barnston (ed.), *Letters from the Crimea and India* (Whitchurch: Herald Printers, 1998), p.125.

was supported by Commander Gordon, RN, of HMS *Sanspareil*, in his response to the Roebuck Committee report made in December 1855:

> A great deal of senseless clamour has been raised because Lord Raglan did not employ his army in making roads. To this Sir de Lacy Evans states that 'No road was attempted because all men, and more than could or ought to have been spared, were in the trenches [and] until the siege was over, no road could be attempted and even then it has taken 10,000 for more than six weeks to complete only from Kadikoi.'[218]

The Engineers reported that improvements in the main roads had been made during January 1855 and wheeled transport could be used increasingly once again, while construction of the railway commenced a short while later (Figure 2.8). Progress was rapid and it became possible to transport supplies as far as Kadikoi on 23 February, and by 26 March they could be delivered to the depot at headquarters. The track was extended to the 3rd Division camp and the Woronzov Road by May and to the Sardinian position in January 1856, by which time it was 19 miles in length.[219]

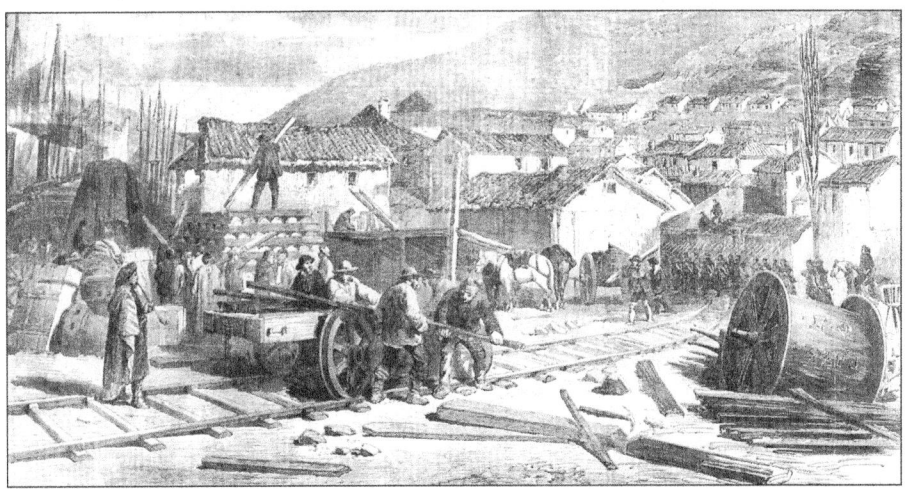

Figure 2.8 Commencement of the railway works at Balaclava. (*Illustrated London News*, 10 March 1855, p.224)

218 W. Gordon, *Balaclava and the Sebastopol Inquiry*, (Dated December 1855; downloaded from Dracobooks, 5 May 2015).
219 For details of the construction and operation of the railway see B. Cooke, *The Grand Crimean Central Railway* (2nd edition) (Knutsford: Cavalier House, 1997). A shorter summary has been provided by A. Vaughan, *Samuel Moreton Peto: A Victorian Entrepreneur* (Hersham: Ian Allen Publishing, 2009), pp.133–5. A map by Captain F. Brine, RE, dated 1857 delineates the final layout of the railway system; TNA: MPH 1/427.

Distribution of stores and equipment: It was the responsibility of the Commissariat to bring supplies to the port but their distribution to the Army was the responsibility of the QMG's department. The scale of rations issued was also decided by the military authorities and could only be changed by them.[220]

For weeks before the hurricane of 14 November Filder had pressed for the 'establishment of supply depots on the upland, but the Army chiefs were naturally still intent on their plans of bombardment, assault, and escape.'[221] It was eventually decided early in 1855 to form a depot in camp near the British HQ where supplies for two weeks could be stored, though bad weather and the state of the roads meant that this objective took longer to achieve than hoped. In the first instant artillery horses and waggons, together with the recently arrived 18th and 39th Regiments, assisted with this initiative,[222] as did Sir Colin Campbell who provided 1,300 men from the Highland Brigade, Marines, and Rifles together with 400 Turks and some horses.[223] The net result of these concerted efforts was that the living conditions of the troops began to improve during January 1855 as food, clothing, and fuel were delivered to the camps in increasing quantities, the sick list began to shorten, and by May 'wood [was] supplied for the most part by the Commissariat [and] forage is obtained without delay at the top of the hill where the rail road terminated.'[224]

A General Order of 28 March 1855 required that applications for the transport of military stores had to be made to the Director General of the LTC by the heads of the 'several Departments of the Army' and that an officer of the LTC would be stationed at each terminus to oversee the loading and discharge of the waggons. However, no ledger detailing the railway's activities has been found in The National Archives and Cooke made no reference to one in his monograph. A surviving return dated 17 April 1855 indicated that the commissariat was allocated 32+10 half waggons, the engineers 6+6 half waggons, and the artillery 22 waggons,[225] while Beatty noted that up to 12 May 1855 the railway had conveyed shot and shell (1,000 tons), small arms (300), commissariat stores (3,600), and miscellaneous items (upwards of 1,000). The railway ultimately had a considerable impact on the British war effort and by the time Sevastopol was occupied it had conveyed to the front 219,723 (92 percent) of 238,610 projectiles, ranging from 8-inch shells to 68-pounder shot.[226]

The experiences of the first winter remained in the minds of Simpson and his successor Codrington and the AWC and the troops spent much time during the autumn of 1855 in constructing roads, which, together with the railway, ensured the

---

220 MacMunn, *Crimea in Perspective*, pp.148–9.
221 MacMunn, *Crimea in Perspective*, p.145.
222 Notes for Colonel Wetherall's history of the war which was never published; TNA: WO 28/199.
223 Campbell to QMG, 6 & 8 January 1855; TNA: WO 28/196.
224 GOC, 2nd Division to AG, 5 May 1855; TNA: WO 28/195.
225 TNA: WO 28/175.
226 Cooke, *Grand Crimean Central Railway*, pp.90, 167 & 171–2.

'plenty' referred to by Maxwell was transported to the camps, and the Army remained well supplied during the rest of time it spent in the Crimea.

Land Transport Corps: The collapse of the Commissariat transport, which was inadequate at the beginning of the campaign,[227] prompted the formation of a military LTC under the command of Raglan.[228] The LTC was authorized by a Royal Warrant dated 24 January 1855 and its functions were to distribute stores (equipment, ammunition, and building materials) and supplies (consumables such as food, fuel, and forage), though sourcing and issuing remained the responsibility of the Commissariat. This seemingly sensible development was not entirely successful and Sweetman suggested that if the 'conditions in the second winter had been similar to the first, it is doubtful it would have provided a better service than the civilian Commissariat.'[229]

The corps eventually numbered over 6,000 men with about 24,000 horses, and in February 1856 it comprised 16 battalions; two with each division and the commissariat, and two for the reserve small arms ammunition.[230] Codrington was of the opinion that the corps should have been formed using 800 men from each division,[231] however, it transpired that only the commissioned officers and NCOs were recruited from the Army with the majority of the men being 'not British' civilians with 'Asiatics' forming the great proportion. The ratio of officers to men was wider than in the Army as a whole, viz. 1:40–1:65 as compared to about 1:25. Sweetman concluded his essay with following succinct paragraph:

> The ineffectiveness of the commissariat's land transport service [...] led to the development of the land transport corps. In turn found unsatisfactory, this new corps was in process of reconstruction as the war closed. Experience [...] emphasized the need for a permanent land transport force [...] under the command of the General Officer Commanding. In this respect the Crimean War was invaluable for the British Army. The Duke of Newcastle maintained that if a land transport corps had been proposed at the commencement of the war [...] it would have been laughed at as an extravagance and absurd. At the close it was not.[232]

---

227 Sweetman, *War and Administration*, pp.45–6. When the Army landed the Commissariat had sufficient carts and pack animals to convey only 80 tons while the appropriation of carts locally increased capacity to 140 tons; Filder's memorandum for HQ, 16 February 1855: TNA: WO 28/199.
228 For a detailed summary of the formation of the LTC, including the problems associated with recruitment and providing equipment etc. see J. Sweetman, 'Military Transport in the Crimean War, 1854–1856', *English Historical Review*, 88 (1973), pp.81–91.
229 Sweetman, *War and Administration*, p.55.
230 Codrington to Panmure, 18 February 1856; TNA: WO 1/382/ff.378–404.
231 Codrington to Panmure, 3 December 1855; TNA: WO 1/380.
232 Memorandum on a Military Train by AG, Horse Guards, 15 October 1856; TNA: WO 123/157.

2.3.2 Harbour facilities

The port at Balaklava was inadequate for the needs of the British Army when first occupied. Its small size presented problems of organization and the lack of storage facilities ashore and the congested state of the roads leading inland resulted in a chaotic situation.[233]

The development and management of the harbour was the responsibility of the Royal Navy and wharves were constructed, initially on the east side and later on the west. They were used where possible for specific purposes, for example, landing ordnance stores, huts or cattle, disembarking troops and embarking the sick and wounded, while others were reserved for the Engineers, Commissariat, and railway. These developments commenced soon after occupation of the town and by January 1855 the Engineers recorded that: 'Much had been done to improve Balaklava. The existing wharves, built during, the previous month, had been considerably enlarged, and new ones had been commenced; at the entrance of the town a pier had been constructed for the embarkation of the sick and wounded, and adjoining another pier was in progress, for unloading the Engineer stores.'[234] Similarly, on 5 May 1855, Captain R. Barnston, a DAQMG, noted that:

> A very nice pier is now being made across the north end of Balaklava harbour, and we hope, with the help of Admiral Boxer, who is wonderfully energetic and particularly civil when properly managed, to make a continuous straight quay all along the east side. Boxer made all the west side himself without any military assistance, and from the great help he has been to us he deserves to be made a peer for making a pier![235]

And, on 18 May 1855, Russell reported:

> Balaklava presents an aspect of extraordinary activity, and the amount of stores of all kinds is beyond conception. When an army has to be fed from beyond the sea, one sees what an all-consuming creature it is. [...] It is to be remarked that much time and labour is lost now and then in consequence of forage being received in bulk instead of bales or sacks. Can anything be imagined more difficult to discharge but straw in bulk? [...] The harbour is, however, now scarcely recognizable [...] vast improvements in the wharfs and quays.[236]

---

233 For correspondence about the management of the harbour when Admiral Boxer was the port admiral see HCPP 1854–55 (512) XXXIV.107: *Correspondence Relative to the State of the Harbour of Balaklava*.
234 H.C. Elphinstone, *Journal of the Operations of the Corps of Royal Engineers*, Part 1 (London: Eyre and Spottiswoode, 1859), pp.79–80.
235 Trevor-Barnston, *Letters*, p.81.
236 *The Times*, 31 May 1855.

The management of the harbour was criticised by several individuals who gave evidence to the Roebuck Committee, and these accounts were justifiably refuted robustly by Commander Gordon, RN, who made it clear in a detailed account of the development and management of the harbour facilities that effective use had been made of the limited space available in the small harbour.[237]

2.3.3 Provisioning the Army

The Commissary General (CG) suggested to HQ that planning for the winter should be considered in August 1854. This advice was seemingly ignored,[238] presumably because it was intended that the attack on the Russians was to be a raid rather than an act of conquest. Clearly Raglan had not anticipated a winter campaign given that Clarendon advised Stratford that Raglan had expressed:

> The most decided opinion against wintering in the Crimea under any circumstances, but how will he get away from it? How [to] embark the two armies with all their guns, stores etc., probably in stormy weather, and with 50 or 60,000 Russians coming upon them like droves of famished wolves? It seems to me [...] that we are on the verge of a monster catastrophe, the only event at all like it [was] the embarkation at Corunna but there our numbers were small and encumbrances light and we had the Spaniards to hold the walls for us.[239]

A Council of War held after Inkerman on 6 November committed the troops to staying in the Crimea, and the next day Burgoyne wrote to the Assistant Inspector-General of Fortifications: 'There is every prospect of our wintering in [...] the Crimea, without towns or villages [...] or any resources but what can be drawn from the sea.'[240] No official announcement of this decision was issued though 'three days after the battle' Raglan 'informed his Commissary General, Mr Filder, that our Army would winter in the Crimea, and desired him to make provision accordingly.'[241] Similarly, he informed Lucan privately on 8 November that he 'might prepare for winter;'[242] while by the 22 November, an assistant surgeon in the RA recorded that: 'We have orders to winter in our present camp.'[243]

Calthorpe, Raglan's junior ADC, recorded that Sir de Lacy Evans had: 'urged upon [Raglan] the utter uselessness, and indeed impracticability, of attempting to hold our present position [...] there was nothing to be done but [...] raise the siege, embark the

---

237 Gordon, *Balaclava*.
238 Filder to Military Secretary, 1 August 1854; TNA: WO 62/13.
239 Clarendon to Stratford, 13 November 1854; TNA: FO 352/37A.
240 Quoted by Sweetman, *Raglan*, p.260.
241 E.B. Hamley, *The Story of the Campaign of Sebastopol Written in Camp*. (Edinburgh: W. Blackwood and Sons, 1855), p.165.
242 Select Committee, 2nd Report, p.302.
243 *Journal of the Royal United Services Institute*, 102 (1957), p.83.

troops [...] and evacuate the Crimea,'[244] while the Prime Minister was informed by his son, who was on the QMG's staff, that he thought that: 'the same advice would be given by every general and officer of experience in this Army, *if his opinion were asked*.'[245]

Raglan had little option, however, as: 'he could not abandon his guns, that he had not transport for half of his army, that he could not leave the French to shift for themselves, and that he could not take such a step without positive orders from home.'[246]

And then came the hurricane of 14 November, and the fate of the Army was sealed. The 'monster catastrophe' predicted by Clarendon came to pass, and all in the Crimea were forced to extemporize the best way they could to cope with the situation.

The destruction of *Prince* and other transports anchored outside Balaklava harbour on 14 November 1854 resulted in the loss of a large quantity of essential stores including clothing, viz. on *Prince*: woollen socks, 35,700; woollen frocks, 53,000; flannel drawers, 17,000; watch coats, 2,500; blankets, 16,100; and rugs, 3,700.[247] Given that a lead time of over two months was required to supply sufficient lime juice to permit dosing each man daily to prevent scurvy (see below) it is obvious that some forward planning by the government must have taken place during the summer to ensure that such large quantities of materiel arrived in Balaklava when they did, and hence it is not surprising that the deficiencies in clothing and other necessaries only began to be made good some weeks later. Details of clothing and other stores sent to the East were published in the form of Parliamentary Papers. Perusal of these documents confirms that enormous amounts of materiel were sent to the East so that the Army was eventually well supplied with what was required.[248]

The details of the number of items issued to each regiment and the other departments were recorded in a ledger.[249] For example, those drawn by the Medical Department, Ambulance Corps, and General Hospital between November 1854 and May 1855 comprised jerseys, 7,933; blankets, 6,412; rugs, 5,057; drawers, 2,854; boots, 1,725; socks, 818; comforters, 650; mits, 282; fur caps, 108; and sheepskins, 104.

Food: The quantities of food needed by the men and animals of the Army were considerable. For example, each day a division of 7,000 men required 3.1 tons of meat

---

244 S.J.G. Calthorpe, *Cadogan's Crimea* (London: Hamish Hamilton, 1979), p.104.
245 A. Gordon to Aberdeen, 17 November 1854; British Library: Add. Ms 42335.
246 A. Gordon to Aberdeen, 9 March 1855; British Library: Add. Ms 42335.
247 Select Committee, 4th Report, p.40.
248 Select Committee, 4th Report, p.40; HCPP 1854–55 (399) XXXII.307: *Number and Description of Articles of Clothing Supplied [...] since 1st Day of October 1854 for the Troops Serving in the Crimea*; HCPP 1854–55 (4) XXXII.631: *Statement of Warm Clothing Lost on Board* The Prince*;* and HCPP 1854–55 (212) XXXII.633: *Return of the Stores Sent to the East from 1st Day of January 1854 to 1st Day of January 1855, with the Totals of Each, the Dates when Sent, and when Arrived in the East.*
249 TNA: WO 28/153.

and 3.1 or 4.3 tons of bread or biscuit, while the divisional animals would consume 6.25 tons of barley and 2.25 tons each of hay and chopped straw.

Under normal circumstances the diet of the men was monotonous and not particularly appetizing or nutritious. It was traditional for them to cater for themselves either singly or in small messes. This was inefficient in terms of manpower and fuel, and hence a move towards catering on a larger scale was an attractive proposition. A General Order of 20 December 1854 stated that it was desirable that the: 'system of messing established by Her Majesty's Regulations should be reverted to, where the regiments are in possession of camp kettles; and the Commander of the Forces desires that, as required by the Regulations, an officer should inspect the messes, and see that the provisions are properly cooked.'

A further development occurred a few months later when Alexis Soyer, sometime head chef at the Reform Club, volunteered to go to the East to advise on the feeding of the troops.[250] His visit received official backing and he arrived at Scutari towards the end of March 1855, where he proved of 'great service to this establishment and when his arrangements are perfected there will be little left to be done.'[251] His 'receipts (*sic*: recipes) have been highly approved' and 'printed by authority of headquarters,'[252] and though Nightingale found his stoves in the hospitals answered 'every purpose of economy and efficiency' she concluded: 'The patients [at Scutari] don't like Soyer's cookery […] nearly so well as ours, and I hear nothing but complaints. But I will not reopen our kitchens yet.'[253] The final sentence may betray a hint of bitterness, not surprisingly perhaps, as the special diet kitchens she had worked so hard to establish had been closed after the development of Soyer's centralized catering facilities.[254]

Before Soyer arrived in the Crimea on 5 May 1855 improvements had been made in some regimental catering facilities by the provision of stone cook-houses and the employment of permanent cooks.[255] Perhaps because of this Soyer anticipated opposition to his visit though 'instead of enemies' he found: 'from headquarters to every camp and regiment, the officers and medical gentlemen have rendered me the utmost assistance, so ready are they to improve the cooking of food for their brave companions in arms. The provisions allowed by the government I consider bountiful, and only require to be applied to the best advantage.'[256]

---

250 For biographies see R. Brandon, *The People's Chef. Alexis Soyer, a Life in Seven Courses* (Chichester: John Wiley, 2004) and R. Cowan, *Relish: The Extraordinary Life of Alexis Soyer* (London: Phoenix, 2007).
251 Cumming to Hall, 4 May 1855; RAMC: 397/F/CO/19/17.
252 Bracebridge, letter; *Lady's Newspaper*, 7 June 1855
253 Nightingale to the Bracebridges, 7 August 1855; Goldie, *Florence Nightingale*, p.144 and McDonald, *Florence Nightingale*, 14, p.211.
254 Cantlie, *A History*, 2, p.148.
255 For example, in the 1st Battalion, Rifle Brigade; G. Fisher, 'Rifleman John Fisher', *The War Correspondent*, 29:3 (2011), pp.10–8.
256 A. Soyer to Editor of *The Times*, 3 June 1855; A. Soyer, *Soyer's Culinary Campaign* (London: G. Routledge & Co., 1856), p.265.

Soyer's stoves, which could be carried in one piece by a mule, could be used by one or two men to cook for a battalion by placing them in a row.[257] They were also found to be 'admirably adapted as regards despatch, cleanliness, and economy.'[258] Soyer was requested to attend a board of general officers to discuss the erection of soup kitchens and the issue of hot meals during the winter.'[259] This proposal was not proceeded with,[260] but his stoves clearly proved their worth as, with some modification they were still in use some 150 years later.[261]

By the autumn of 1855 the infrastructure in the camps had been developed further and at this juncture Hall reported on the stoves to the War Office in a practical, if slightly less enthusiastic manner than some other commentators:

> Most of the kitchens in camp are substantially built with coppers and stoves set, and [...] as many saucepans and kettles as they require so they are better off than if they were supplied with M. Soyer's stove kettle alone. [...] many regiments are supplied with Feetham's stove which is more portable and better adapted for the hospital purpose than Soyer's. [...] if the army takes the field camp kettles and A and B canteens would all that could be carried [...] and M. Soyer's stoves would have to be left behind. M. Soyer's stoves would be a long time clearing its expense in the saving of fuel, as that is not generally an item of expenditure with an army in the field.[262]

Hall issued a Medical Department Memorandum on the composition of hospital diets on 27 January 1856 and this included three of Soyer's recipes for making soup which 'may not be unacceptable to those medical officers who have inexperienced hospital chefs.'[263] Shepherd concluded that: 'There is no evidence that the medical officers viewed [Soyer's] reforms unfavourably,' but added the caveat that 'It may well be that they were more ready to accept advice from a man, rather than from Nightingale. [...] Soyer had been sent out officially and was well known to so many people of influence at home [and also in the Crimea no doubt].'[264]

It cannot be determined if the troops would have enjoyed better health if Soyer's culinary reforms had been introduced before the Army left for the East but by the spring of 1855 the government was probably relieved to sanction a famous chef to

---

257 IGH Alexander's evidence to the Royal Commission, 25 May 1857; Royal Commission Report, pp.86–7.
258 Dr. G. Taylor to Soyer, 5 July 1856; Soyer, *Culinary Campaign*, p.417.
259 AG to Soyer, 1 September 1855; TNA: WO 28/123.
260 QMG to Soyer, 7 October 1855; TNA: WO 28/139.
261 Soyer's camp kitchen is depicted in the *Illustrated London News*, 22 September 1855.
262 Hall to Deputy Secretary for War, 19 November 1855; RAMC: 397/F/CO/1/2/3606.
263 RAMC: 397/F/CO/1/3.
264 Shepherd, *Crimean Doctors*, 1, p.370.

advise on nutritional matters, and thus hopefully prevent problems with catering occurring during the rest of the campaign.

Irrespective of the problems encountered during the first winter matters were rectified and when the Supplies Commissioners left the Crimea in early June 1855 they noted that: 'supplies of food to the army [...] were abundant, and the diet of the soldier [is] better than [...] in any former campaign,'[265] though they did point out that: 'It [is] a defect in [the] British Army, that no one is responsible for the fitness of the diet supplied to the troops,' and they recommended that a staff officer should attend to 'the supply of the Army' thus making the best use of supplies available, especially locally. There is no evidence that this policy was put into effect in the Crimea; possibly because supplies of all kinds were freely available when the recommendation was made.

Clothing: The losses on *Prince* and other vessels began to be made good towards the end of the year when 'blankets and other warm clothing were pouring in'[266] although their issue was initially hampered by a want of store room and sufficient unpackers and issuers.[267] In the first week of January Hall was able to recommend to regimental surgeons that they apply to the QMG's store at Balaklava for blankets and warm clothing as there was plenty for both sick and well.[268] By the middle of the month 'warm clothing is now being carried up in larger quantities to be divided amongst the troops,'[269] Dr G. Lawson wrote home that things were beginning to improve, though very slowly at first. Warm clothing had already arrived 'in enormous quantities', and 'a daily inspection of the men is now ordered' to see they really have the warm clothing that has been issued to them.'[270] The Engineer's journal recorded on 18 January that: 'Vast quantities of warm clothing [...] had been disembarked, and [...] almost every man had been supplied with a second blanket, a jersey frock, flannel drawers and socks, and with some kind of winter coat, in addition to the ordinary great coat;'[271] and the AG reported: 'The warm clothing has been a great comfort; the sheep skin coats especially, and the buffaloe [sic] skins in the field hospitals' though it was not possible to 'make much progress in getting the men off the ground [and] the boots sent are much too small.'[272]

265 Supplies Commission Report, pp.14–5.
266 L.G. Heath, *Letters from the Black Sea during the Crimean War, 1854–1855* (London: Richard Bentley, 1873), p.125.
267 DAQMG, Balaklava to QMG, 28 December 1854; TNA: WO 28/196.
268 Hall to PMO, 2nd Division, 7 January 1855; Royal Commission Report, Appendix LXXIX, p.112.
269 Special correspondent, 20 January; *Daily News*, 3 February 1855.
270 V. Bonham-Carter and M. Lawson, *Surgeon in the Crimea* (London: Military Book Society, 1968), p.150.
271 Elphinstone, *Journal*, pp.79–81.
272 Estcourt to AG, Horse Guards, 20 January 1855; National Army Museum: 1962-10-95-2.

The House of Commons was subsequently informed by Mr Monsell, MP, on 3 March that between November 1854 and January 1855 the Ordnance had sent out about 2,000 tons of warm clothing to the Crimea,[273] and this had been augmented by clothing obtained more locally, for example, a steamer left Trieste on the 30 December with a cargo including 17,156 fur coats. 24,900 fur caps, 64,000 pairs of gloves, 11,800 woollen shirts, 18,000 woollen drawers, 2,500 woollen socks, and five wooden houses.[274]

Fuel: The area of the Crimean peninsula occupied by the allies was not well wooded and the shortage of timber for fuel soon became a serious problem, and thereafter all categories of fuel had to be imported and transported to the camps. It had not been usual practice for the Commissariat to provide troops with fuel, except when in barracks, and hence no provision for this had been made in advance of the invasion. Raglan subsequently ordered the CG to provided fuel for the Army on 11 November, though it was not until the end of December that 'the troops in and near Balaklava received rations of fuel' while until the onset of spring 'the want of land transport made it impossible to carry it to the front, except in small quantities for use in hospitals.'[275].

The provision of fuel resulted in a 'considerable addition to the duties of the Commissariat' since the whole requirement had to be imported, landed at Balaklava and carried up to camp. The scale of the task can be gauged from the CG's estimate of the amount of fuel and light required during December 1854 to meet the requirements stipulated in a General Order of 28 May 1854, viz. charcoal, 481 tons/month and 300 pack animals per day; coal, 963 and 360, and wood, 1,927 and 720 respectively.[276]

Housing: The shortage of adequate living accommodation had serious repercussions for both sick and well during the months after the invasion, particularly as preference was given initially to accommodating horses and mules under cover rather than the sick, a policy understandably deprecated by Hall.[277]

The provision of huts became a priority once it was decided to over-winter in the Crimea.[278] Contracts were entered into in England while locally the QMG instructed the CG to purchase timber and other building materials.[279] The first of several consignments of loose boarding etc. sufficient for 10,000 men and 3,500 horses arrived from

---

273 *Hansard*, 5 March 1855.
274 Earl of Westmorland, the Ambassador in Vienna, to Mr Colquhoun, the Vice-consul, Varna, 30 December 1854; TNA: WO/28/155.
275 Supplies Commission Report, pp.10–11.
276 Filder to Raglan, 9 December 1854; TNA: WO 28/193.
277 QMG to CRE, 25 November 1855; TNA: WO 28/196 and Hall, diary entry, 1 December 1954; RAMC: 524/15.
278 The report of the Supplies Commissioners includes an overview on accommodation; Supplies Commission Report, pp.33–6 & 284–8.
279 QMG to Filder 7 November 1854; TNA: WO 28/198.

Black Sea ports and elsewhere on 25 November,[280] while the first of several ship loads of huts arrived from England on 25 December (Figure 2.9).

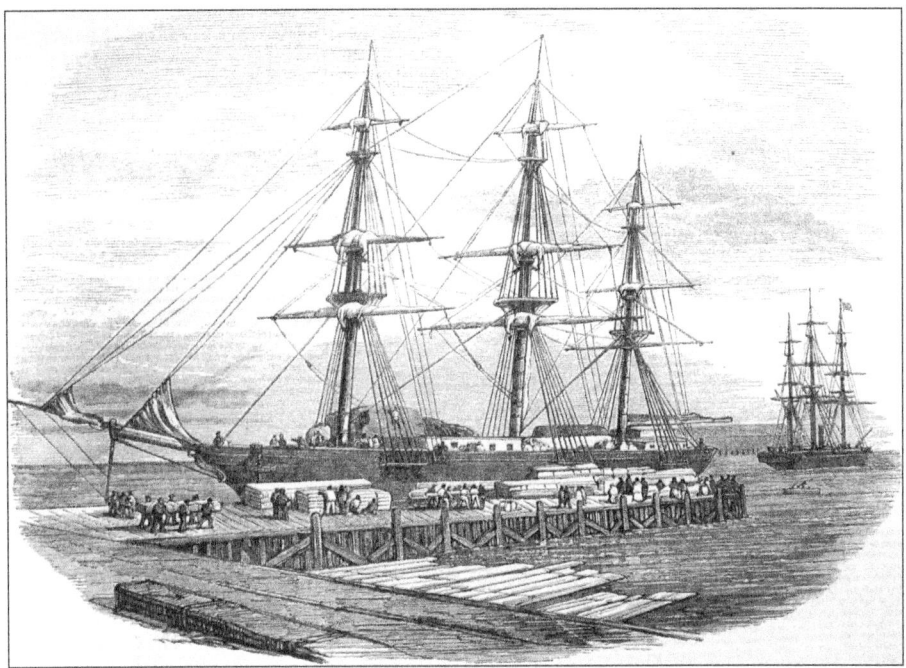

Figure 2.9 Shipment of wooden barracks, on board "The White Falcon", at Southampton, for the French Army in the Crimea. (*Illustrated London News*, 3 February 1855, p.105)

The unloading of this bulky material increased congestion in the harbour area. The huts were heavy and 250–300 men were required to man-handle a hut for 25 up to the camps for want of wheeled transport and pack animals,[281] while construction using sawn timber was hampered by the shortage of skilled labour.

Regimental hospitals were originally housed in bell tents and marquees but huts became increasingly used. The 'more seriously ill were being retained in regimental hospitals instead of being evacuated to Scutari'[282] by March 1855, though provision for the well proved more variable.[283] Hut building continued during the remainder

---

280 Supplies Commission Report, p.34. See *Illustrated London News*, 13 January and 3 February 1856 for the wood for barracks on the docks at Trieste and Southampton respectively..
281 This is in contrast to I.K. Brunel's prefabricated hospital erected at Renkioi; the components of which could be carried by one man or two.
282 Shepherd, *Crimean Doctors*, 1, p.295.
283 Supplies Commission Report, pp.38 & 284–8.

of 1855 though 4,000 men were still accommodated under canvas by its end, albeit all were in double tents with wooden floors,[284] while, not unexpectedly officers were generally better accommodated than the men.[285]

The provision of huts proved a massive undertaking. The number sent from England numbered 4,550.[286] About 38 miles of planking were imported,[287] and as late as the spring 1856 75 miles of roofing felt was sent to the Crimea to effect repairs.[288] Huts were certainly better than tents but they were not an unalloyed success as they could become hot in the summer and the ventilation was not always adequate. In addition, they could prove unstable in windy weather unless appropriately strutted[289] and were a greater fire risk than with tents.[290] Many required regular maintenance as they were constructed from poor materials, and the failure to undertake this proved a recurrent cause of complaint from medical officers. This was supported by Codrington who notified Panmure towards the end of 1855 that: 'of 640 huts including hospitals […] only 100 are reported watertight. The old ones all want fresh covering, the best of the new ones leak badly at the joints, the thin single-board roofs of the smaller new ones are still worse, and felt is only just arrived.'[291]

Codrington informed Panmure in May 1856 that the Russians had no wish to purchase huts on the plateau and so they were being sold to individuals or used for firewood.[292] Some of the best huts were taken to Malta,[293] while a General Order dated 22 May required that each regiment 'will leave the camp perfectly clean, the huts empty, temporary stables and kitchens levelled, dug out tents and latrines filled up.'[294]

Some days later Codrington suggested to Panmure that the Russian government will no doubt seize every hut 'on our quitting' and if it was not an 'undignified dog-in-the-manger proceeding, what a magnificent bonfire the whole camp would make!' In his reply of 23 June Panmure opined that 'if the Russians do not buy our huts, or have the decency to ask for them civilly' he could 'see no reason why a farewell bonfire might not be made of them.'[295] That this happened was confirmed by Assistant

---

284 Journal of Proceedings, 30 December 1855; TNA: WO 28/143.
285 For a comprehensive review see C. Cohen, 'Accommodating Officers', *The War Correspondent* 34:2 & 34:3 (2017), pp.38–48 & 36–48 respectively.
286 HCPP 1857 Session 2 (267) XXVII.155: *The Number of Huts Supplied to the Ordnance or War Departments during the Years 1854–55 and 1855–56*. These comprised those for officers, 788; soldiers, 3,154; cook houses, 4; hospitals, 317; stables, 260; and stores, 27.
287 QMG to CRE, 19 July 1855; TNA: WO 28/138.
288 Undersecretary of War to Smith, 17 March 1856; Smith, *Précis of Letters*.
289 Burgoyne to QMG, 18 January 1855; TNA: WO 28/197.
290 DAQMG, Balaklava to QMG, 11 May 1856; TNA: WO 28/136.
291 Codrington to Panmure, 29 November 1855; TNA: WO 1/380.
292 Codrington to Panmure, 13 May 1856; TNA: WO 1/384.
293 Circulars to GOC Divisions and HoDs, 19 & 28 May 1856; TNA: WO 28/140.
294 TNA: WO 28/131.
295 Douglas and Ramsey, *The Panmure Papers*, 2, pp.249 & 258.

Surgeon Greig who counted 'no less that ten fires blazing all over the camp' on the night of 14 June 1856.[296]

Lime juice: Nowhere is the relationship between supply and health more obvious than in the case of scurvy. This deficiency disease was noted first towards the end of October 1854 (see Section 5.4) and local available supplies of lime juice were landed shortly afterwards. Immediately Smith heard the news in mid-November he arranged for large volumes of juice to be forwarded to the Crimea but despite pressing the point to the military authorities it was not until the beginning of February 1855 that sufficient quantities arrived for the troops to receive a prescribed amount each day. This proved beneficial and it was decided to continue prophylactic dosing for the duration of the campaign, with the result that in the autumn of 1855 about two tons of juice was required daily to meet this need.

2.3.4 *Royal Navy*

A detailed assessment of victualling the Royal Navy is outside the scope of this monograph. Unlike the Army, which traditionally obtained supplies from local sources when on campaign, the naval authorities had to provide the ships with all their needs for long sea voyages during which additional supplies may not be readily available. The responsibility for this task resided with the Comptroller of Victualling and Transports, with the principal victualling yards in England being located adjacent to the Royal Dock Yards in Deptford, Portsmouth and Plymouth.[297] These facilities were extensive and had bakeries, breweries, mills, slaughterhouses, and a cooperage for the making of barrels. The yards also stocked or manufactured other foodstuffs.

A victualling yard had also been built in the Malta dockyard in 1845; the Malta Maritime Museum is now housed in the former bakery building.

2.3.5 *Concluding remarks*

Raglan pointed out to Newcastle at the end of January 1855 that: 'the organization of the British Army, which is framed for stationary service in the colonies, or for home duty, is undoubtedly defective for operations in the field.'[298] How right he was. These shortcomings, coupled with a combination of bad weather, a lack of wheeled transport, and the deterioration of rudimentary rural roads, resulted in substantial difficulties in bringing the 'plenty' in Balaklava harbour to the camps during the winter 1854–55. This combination of circumstances, coupled with the effects of the losses of stores sustained during the storm of 14 November, together with the failure to make timely provision of adequate shelter, proved catastrophic. Collectively these oversights

---

296 D. Hill, *Letters from the Crimea* (Dundee: Dundee UP, 2010), p.200.
297 For a summary of the activities on the yard in Deptford see S. Littledale, 'Deptford's Navy Victualling Yard', *Magazine of the Friends of The National Archives*, 28:2 (2017), pp.7–10.
298 Raglan to Newcastle, 31 January 1855; TNA: WO 33/1/17/55.

overwhelmed the limited resilience of the army supply system and thus contributed directly to the excessive losses from disease described in Chapter 5.

In his evaluation of the organization and performance of the Commissariat Sweetman concluded, inter alia, that the 'numerical strength and the experience of Filder's force were unsatisfactory,' and the events of the first winter 'cruelly exposed the dangers of relying on the existing contract system' and of obtaining 'waggons of the country [and] supplies from the theatre of war.' The net effect was that the limitations of the systems of management, which were excessively complex and rigid, were 'severely exposed' and the department resembled 'Charles Dickens' Circumlocution office.'[299] Nevertherless, despite these short comings MacMunn concluded that by general agreement Filder did reasonably well in supplying the Army until the Hurricane of 14 November and the following failure of supply was not Filder's fault.[300] In fact, Maxwell made it clear that up to this point the Commissariat had sufficient carts and pack animals to transport about 130 tons which would have been more than sufficient if conditions had not deteriorated.[301]

Wars are won or lost through logistical strengths and capabilities. For example, the loss of the American colonies can be attributed largely to a logistics failure.[302] MacMunn was of the opinion that: 'complete failure in the preparation during the ample months of waiting, is the marvel of the period. [and] The failure to provide that large number of officers needed for [...] the line of communications [...] is an equally clear sign of the War Office and Horse Guards inability to envisage the problem.'[303]

While the difficulties experienced in the Crimea did not lead to a strategic failure, they were disastrous enough, and thus it was the tenacity of those on the ground who did much to rectify matters. Their perseverance, coupled with improvements in the roads, the rationalization of land transport, and particularly the construction of a railway network, ensured that the necessaries for life were eventually brought to the camps on a regular basis, and the health of the troops improved considerably to give the Victory over Disease of 1856 to which reference has already been made.

---

299 Sweetman, *War and Administration*, pp.41–59.
300 MacMunn, *The Crimea in Perspective*, pp.148–9.
301 Anon [Maxwell], *Whom Shall We Hang?*, pp.142–8.
302 See R.A. Bowler, *Logistics and the Failure of the British in the America 1775–1785* (Princeton: University Press, 1975) and Christopher, *Logistics and Supply*.
303 MacMunn, *The Crimea in Perspective*, pp.241–2.

3

Provision of hospital facilities

The regiment was the principal component of the army and was essentially a self-contained unit. It was equipped to provide primary health care for the troops including hospital facilities when stationary; the provision of which was the responsibility of the Commanding Officer. However, in the case of the Crimean campaign the rapid lengthening of the sick list during 1854 necessitated the need for general hospitals to assist with the treatment of additional patients. The development of these facilities in Turkey, the Crimea, and elsewhere are discussed in this chapter.

The policy of developing general hospitals was not universally accepted as overcrowding was recognized in the Peninsular War as being an 'artificial cause of the destruction of armies' because the 'effect of accumulation evidently corrupts the air, and this generates an artificial malignancy' and 'relapses are the leading cause of mortality.'[1] It was also recorded that soldiers 'sent to general hospitals [were] rarely restored to [their] corps during the campaign.' Regimental hospitals were thus preferred because 'not collecting soldiers into one spot reduces the chances of contagion.' and 'the average duration of sickness is always less in regimental hospitals.'[2] However, as Martineau pointed out, there was a need for general hospitals as regimental hospitals would not have the capacity to cope with a 'virulent epidemic, or after a sanguinary battle.' It would, however, be necessary for their provision to be planned in advance and their function properly defined.[3]

Shortly after war was declared Smith suggested that hospital accommodation should be developed on healthy islands in the Black Sea or Greek archipelago.[4] No action was taken at that time and Cantlie suggested that the responsibility for this

1 Jackson, *Remarks*, pp.345–6.
2 W. Fergusson, *Notes*, p 60.
3 Martineau, *England and Her Soldiers*, pp.89–90.
4 Smith to Military Secretary, 11 May 1854; Smith, *Précis of Letters* and Royal Commission Report, Appendix LXXIX, p.7 with an extract in *The Lancet*, 21 April 1855. Smith mentioned that the French had arranged for hospital facilities at Candia (now Iráklion) in Crete.

omission in forward planning must rest with the Military Secretary, the Commander-in-Chief, Viscount Hardinge, or the Secretary for War, the Duke of Newcastle; and not the Army Medical Department.[5]

Nine general hospitals were in operation in Turkey and the Crimea for varying lengths of time between June 1854 and June 1856. Table 3.1 indicates when they were open and Maps 3.1 & 3.2 gives their location. The regimental hospitals were accommodated in bell tents and/or marques in the early months but as the campaign progressed huts were in general use.

Table 3.1 The months during which the hospitals of the Army of the East were in operation, April 1854–June 1856

Hospital[*]	1854			1854–55						1855–56		
	A–M	J–S	O–N	D–J	F	M	A–M	J–S	O–N	D–A	M	J
Regimental hospitals	•	•	•	•	•	•	•	•	•	•	•	•
I Scutari		•	•	•	•	•	•	•	•	•	•	•
II Varna		•	•	•								
III Balaklava General			•	•	•	•	•	•	•	•	•	•
IV Abydos				•	•	•	•	•				
V Smyrna					•	•	•	•	•			
VI Castle General						•	•	•	•	•	•	•
VII Camp General							•	•	•	•		
VIII Monastery								•	•	•	•	
IX Renkioi									•	•	•	•
Number operational	1	3	4	5	5	6	7	8	8	7	6	5

* Details of the hospitals of the cavalry and infantry regiments are included in the *Medical and Surgical History*, 1, while the tables for the general hospitals, designated I–IX, form an appendix in the *Medical and Surgical History*, 2.

The need for convalescent hospitals relatively near the front became obvious soon after hostilities ocmmenced. These would cater for patients likely to 'recruit their health' in reasonable time and hence Hall recommended in the first instance that they should go to Malta 'for a change of air,' and only invalids should be sent to England.[6]

---

5   Cantlie, *A History*, 2, pp.54–5.
6   Hall to Raglan and QMG, 27 October and Hall to Menzies, 28 October 1854; RAMC: 397/F/CO/1/1/819, 820 & 842, and Royal Commission Report, Appendix LXXIX, p.103.

Provision of hospital facilities 99

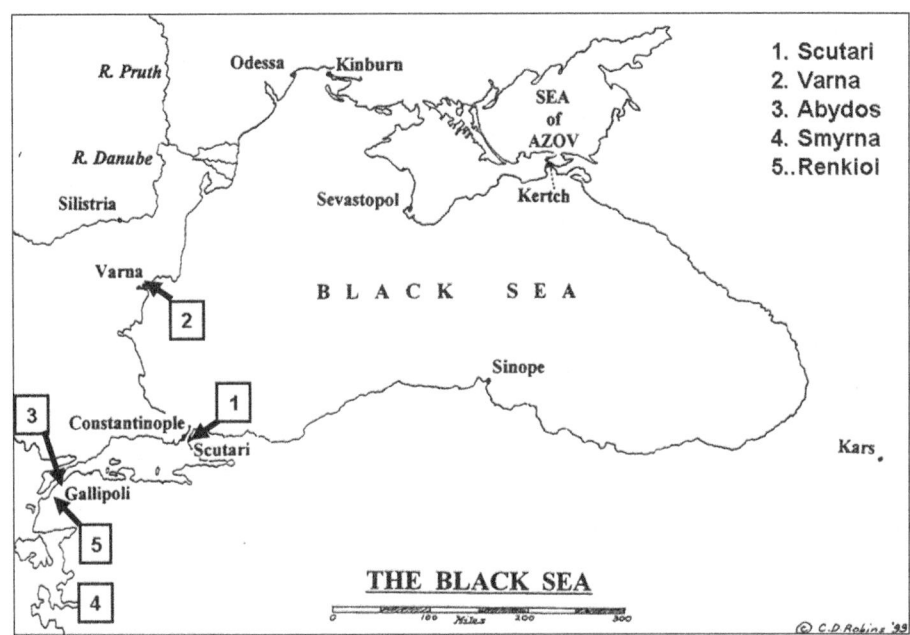

Map 3.1 Location of the general hospitals in Turkey and Bulgaria.
(Map by Colin Robins, used with permission)v

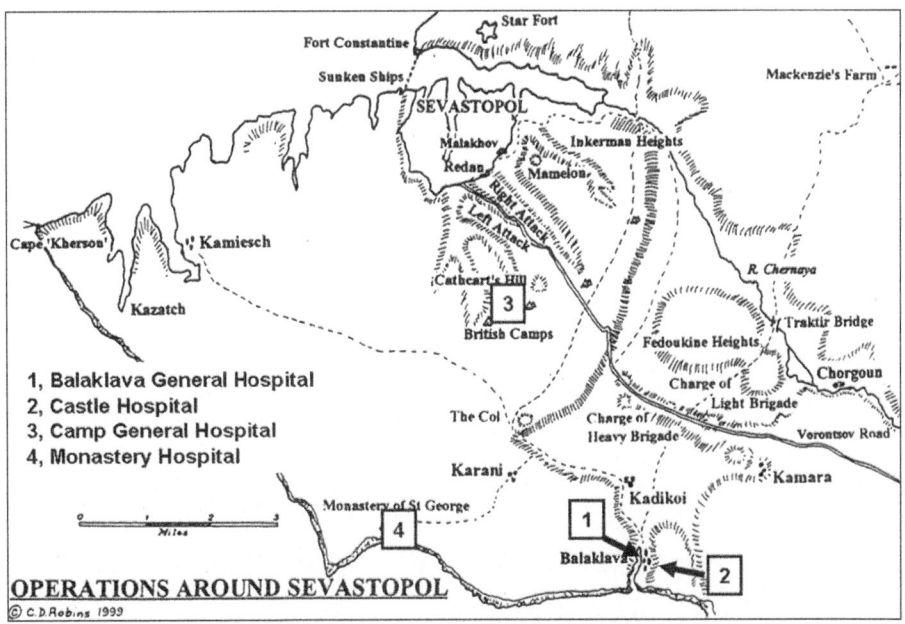

Map 3.2 Location of the general hospitals in the Crimea.
(Map by Colin Robins, used with permission)

This policy was authorized by Raglan[7] thus releasing space in the general hospitals for acute cases.[8]

The early development of sanatoria was hampered by a shortage of manpower, as 'medical staff must be provided, as also hospital orderlies, and a military commander, and a detachment capable of bearing arms to enforce order [...] but I [Raglan] have not a notion whence the officers could be taken [as] there is a great want of them at Scutari.'[9] This dilemma was echoed a year later by the PMO, Scutari who informed Smith that the 'hospital at Smyrna will require a large staff; none can be spared from here.'[10]

The need to provide military and medical staff on hospital transports exacerbated the shortage of land-based manpower.[11] Additionally, the piecemeal movement of patients presented the military authorities with administrative problems, particularly in the early stages, as it proved difficult to keep track of their whereabouts, despite a General Order of 18 December 1854 that stipulated that Purveyors were 'strictly ordered to communicate to regiments [...] the death, or removal to England, of any soldier.'[12]

Gozo appeared to be the only hospital developed specifically for convalescents while Corfu, Rhodes, Sinope, and other sites were considered as potential locations, but none were utilized. Additional accommodation for convalescents was subsequently provided in the general hospitals at Scutari and Kuleli while civilian hospitals at Smyrna and Renkioi only came into use when the health of the Army had much improved, and hence some of the patients sent there would have been close to becoming convalescents when they arrived.[13]

3.1 Turkey

The first General Hospitals to be occupied at Scutari were a Turkish General Military Hospital and the Turkish Barracks. This had to be adapted for hospital use though it never proved entirely fit for purpose.[14] Other buildings that were utilized included a

---

7   Hall to Cumming, 10 November 1854; RAMC: 397/F/CO/1/1/892.
8   PMO, Scutari to Hall, 10 November 1854; Smith, *Précis of Letters*. In the event *Emeu*, HMS *Arethusa*, *Blake*, *Trent*, *Jura*, and *Ripon* disembarked invalids at Malta between 17 November and 31 December 1854; TNA: WO 15/1187.
9   Raglan to Newcastle, 10 January 1855; TNA: WO 1/370/747–752.
10 PMO, Scutari to Smith, 25 January 1855; Smith, *Précis of Letters*.
11 Estcourt to the AG, Horse Guards, 3 February 1855; National Army Museum: 1962-10-95-2.
12 TNA: WO 28/130. The order was restated on 8 January 1855 as it had not been fully implemented.
13 Hall to QMG, 15 October 1855; RAMC: 397/F/CO/1/2/3412.
14 The performance of these two facilities was not presented separately in the *Medical and Surgical History* and hence no comparison is possible.

Pavilion which formed part of the Barrack Hospital and housed officers and which was closed towards the end of 1855 to reduce expense, parts of a Palace at Haidar Pasha, the Harem of which was destroyed by fire in early 1856,[15] and a barrack on the shores of the Bosphorus at Kuleli.

The hospital facilities were in operation from June 1854 until June 1856 and during that time 43,288 NCOs and men were admitted of whom 5,432 (12.5 percent) died.

3.1.1 Scutari and Kuleli

Stratford informed Raglan on 31 August 1854 that the General Hospital and the barracks at Scutari and Kuleli would be cleared by the Turkish authorities and made available for the British Army[16] (Figures 3.1 and 3.2).[17] The buildings were subsequently used for patients from the Crimea and the local military depots, though with time some facilities were developed for convalescent soldiers.

In order to reduce pressure on hospital accommodation, men sufficiently recovered were returned to the front from the beginning of November 1854, while effective men and convalescents would be moved to Kuleli from the Barrack Hospital if large numbers of sick and wounded arrived.[18] Convalescents were also employed as hospital orderlies while others guarded wounded Russians,[19] or were sent to the depot, located initially in the Barrack complex, or to vessels moored at the mouth of the Golden Horn.

Huts were erected in the quadrangle of the Barrack Hospital and, although Cumming, the PMO, did not 'approve of their situation', he intended to 'occupy them with convalescents [...] which will thin the wards and corridors,'[20] and thus allow the walls of the wards to be whitewashed.[21] However, one of the perceived 'evils' of housing convalescents adjacent to a town was the men had access to grog shops and some relapsed and had to be 'sent back to their wards.'[22]

Some weeks after the invasion a Turkish frigate, and *Bombay*, a fine Indiaman, were moored in the Golden Horn and fitted up for convalescents,[23] as reported by Hall and Sillery, the commandant:

---

15 PMO, Scutari to Smith, 29 November 1855; Smith, *Précis of Letters* and PMO, Scutari to Smith, 7 February 1856; Smith, *Précis of Letters*.
16 TNA: WO 28/197.
17 For other illustrations of the Barrack hospital see the *Illustrated London News*, 1 July 1854, p.626 and 15 December 1854, p.625.
18 Sillery to AG, 9 & 15 November 1854; TNA: WO 28/186
19 Paulet in answer to letter from the AG, 24 December 1854; TNA: WO 278/186.
20 Cumming to Smith 22 February 1855; Smith, *Précis of Letters* and Royal Commission Report, Appendix LXXIX, p.36; and HCPP 1854–55 (449) XXXIII.361: *Official Reports on the Hospitals at Scutari, Kululee, Abydos, and Smyrna, since February Last*, p.26. (Hereafter: Reports on Hospitals in Turkey).
21 Cumming to Hall, 2 March 1855; RAMC: 397/F/CO/19/9.
22 *Medical Times and Gazette*, 26 May 1855.
23 *Illustrated London News*, 11 November 1854 includes an engraving of the Turkish hulk used as the hospital ship.

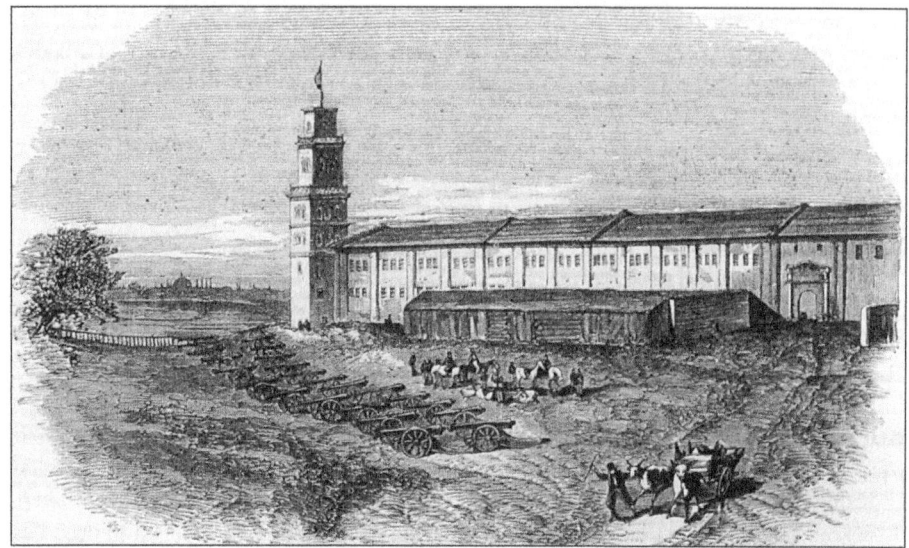

Figure 3.1 The British hospital, Scutari (From a sketch by Julian Portch. *Illustrated Times*, 8 December 1855)

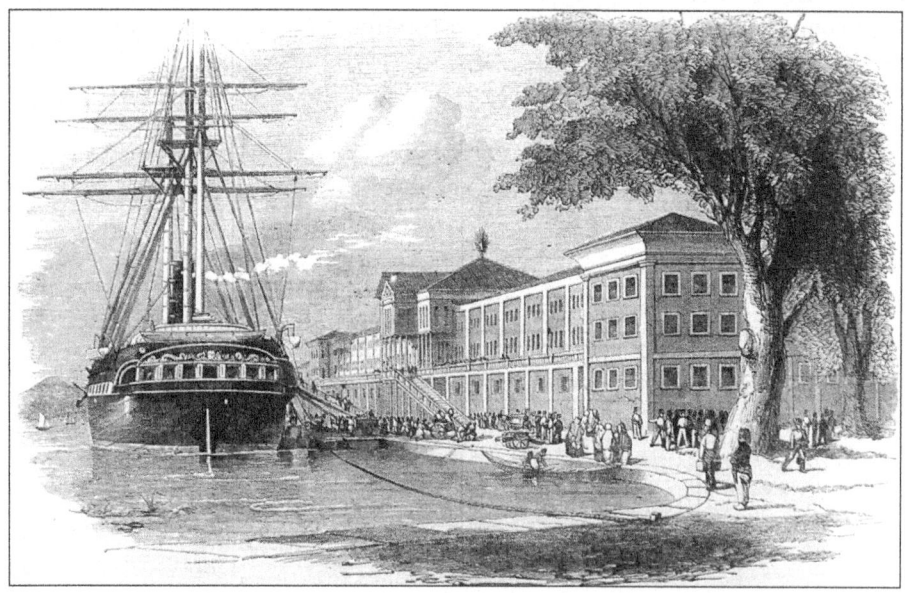

Figure 3.2 The Kukeieh (*sic*) Barracks, Constantinople – The Royal Artillery disembarking. (From 'The Jason'. *Illustrated London News*, 16 September 1854, p.260)

Hall: Today we [...] move 500 convalescents onto an old line of battle ship [...] fitted up and moored within the Seraglio point, and in a day or two we shall be able to despatch 170 invalids to England [...] and 50 women whose husbands have either died or been killed in action, and who, poor creatures, are an embarrassment to us in the way of accommodation.[24]

Sillery: We sent about 400 men on board the hospital ship yesterday, all convalescents, all improving. I sent one officer, three sergeants, three cooks, and 10 orderlies. [...] a naval assistant surgeon in medical charge. [...] I think the ship very comfortable [...] all can sit down for their meals.[25]

The Hospital Commissioners subsequently considered it 'inexpedient to send convalescents on board ship' as the confinement was 'prejudicial both to their health and spirits.' Although initially intended for convalescents the two hulks had effectively become floating hospitals by the time they were inspected by the Sanitary Commissioners, who likewise found them unsatisfactory,[26] and they had ceased to be used for this purpose by the spring of 1855.[27]

Herbert reported to Smith that he had heard from both Cumming and Maxwell that 'Scutari is fast getting into order, but [the hospital is] full, and we must organize another hospital as soon as we can.'[28] Permission to utilize the barracks at Kuleli was obtained from the Porte in December 1854 and the first patients were admitted the following month.[29] The 'fine riding-school' was subsequently used as a convalescent hospital for 180 men.' 'It was 'contiguous to the Bosphorus [and] proved very healthy'.[30] It was seemingly 'much admired' and 'kept in beautiful order.'[31] It was later

---

24 Hall to Raglan, 5 October 1854; National Army Museum: 1968-07-293 but no copy in RAMC: 397/F/CO/1/1.
25 Sillery to AG, 4 October 1854; TNA: WO 28/186. Hall and Sillery were referring to the Turkish frigate as *Bombay* did not arrive until later with: '460 sick, mostly convalescents who would soon be fit for duty'; Sillery to AG, 11 October 1854.
26 For the Commissioners report to Admiral Gray and his response dated 17 & 18 March 1855 respectively, see TNA: FO 195/452 (longhand copy) and TNA: WO 33/1/24/55 (Cabinet paper), with a summary in Sanitary Commission Report, pp.27-8.
27 Hospital Commission Report, p.47. On 23 March 1855 Cumming informed Hall that '*Bombay* has been emptied [...] The Turkish hulk will also if possible be vacated;' RAMC: 397/F/CO/19/14. Paulet also informed Panmure that he had 'caused the Turkish hulk [...] to be cleared [...] *Bombay* convalescent transport-ship has also been cleared [...]'; Reports on Hospitals in Turkey, pp.22-3.
28 Herbert to Smith, 24 December 1854; Select Committee, 4th Report, pp.343-4.
29 Paulet to AG, 20 December 1854; TNA: WO 28/186. Incidentally, the demand for accommodation near the Bosphorus resulted in few suitable buildings remaining available for hospitals or stables; Stratford to Clarendon, 17 January 1855; TNA: FO 78/1070.
30 Paulet to Panmure, 25 April 1855; Reports on Hospitals in Turkey, p.22.
31 A Lady Volunteer [Frances M. Taylor], *Eastern Hospitals and English Nurses* (London: Hunt and Blackett, 1856), 2, pp.273-5.

retained for the British Army when the principal buildings were handed over to the British German Legion during November 1855.

Thirteen regiments of the Cavalry Division relocated to Turkey in November and December 1855. The Hussars Brigade was quartered at Ismid and they established hospital facilities there and did not utilize those at Scutari.

By March 1856 a correspondent was able to write: 'Our hospitals at Scutari continue in the best possible state containing scarcely any patients. [...] This is all the more gratifying when we consider the condition of our poor allies the French, in their hospitals across the Bosphorus.'[32]

3.1.2 Abydos

F.W. Calvert, the Consul on the Dardanelles, organized hospital facilities at Abydos with 400 beds to cater for the troops when they first arrived in 1854 (Figure 3.3).[33] Hall advised Raglan in June that a lazaretto there would make a suitable hospital,[34] and Dr Jameson was instructed to form a general hospital during October.[35] *Kangaroo* and *Emeu* arrived on the 6 and 25 December with 207 and 142 patients respectively with *Robert Lowe*, *Brandon*, and *Melbourne* bringing 316 more during February and April 1855.[36]

The hospital proved 'an out of the way place, very inconvenient,'[37] and it became used more for convalescents,[38] although by August it was 'almost empty and scarcely required', with only 32 men remaining to be repatriated.[39] It was no longer needed by the Army in October[40] and Panmure approved that military medical personnel could be replaced by civilians from the hospital at Renkioi, though with Captain Segrave in military command.[41]

Storks, Paulet's replacement, favoured transferring convalescents awaiting discharge from Renkioi to Abydos as they could be 'kept under closer discipline' than 'they are likely to be at Renkoy (*sic*).'[42] On the other hand, Hall recommended sending them to Scutari 'where facilities for their reception already exist.' In Hall's opinion Renkioi was

---

32 Shepherd, *Crimean Doctors*, 2, p.529.
33 Evidence given on 31 May 1858; HCPP 1857–58 (482) VIII.1: *Select Committee on Consular Services*, p.220.
34 Hall to Smith, 23 June 1854; Smith, *Précis of Letters*. A lazaretto was a reception centre for those in quarantine.
35 Hall to Jameson, 19 October 1854; RAMC: 397/F/CO/1/1/826.
36 *Medical and Surgical History*, 2, p.478. *Kangaroo* then sailed to Marseilles; TNA: ADM/7/576.
37 Cumming to Hall. 28 July 1855; National Army Museum: 2007-07-16-43.
38 Smith to PMO, Scutari, 10 May 1855; Smith, *Précis of Letters*.
39 PMO, Scutari to Smith, 16 & 30 August 1855; Smith, *Précis of Letters*.
40 Hall to QMG, 15 October 1855; TNA: WO 28/140.
41 Parkes to QMG, 22 September1855; TNA: WO 28/140; Panmure to Storks, 13 October 1855; TNA: WO 6/71; and Scutari District Orders, 15 October 1855; TNA: WO 28/103.
42 Storks to QMG, 25 October 1855; TNA: WO 28/186.

Provision of hospital facilities 105

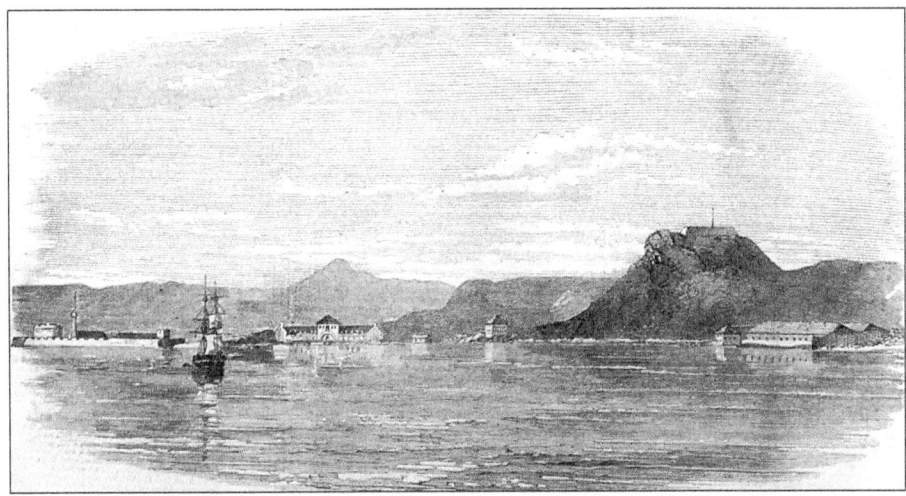

Figure 3.3 The English Hospital at Abydos. (*Illustrated London News*, 6 January 1854, p.244)

'little more than a convalescent station' because 'its distance from the Crimea rendered it unfeasible to send acute cases,'[43] and 'with the exception of the Land Transport Corps, which had been most injudiciously recruited, no serious disease prevailed.'[44] Hall's opinion appears to have prevailed and Storks was instructed to send convalescents from Renkioi to Scutari and not Abydos.[45] The hospital was subsequently turned over to the French,[46] although a wharf was retained for the use of a LTC depot.

3.1.3 Smyrna
There was a small British hospital in Smyrna which provided for expatriates and sailors using the port but it was too small for military purposes. Clarendon ordered Stratford to procure additional hospital accommodation[47] and accordingly a Staff Surgeon and a Commissariat officer were sent to Smyrna to seek suitable facilities for a convalescent hospital.[48] They recommended a Turkish barrack located near the shore, and close

43 Hall to QMG, 15 October 1855; RAMC: 397/F/CO/1/2/3412.
44 J. Hall, *Observations on the Difficulties Experienced by the Medical Department of the Army, During the Late War in Turkey, by Sir John Hall, M.D., K.C.B., Principal Medical Officer of that Army*. Unpublished versions in RAMC: 397F/RT/2 and TNA: WO 33/3B. (Hereafter: Hall, *Observations*.)
45 QMG to Storks, 22 October 1855; TNA: WO 28/192
46 Stratford to Clarendon, 1 October 1855; TNA: FO 78/1088. The French had earlier expressed an interest in the facilities and were assured they would not be used by General Beatson's Irregular Cavalry; Paulet to Stratford, 24 August 1855; TNA: FO 195/452.
47 Newcastle to Raglan, 11 December 1854; TNA: WO 6/70/712 and Cabinet paper; Wiltshire and Swindon History Centre: 2057/F8/III/C/65.
48 Departmental Order issued by the PMO, Scutari, 20 December 1854; TNA: FO 195/452

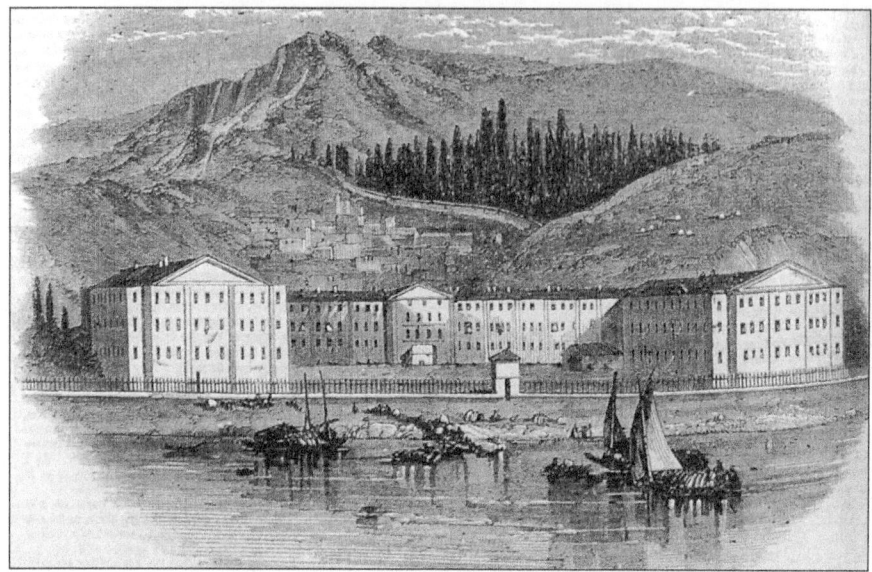

Figure 3.4 The hospital at Smyrna (From a sketch by Julian Portch. *Illustrated Times*, 24 November 1854, p.396)

to an 'abundant market'.[49] The building comprised a casement, which was deemed unsuitable for patients, and two upper stories which could accommodate 520 patients with safety,[50] as well as a large number of attendants. (Figure 3.4). Quarters were available nearby for the medical staff.[51]

The hospital opened on 15 February 1855 and was staffed by military medical officers until replaced by civilians during the course of March. Six hospital transports sailed there from Balaklava between 3 and 16 February, and, although all called at Scutari to disembark the worst cases,[52] it soon became over crowded,[53] necessitating a request for additional accommodation in a nearby barrack and lazaretto.[54]

---

49   FO 195/456. Staff Surgeon Moorhead's report is reproduced in Smith, *Précis of Letters*, 1, Appendix III. The barrack building is depicted in *Illustrated London News*, 1855, I, p.472.
50   It was suggested that there would be 2,000 beds; *The Lancet*, 27 January 1855
51   Hospital Superintendent to Panmure, March and 14 April 1855; Reports on Hospitals in Turkey, pp.54–6.
52   These comprised *Adelaide* (173 men), *Emeu* (155), *Melbourne* (151), *Brandon* (120), *Medway* (196), and *Tynemouth* (301). Of these 11 died during the voyage across the Black Sea and 96 were disembarked at Scutari; *Medical and Surgical History*, 2, pp.469–470 & 479. Incidentally, Cumming, the PMO, pointed out to Smith on 28 April 1855 that the policy of disembarking the worst cases at Scutari would result in fewer patients dying at Smyrna; Reports on Hospitals in Turkey, p.46.
53   *Medical Times and Gazette*, 24 March 1855 based on information dated 3 March.
54   Paulet to Stratford, 21 February and Storks to Stratford, 1 March 1855; TNA: FO 195/452.

It was suggested before the hospital opened that, notwithstanding the shortage of medical staff, it should not be used solely for convalescents as these were relatively few patients compared to the number of sick needing treatment.[55] Initially there was a bias towards the less seriously ill, since during the first 2½ months to the end of April the ratio of deaths to admissions was 12 percent as compared to 28 percent in the Scutari hospitals.[56] Thereafter the ratio was much reduced to two percent,[57] thus confirming that Smyrna became a 'convalescent station', as was originally envisaged.[58] A sensible policy given that the long voyage from the Crimea 'should not be thought of' both for those in 'the trying state of a severe disease [or] severe surgical cases.'[59, 60]

Paulet visited Smyrna in June and told Raglan privately that 'a civil hospital [was in no way] advantageous; it is very expensive, and it certainly does not improve the discipline of our soldiers.' He continued by saying that both Smyrna and Abydos 'required many things doing for [the soldiers'] comfort' and 'we have comfortable accommodation for nearly 3,000 sick [at Scutari]' though he suggested that 'the distant hospitals should be kept in case of [increased demand, although it involved] a great deal of trouble when men are at a distance, and Smyrna lays quite out of the regular line of ships from and to England.'[61]

Incidentally, Panmure informed Paulet during March that the high summer temperatures at Smyrna may hinder recovery[62] and that this may account in part why there were no sailings from Balaklava after *Sydney* and *Brandon* departed at the end of April until *Severn* and *Imperador* left on 26 October 1855, although both called first at Scutari.[63] This would appear to be in response to an instruction from the Deputy Secretary since Hall informed Storks that: 'His Lordship's [Panmure] orders will be complied with, when the hospital ships now fitting are ready for the reception of sick but the distance of Smyrna and Renkioi is a drawback to their

---

55 Dr R. Lawson to Smith, 28 January 1855; Smith, *Précis of Letters*.
56 Enclosure of the cemetery with masonry for £93/-/12d was authorized; Panmure to Storks, 15 September1855; TNA: WO 6/71.
57 The principal causes death were diarrhoea or dysentery (67 cases), fever (38), frostbite (18), scurvy (14), and respiratory disease (11); *Medical and Surgical History*, 2, General Hospital Returns VIII.
58 For example, Herbert to Cumming, 5 January 1855; Wiltshire and Swindon Record Centre: 2057/F8/III/C/15.
59 *The Lancet*, 24 February 1855 and *Medical Times and Gazette*, 23 August 1855.
60 Dr Spencer Wells, a naval surgeon employed in a civilian capacity, noted in a letter dated 16 June 1855 that the 'length of the voyage from Balaklava to Constantinople is generally about thirty hours. It is about fourteen hours further to the hospitals on the Dardanelles, and another sixteen or eighteen hours to Smyrna'; *Medical Times and Gazette*, 30 June 1855.
61 Paulet to Raglan, 22 June 1855; TNA: WO 28/186.
62 Panmure to Paulet, 5 March 1855; TNA: WO 6/70. Incidentally, Nightingale considered it would be untenable within a month of her writing to Herbert on 26 March; McDonald, *Florence Nightingale*, p.172.
63 *Medical and Surgical History*, 2, p.479.

usefulness and if they are to be occupied an additional quantity of sick transport will be required.'[64]

Hall also suggested to Smith that the reasons the Deputy Secretary gave for sending patients to Smyrna 'would amuse you [...] It was not that they were requiring accommodation, but the expensive civil establishment employed by government might have occupation.'[65]

At the end of October Storks informed the QMG [Airey] that the Secretary of State's instructions had been put into effect and the transfer of 377 and 215 patients to Smyrna and Renkioi had resulted in 2,228 beds being available at Scutari.[66] Smith was subsequently informed of these developments,[67] and there the matter rested as the hospital closed at the end of the month and was handed over to the British Swiss Legion which was based in Smyrna from the beginning of December 1855 until the end of the war.

The development of the hospital at Smyrna was essentially a political initiative, first mooted quite reasonably when matters were pressing, and Newcastle, the minister at the time, seemingly intending that it should be used for convalescents.[68] His successor, Panmure, thought differently as he considered that the civilian medical staff should obtain worthwhile practical experience, particularly as they had become his responsibility following Smith's refusal to be involved on the grounds that it was a civilian and not a military undertaking.[69]

Panmure's aspirations for success resulted in a tendency for him to interfere in the day to day running of the Army; a style of management that was generally unwelcome. For example, Brevet Major G.L. Goodlake wrote home on 10 January 1856: 'Panmure sends out insulting rubbishing idiotic messages, which are ludicrous and ridiculous. I don't believe Codrington could send 500 men anywhere without being obliged to telegraph home to know if he might do so.'[70]

The Medical Department was not spared similar interference as evinced by a letter sent to Hall by the Deputy Secretary on 30 March, which suggested Panmure had adopted a policy diametrically opposed to the one promulgated during Aberdeen's administration:[71]

64　Hall to Storks, 9 October 1855; RAMC: 397/F/CO/1/2/3340. There is no despatch from Panmure on this matter in TNA: WO 6/71.
65　Hall to Smith, 10 November 1855; S.M. Mitra, *The Life and Letters*, pp.401–2. Hall suggested that the Deputy Secretary had intervened to avoid awkward questions in Parliament; though there is no record any were posed.
66　Storks to QMG, 30 October 1855; TNA: WO 28/186.
67　Undersecretary to Smith, 5 November 1855; Smith, *Précis of Letters*.
68　Diary entry following a visit, 13 July 1855; University of Nottingham, Ne/2F/10/1.
69　For example, Smith to Military Undersecretary, 23 Mar 1855; Royal Commission Report, Appendix LXXIX, p.45 and Smith to Deputy Secretary, 16 June 1855; Smith, *Précis of Letters*.
70　M. Springman, *Sharpshooter in the Crimea* (Barnsley: Pen & Sword Military, 2005), p.166.
71　TNA: WO 28/176. The letter was probably a response to a complaint from Meyer, the medical superintendent, who 'considered it essential' that they should receive a 'fair

[In] organizing the civil hospital at Smyrna it was expressly stated that the successful realization of the plan will very much depend upon the class of patients to be admitted. If the hospital were [...] for chronic cases and convalescents the best men would be deterred from undertaking the duties of physicians and surgeons. [It is] essential that the civil hospital should [...] receive its fair proportion of all cases including wounded directly from the Army. [...] Lord Panmure [instructs] you to charter ships direct to Smyrna which will carry the sick thither without [stopping] in the Bosphorus,[72] [...] Colonel Storks, the commandant at Smyrna, has been instructed to report to you the number of available beds from time to time.[73]

Hall forwarded the letter to the QMG and informed him that he had been directed to charter ships to convey sick direct from the Crimea to Smyrna. He continued: 'at present we are not particularly pressed for hospital accommodation,[74] but if we were I neither know the number of beds they have in the hospital at Smyrna, nor if I did could I obtain the tonnage for the sick. I submit this letter, therefore, for consideration in case a necessity should arise for sending sick down to Smyrna.'[75]

Heath, the AoT, also pointed out that 'the vessels would have to be steamers of which there are none at present available for charter in this part of the world.' He continued:

Between 1 and 18 April about 600 sick have been sent [...] to Scutari.[76] The six hospital steamers can convey rather more than 700 in each 10 consecutive daily period;[77] [...] as every individual sent to Smyrna will be a deduction from the number for Scutari [...] I would propose that [...] the two smaller steamers should be appropriate to that service. There would then remain sufficient transport for 500 patients every ten days to Scutari [and] about 100 men a week could be sent to Smyrna.[78]

  proportion of all cases included wounded directly from the Army;' see Cantlie, *A History*, 2, p.169.
72 Hall's authority did not extend to chartering transport vessels, and hence it is perplexing why this was suggested.
73 The last paragraph on the original document was marked in pencil in the margin: '!!!'. See Smith, *Précis of Letters*, 1, Appendix XV for the text.
74 It should have known in London by the third week of March that 1,300 beds were available at Scutari; Paulet to Panmure, 8 March 1855; Reports on Hospitals in Turkey, p.1. Incidentally, on 13 May Cumming informed Hall that there were 1,900 beds spare; National Army Museum: 2007-07-16-27.
75 Hall to QMG, 15 April 1855; RAMC: 397/F/CO/1/2/1839 and TNA: WO 28/176.
76 During this period *Sydney* (98 patients), *Brandon* (111), *Ottawa* (120), and *Severn* (180) sailed to Scutari; *Medical and Surgical History*, 2, p.471.
77 These vessels comprised *Australian, Brandon, Melbourne, Ottawa, Severn,* and *Sydney*; Smith, *Précis of Letters*, 1, Appendix XV.
78 Heath to QMG, 19 April 1855; TNA: WO 28/176.

Heath's letter was referred to Hall who reiterated that he 'did not know what number of spare beds there are at Smyrna, and he would not wish to recommend sick men to be sent there until this was ascertained.' He clearly considered the policy was unnecessary as there were '747 spare beds at Scutari.'[79] Hall subsequently replied to the Deputy Secretary on 24 April and informed him that he was not:

> aware that the Smyrna Hospital had been established for the treatment of acute cases of disease, as it is rather too distant [...] for that purpose, [...] my impression was that it was [for] those [...] not improving. [...] I am of the opinion Smyrna will not be found a desirable locality either for fever cases or wounded men in the summer and autumn. With respect [to] me chartering ships for the conveyance of the sick direct from Balaklava to Smyrna [...] I have no means of carrying out the measures [as all ships are controlled by] the Admiral Superintendent.[80]

The authorities in the Crimea responded in a limited manner to Panmure's wishes by sending *Brandon* and *Severn* to Smyrna on the 26 and 29 April with 99 and 97 patients respectively.[81]

When Smith received copies of this correspondence he informed the Deputy Secretary that ordering ships for Smyrna not to stop on the Bosphorus was 'most objectionable' as if done regularly 'individuals will have to encounter [...] suffering which would not fall their lot if the vessels touch at Scutari [...] This measure [...] is alike required for the cause of humanity and for the good of the public,' although he did concede that the hospital should not be solely for 'slight or chronic cases.'[82]

The issue did not end there, however, because a month later the Deputy Secretary requested Smith 'to give an opinion whether the ships should stop at Scutari while quarantine laws still operate and as the hospital arrangements at Balaklava are now intended to provide for all acute and urgent cases and so it would seem less necessary for the vessels to stop at Scutari where probably only convalescents will be sent.'[83]

---

79 Hall to QMG, 20 April 1855; TNA: WO 28/176. Cantlie, *A History*, 2, p.170 considered that Hall's logic 'was unanswerable' but Meyer was 'annoyed, and made the invidious suggestion that Smyrna was not used because the Army medical officers were envious of its high standard compared with their own military hospitals.'

80 Hall to Deputy Secretary, 24 April 1855; RAMC: 397/F/CO/1/2/1832 and Smith, *Précis of Letters*, 1, Appendix XV. The back of the Deputy Secretary's letter was annotated by the QMG 'Refer this correspondence to Dr Hall, who will now have the means of reply to the Deputy Secretary for War.'

81 Hall to Deputy Secretary, 4 May 1855; RAMC: 397/F/CO/1/2/1832. It was not recorded whether the vessels called at Scutari or not.

82 Smith to Deputy Secretary, 5 May 1855; Smith, *Précis of Letters* and Royal Commission Report, Appendix LXXIX, pp.52–3. Incidentally, Smith had already recommended to the Deputy Secretary on 23 May that vessels for Smyrna should touch at Scutari; Smith, *Précis of Letters*.

83 Deputy Secretary to Smith, 6 June 1855; Smith, *Précis of Letters*.

To this Smith stated that he was unaware that vessels touching at Scutari would be subject to quarantine at Smyrna, but he thought that 'even that would be a less evil than passing Scutari without calling there.'[84]

Shortly after the war ended the Deputy Secretary appeared to do a U-turn when he conceded that though the selection of the patients for the civil hospital was in 'the hands of the medical men' in the Crimea 'special direction had been given on the type of patient selected' but the 'altered state of things that ensued quite prevented that being acted upon, and the large extension of hospital accommodation in the Crimea has prevented so a large a number being sent to either of the civil hospitals as was originally contemplated,'[85] thus vindicating Hall's objection to the instructions from London which he made on both practical and humane grounds

There is no assessment of the hospital at Smyrna in the *Medical and Surgical History* though contemporary accounts were published, one by a physician and another by a lady nurse.[86]

3.1.4 Renkioi

The decision to construct a prefabricated hospital designed by I.K. Brunel was taken in London during February 1855. Dr E. Parkes, the nominated civilian superintendent, was informed that it was Panmure's wish that he should be wholly 'responsible for the efficiency of the hospital [...] to be established on the shores of the Bosphorus [at] a site chosen by you,' after taking into account the information collected by Paulet.[87] No evidence has been found that Raglan and Hall heard of this plan officially though Hall assured Parkes of his support on 23 April: 'If there is anything I can do to assist you, or forward the object you are sent out to accomplish, I shall be very happy, and you may command my services.'[88] Hall wrote again to Parkes a few months later and made the following, frank, but not unfriendly comment: 'I regret its distance from us will militate against your usefulness, but with my good wish for the success of your undertaking.'[89, 90]

Parkes failed to find a suitable site on the Bosphorus and decided on Renkioi, apparently on the recommendation of the Consul on the Dardanelles.[91] The first prefabricated components arrived on 17 May and by 14 July, when Newcastle passed

---

84 Smith to Deputy Secretary, 11 June 1855; Smith, *Précis of Letters*.
85 Paraphrased from the Deputy Secretary's evidence to the Select Committee on the Army Medical Department, 18 June 1856; *Select Committee on the Medical Department*.
86 HCPP 1857 Session 1 (0.51) IX.673: *Report on Smyrna by George Rolleston, Late Assistant Physician to the British Civil Hospital at Smyrna* and A Lady [Martha Nicol], *Ismeer, or Smyrna and its British Hospital in 1855* (London: James Madden, 1856).
87 War Office to Parkes, 4 April 1855; TNA: WO 43/991.
88 Hall to Parkes, 23 April 1855; RAMC: 397/F/CO/1/1/1894.
89 Hall to Parkes, 13 August 1855; RAMC: 397/F/CO/1/2/2925.
90 For accounts see Toppin, 'British Hospital' and Silver, *Renkioi*; and TNA: WO 43/99 for contemporary letters and reports.
91 *Select Committee on Consular Services*, pp.22.

by, it was ready for 300 patients, although the design was for 3,000. The number had increased to 500 by mid-August at which time Panmure made it clear that the hospital should not receive Sardinian patients but should be 'kept as a reserve for the sick and wounded of the British Army.' He also recommended that patients should be sent there from Scutari, even if there was surplus accommodation, as this would keep the 'establishment in working order and so prepare it for the heavier labours which may be anticipated in the ensuing winter.'[92] Neither suggestion was unreasonable given that the siege was still in progress, although it was October before the first of 1,300 admitted during the first five months of operation arrived. Thereafter only 30 new patients arrived before the hospital closed at the end of June 1856 (Figure 3.5).

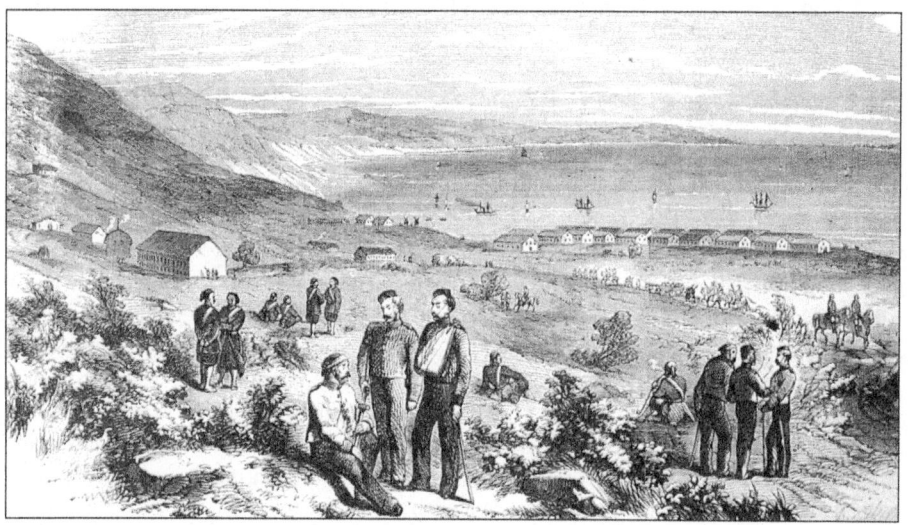

Figure 3.5 The British hospital at Renkioi. (*Illustrated Times*, 1 December 1855, p.412)[93]

Newcastle considered locating a hospital at Renkioi was a 'very questionable experiment [as] its distance from any town of any importance almost fatal for a hospital of such magnitude.' He considered that its 'only special advantage is an abundant supply of good water' and that the whole 'affair looks to me like a crochet. [...] I am sure it will be expensive;' and on this Hall agreed when he wrote after the war:

> The personal pay of the medical and purveying departments amounted to 15,378*l*., and of the whole establishment to 24,930*l*. per annum, exclusive of

---

92 Panmure to Storks, 25 August 1855; TNA: FO 6/71.
93 The hospital received patients by sea on ten occasions between 2 October 1855 and 10 February 1856; *Medical and Surgical History*, 2, p.480.

the pay of the military staff, the diets and store expenses of the patients to say nothing of the heavy expense of erecting this magnificent establishment, which was placed at too great a distance from the seat of active operations to be of much use to the Army; and this defect was pointed out from the very first.[94]

Bryce, a civilian surgeon, visited the hospital and was impressed though made the point that it had never had the chance to prove its worth: 'save for humanity sake one could have wished that the requirements of the service had fairly tested the merits of the *civil* hospital [where] nothing which high professional sagacity could devise, and engineering skill accomplish, was left undone to make the establishment perfect of its kind.'[95] There was no assessment of the hospital in the *Medical and Surgical History* though after the war Parkes published and account of its operation.[96]

3.1.5 French hospitals
Bryce also visited the French hospitals on the Bosphorus during the spring of 1856 and found that 'The first general view of the *Hôpital de Pera* disappoints and grieves the visitor' and 'in a medical sense, the state of the individual sick was very bad – that is, the prognosis was against recovery', and hence in complete contrast to what obtained in the British hospitals.[97]

3.2 Bulgaria

In early June 1854 Dr Dumbreck reported that the building selected for the General Hospital in Varna was in a 'defective condition' and 'overrun with vermin' and that he was 'at a loss to know in what manner provision could be made for the treatment of the sick unless something is done to mitigate the serious objections [...] referred to.'[98] Some days later he submitted suggestions for improvements in the ventilation, drainage, storage, and warming the hospital to Brigadier W.B. Tylden, RE.[99] 2nd Class Staff Surgeon T.P. Matthew, supported Dumbreck concerns with respect to the state of dilapidation, want of ventilation, drainage, and facilities for surgery, cooking etc. and he also stressed the need for hospital orderlies.[100] Matters appeared to have

---

94 Hall, *Observations*. There is a marginal note in the draft version: 'Each patient cost for medical attendance £18/14/10d.'
95 Bryce, *England and France before Sebastopol*, p.22.
96 Parkes, *Renkioi Hospital*.
97 Bryce, *England and France before Sebastopol*, pp.40–73.
98 Dumbreck to General Brown, 6 June 1854; Royal Commission Report, Appendix LXXIX, p.260. See also *Medical and Surgical History*, 2, p.9 for a description of the building.
99 Dumbreck to Tylden, 16, June 1854; Royal Commission Report, Appendix LXXIX, pp.260–1.
100 Matthew to Hall, 19 June 1854; Royal Commission Report, Appendix LXXIX, p.190.

improved to an extent as Dumbreck was able to report that the 'General Hospital is fairly well established but pressed for room, as only part is fit for patients. [...] The sick are well cared for, and want for nothing. [but] he hears nothing of the Ambulances and the Hospital Corps; both very much required [...] as medical officers suffer very much from want of domestic aid,[101] while a General Order dated 4 July 1854 required the 3rd Division to provide orderlies and attendants in the hospital.

The lengthening sick list put pressure on the regimental and general hospitals and Hall informed Smith that Raglan had authorized the use of a transport ship to accommodate 110 patients;[102] while a memorandum issues by Dr W. Linton, the PMO of the 1st Division, recommended discharging patients who can either attend daily or do light duty in order to relieve space in the hospital.[103]

At the end of August the General Hospital had 350 beds while 'light cases' and convalescents were encamped at the south side of Varna bay,[104] while nearly two weeks before the invasion Hall informed the PMO, Scutari that *'Bombay* and *Mercia* will bring 400 and 250 convalescents.'[105] He continued: 'We have had an enormous number of sick thrown on our hands [...] and have been much pressed to provide for them' and by pointing out that Raglan wished to 'gradually get the sick away' and 'they will be sent down when [...] convalescent, and opportunities for transport present.'[106]

When the Army left Bulgaria for the Crimea the military authorities seemingly acted irresponsibly with respect the sick personnel that necessitated Hall to report to Smith that:

> It would scarcely be credited that the first intimation I had of the march [of troops] into Varna was the deposit of their sick by the hundred in the hospital square of that place. No adequate provision had been made for their reception, nor could it be done in a moment. The divisions [...] literally left their sick [...] on the beach [...] and I had to form two encampments [...] in addition to the General Hospital, for the accommodation of about 2,000 sick that were left behind.[107]

The General Hospital was operational from June–November 1854 and an Invalid Depot from August 1854–January 1855. The number of patients treated in these

---

101 Dumbreck to Smith, 23 June 1854; Smith, *Précis of Letters*.
102 Hall to Smith, 24 July 1854; RAMC: 397/F/CO/1/1/397.
103 Royal Commission Report, Appendix LXXIX, p.154.
104 Hall to Smith, 29 August 1854; RAMC: 397/F/CO/1/1/665.
105 Hall to Smith, 4 September 1854; Smith, *Précis of Letters*. Hall estimated that about 2,000 sick remained in Bulgaria.
106 Hall to PMO, Scutari, 2 September1854; RAMC: 397/F/CO/1/1/682. Incidentally, Cantlie, *A History*, 2, p.42 implied incorrectly that Hall ordered these vessels to Scutari; it was the Royal Navy that controlled the movement of transport vessels.
107 Hall to Smith, Confidential letter, 20 November 1854.

establishments were 1,914 and 927 respectively of whom 282 (15 percent) and 92 (10 percent) died. Cholera had been diagnosed in the British Army in June and 197 cases were admitted to the General Hospital of whom 148 (75 percent) died.

On 13 October Hall requested that the patients remaining in Bulgaria should be sent to the hospital in Abydos 'if a ship could be despatched to Varna at an early opportunity, the interests of the Public Service would be promoted.'[108] This objective was not achieved until some months later when the hospital at Abydos opened in December.

3.3 Crimea

Hall landed at Calamita Bay on 17 September and Cantlie pointed out that he:

> Must have felt desperately worried at the medical arrangements. The lack of transport dominated everything. It was a hazardous policy for an army to enter a hostile country in the face of an enemy of unknown strength without the means of transporting its own food and equipment. [...] the Commander-in-Chief now made a decision which dealt the medical arrangements a devastating, nay, a mortal blow. No Regimental hospital equipment of any kind was to be allowed, and the surgeons had to depend on one bell tent for use as an aid post, a pair of panniers, and a small box of medical comforts. [...] that the Army on Lord Raglan's deliberate orders, took the field without a single hospital bed. And this at a time when cholera was hourly claiming its victims! This calculated neglect must have sealed the fate of many.[109]

It might have been desirable if Hall had organized a general hospital near the shore after the battle of the Alma but Cantlie concluded that in the circumstances: 'he had little alternative but to evacuate the sick and wounded without delay,'[110] prior to the Army marching south towards Sevastopol.

Hall's medical strategy in the first instance was to 'Treat the sick and wounded as far as possible in the Regimental hospitals; to open a General hospital at Balaklava for the overflow; and to evacuate the surplus to the base hospitals at Scutari.' However, the commanding officers of regiments were unable to set up hospitals for their men until the Army became stationary and this objective was hampered further because the 'Regimental medical officers do not know what had become of their stores,' while Hall's intention of opening a general hospital at Balaklava was hindered by the difficulty of finding a building large enough.[111]

---

108 Hall to Boxer, 13 October 1854; RAMC: 397/F/CO/1/2/791.
109 Cantlie, *A History*, 2, p.47–8.
110 Cantlie, *A History*, 2, p.55.
111 Cantlie, *A History*, 2, pp.66–7.

Inadequate living accommodation in the months following the invasion had serious repercussions for both the sick and well and, particularly as preference was given initially to accommodating horses and mules undercover rather than the sick, a policy understandably deprecated by Hall.[112] Nevertheless facilities did develop in the Crimea as the campaign progressed and this meant that those wounded in action and seriously ill patients, as well as convalescents and 'light cases', such as ophthalmia, could be cared for locally and were thus spared the 'evils of the voyage to Scutari, or the longer passages to Abydos and Smyrna.'[113]

3.3.1 General hospitals
Balaklava General Hospital: The first of the general hospitals opened on 27 September 1854 in a former school and it soon proved too small to accommodate sufficient beds.[114] In due course capacity was increased using marquees, and later by constructing wooden huts. (Figure 3.6) The slow progress frustrated Hall who wrote the following to the QMG on 7 December 1854:

> I [...] call attention to the want of hospital accommodation in Balaklava and the unfinished state of the new building at the General Hospital. [...] It is of the most vital importance to obtain better cover for the sick in camp [because] medical treatment is in a great measure counteracted by the dampness exposure they are subjected to in the wet weather, as the bell tents, in which many of them are necessarily placed for want of hospital marquees, are thin and the rain beats thro' them.[115]

Inevitable there was some rearrangement in hospital accommodation from time to time which probably went unrecorded in formal documents, for example, Hall informed Smith in a private letter dated 19 March 1855 that he was: 'endeavouring to make arrangements for the accommodation of the wounded and I shall get some spare huts near Balaklava, lately occupied by the 39th Regt, to put the Croats and sailors into, who are now accommodated in the General Hospital and that will give us four extra huts for the troops.'[116]

Spencer Wells, a civilian surgeon, visited the Crimea during June 1855 and noted that the hospital comprised: 'an old stone house with tiled roof, and wooden huts' but

---

112 QMG to CRE, 25 November 1854; TNA: WO 28/196 and Hall, diary entry, 1 December 1854; RAMC: 524/15.
113 News item, 2 April; *The Times*, 18 April 1855.
114 For a description of the premises and its short comings see Hospital Commission Report, p.44.
115 Hall to QMG, 7 December 1854; RAMC: 397/F/CO/1/2/1046; TNA: WO 28/196; and the Supplies Commission Report, Appendix, p.162. Hall wrote again on the same topic on 19 December 1854; RAMC: 397/F/CO/1/2/1183.
116 Wellcome Library: MS 8520, ff.307–10.

he considered that it was 'very badly situated, near the head of the harbour, some 40 or 50 feet above the sea-level.'[117] Nevertheless, conditions were improved with time so that between October 1855 and the final evacuation of the Crimea there were 27 (two percent) deaths amongst 1,363 patients admitted.

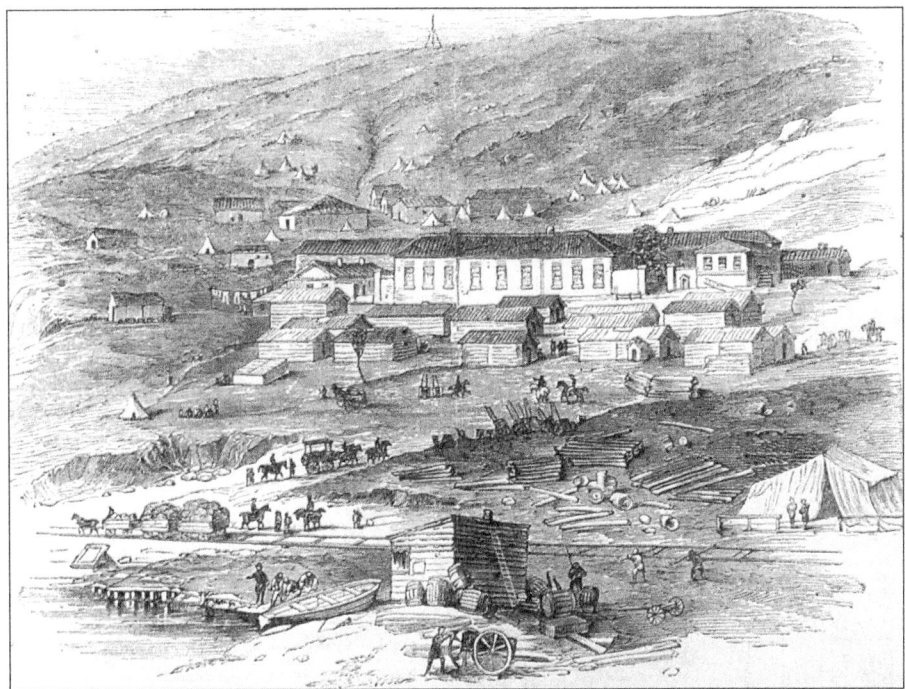

Figure 3.6 Hospital and the quarters of the medical staff, Balaclava harbour. (From a sketch by Julian Portch, *Illustrated Times*, 11 August 1855, p.149)

Castle General Hospital: The hutted hospital was 'situated above the town of Balaklava, at a height of 300 feet above the sea,' but, as Spencer Wells pointed out: 'The access is very difficult. Wounded men have to be carried up a very steep, rugged path, on one side of a ravine.' (Figures 3.7, 3.8, and J) The hospital eventually comprised 28 huts with 590 beds though the maximum number occupied was 348 with an average occupancy of 310.[118] It opened on 3 March 1855 and when it closed on 30 June 1856 2,554 patients had been admitted of whom 96 (3.75 percent) died.

---

117 T. Spencer Wells to editor, 16 June 1855; *Medical Times and Gazette*, 30 June 1855, pp.648–50.
118 For a description of the hospital see *Medical and Surgical History*, 2, pp.255–6.

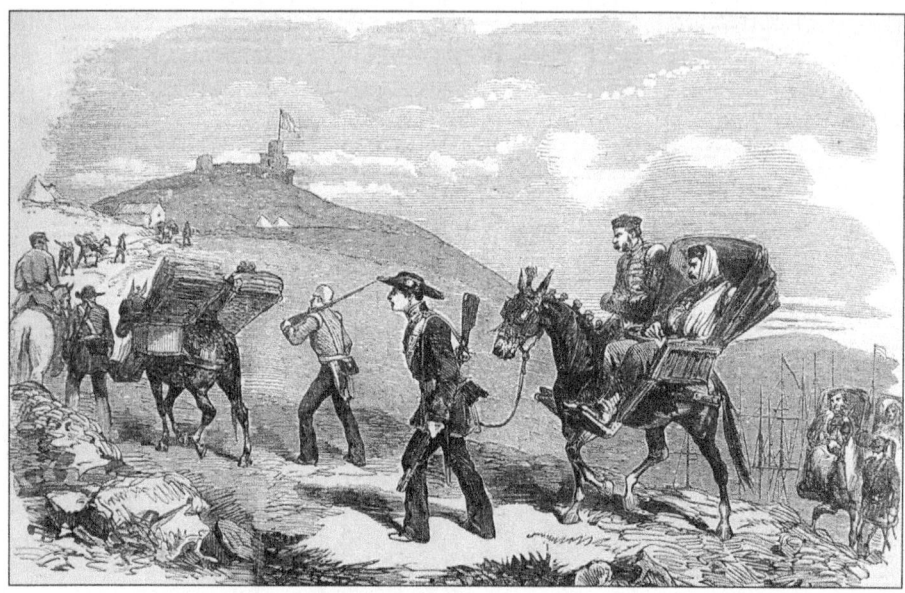

Figure 3.7 New ambulance transport service. (*Illustrated London News*, 4 August 1855, p.156)

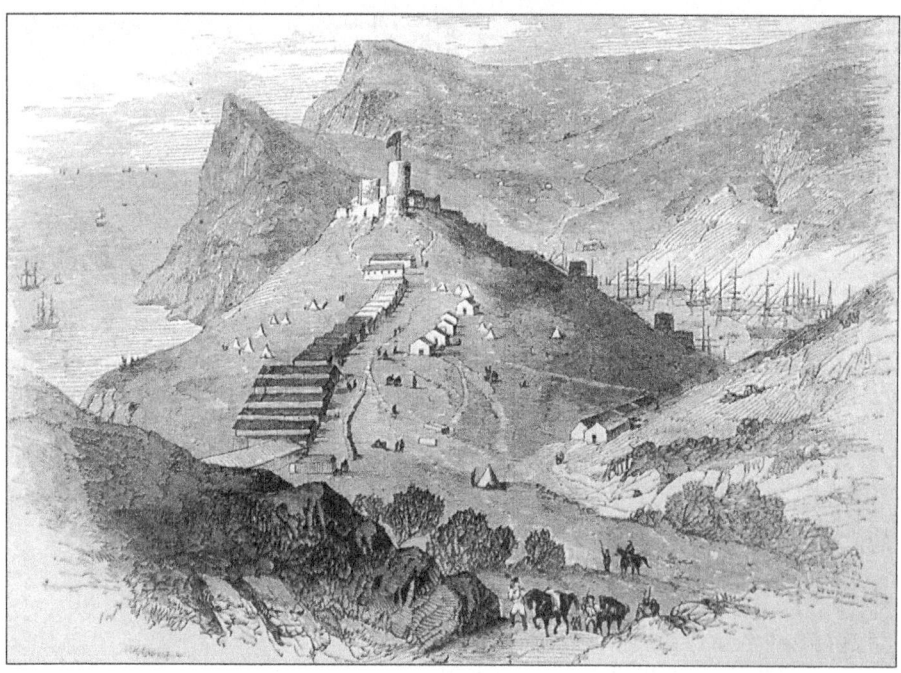

Figure 3.8 The new sanatorium, or Castle Hospital, at Balaclava. (From a sketch by Julian Portch, *Illustrated Times*, 11 August 1855)

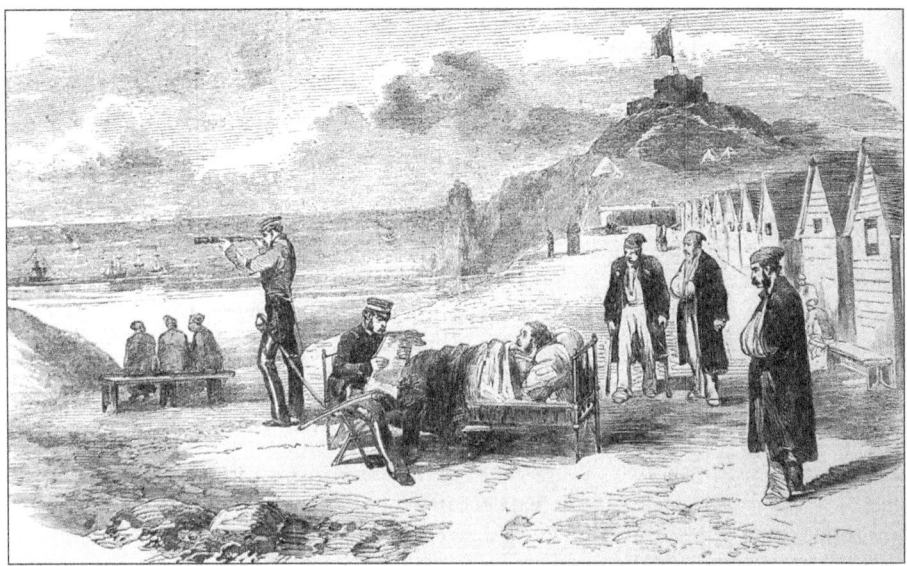

Figure 3.9 The new Castle Hospital at Balaclava. (*Illustrated London News*, 28 July 1855)

It was anticipated that wounded men would recover better in the Castle Hospital than at Scutari,[119] and though Hall had to complain about the slowness of its construction,[120] Russell noted within a few weeks of it opening that it was 'becoming a great curative establishment, and promises to afford great benefits to our sick and wounded men.'[121] Men with disease were admitted during the first month but the policy changed in early April and between then and the end of October wounded soldiers accounted for 1,805 (92 percent) of 1,966 admissions, of whom 80 (4.5 percent) died, as compared with 25 percent in the Camp General Hospital which received casualties direct from the front. Thereafter, men with disease predominated and provided 317 (93 percent) of 340 admissions. None of these died which suggests the hospital continued to be used for convalescents, as originally intended.[122]

Camp General Hospital: The hospital was closest to the front and it was 'almost entirely surrounded by camps'; though in this respect it 'was no worse off than the regimental hospitals.' It opened on 1 April 1855 and made use of accommodation previously been used to house soldiers. It comprised 'at first 22, and afterwards 26 huts with a total capacity of 365 patients.' In all 1,083 patients were treated before it closed

119 Hall to Smith, 10 March 1855; RAMC: 397/F/CO/1/2/1605 and Smith, *Précis of Letters*.
120 Hall to QMG, 27 March 1855; RAMC: 397/F/CO/1/2/1716 and Royal Commission Report, Appendix LXXIX, p.120.
121 Despatch, 2 April, *The Times*, 18 April 1855.
122 *Medical and Surgical History*, 2, General Hospital Returns IV.

13 months later; of these 730 (67 percent) were from gunshot wounds, of whom 184 (25 percent) died.[123]

Monastery General Hospital: Cossack Bay, near the entrance to Balaklava harbour, was inspected in March 1855 as a potential site for a convalescent hospital. Hall, however, recommended expansion at the Castle as it was a good site with an abundant supply of water and it would 'economise our resources'.[124] The need for additional hospital accommodation was considered further the next month when Hall expressed his preference for 'uncontaminated sites' such as the plateau to the west of the entrance of Balaklava harbour or the neighbourhood of the Monastery,[125] which was eventually chosen. Cossack Bay was reconsidered in May, and Hall pointed out that landing would be difficult if a southerly wind caused a swell, though he conceded that there would be less trouble in transporting stores there than to the Monastery.[126] The Monastery, which opened on 21 July 1855, never became a convalescent hospital in the strict sense although during the first five months from July 1855 the ratio of deaths to admissions was 25 (five percent):508 suggesting a selection in favour of the less seriously ill. After this time the policy changed and ophthalmia accounted for a nearly three-quarters of the admissions although there were three deaths among the other 107 patients.[127]

Balaklava Harbour: Officers went on board ship in the harbour for the 'recruitment of the health' but it was not until the summer of 1855 that Panmure desired 'that arrangements should be made with the naval authorities that [...] accommodation may be prepared on board ship [...] as floating hospitals for 500 to 600 men.' The Port Admiral was requested to 'name vessels for this service,' and to take care that sufficient room was allowed between cots for medical officers to attend the patients. Several vessels were fitted up within a few days despite a shortage of carpenters, and provided for 921 patients, together with 426 additional beds in the hospitals.[128] It has not been established how much use was made of these vessels though some were later employed on the shuttle service to Turkey (see Section 4.2.4).

---

123 For a description of the hospital including the means of refuse disposal and water supply see *Medical and Surgical History*, 2, p.255.
124 Hall to QMG, 7 March 1855; RAMC: 397/F/CO/1/2/1591 and Royal Commission Report, Appendix LXXIX, p.117.
125 Hall to QMG, 25 April 1855; 1855; RAMC: 397/F/CO/1/2/1923, RAMC: 397/M1/15, and Royal Commission Report, Appendix LXXIX, p.121.
126 Hall to QMG, 5 May 1855; RAMC: 397/F/CO/1/2/2008.
127 *Medical and Surgical History*, 2, General Hospital Returns VI.
128 QMG to Admiral Lyons, 30 March; QMG to Boxer, 30 March & 1 April; DAQMG to QMG, 4 April, and AQMG to QMG, 10 April 1855; TNA: WO 28/192. The vessels included *Ottawa* (100 berths), *Severn* (140), *Australian* (100 if not full of platforms), *St Hilda* (91), *Wm Jackson* (110), *Orient* (110), *Robert Lowe* (100), *Poietiers* (100), HMS *Leander* (50), HMS *Wasp* (20), and *Ottawa* (100).

Naval General Hospitals: There was a general hospital on the marine heights about 100 feet above the Castle hospital and another on the other side of Balaklava harbour which was erected in May 1855 to replace HMS *Diamond* that had been moored in harbour and used when the Naval Brigade commenced serving ashore. Patients requiring longer periods of convalescence were sent to a naval hospital on the European side of the Bosphorus at Therapia (see Figure 3.10).[129]

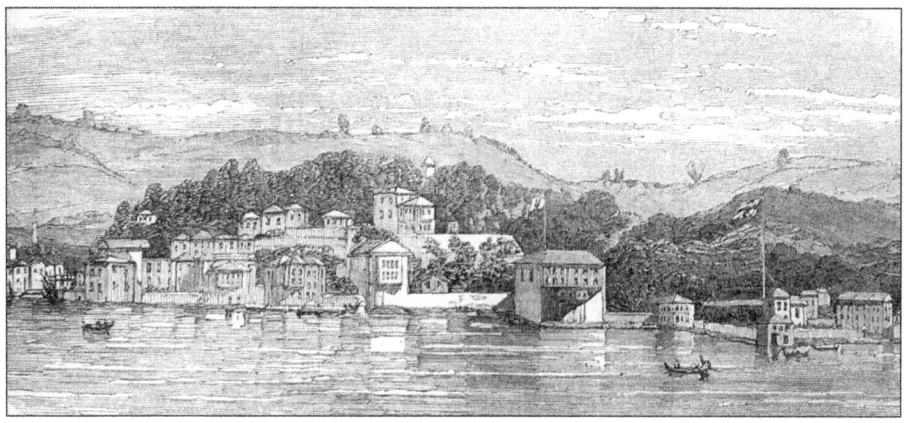

Figure 3.10 Therapia, sketched from the Asiatic bank of the Bosphorus. (*Illustrated London News*, 6 August 1853, p.97)

3.3.2 Regimental and divisional hospitals

Each cavalry and infantry regiment had a complement of surgeons and assistant surgeons and it was the responsibility of the Commanding Officer to provide hospital facilities for the troops, at least when the regiment was stationary. Following the invasion of the Crimea these hospitals were housed in bell tents and marquees and initially conditions could be extremely unsatisfactory for both the patients and the medical staff, while the facilities available for preparing food were frequently inadequate.

Hall was anxious that the first available huts should be used for hospital accommodation and towards the end of December 1854 a few had been erected, and by the middle of March the difficulties encountered in regimental hospitals had been largely overcome and the 'more seriously ill were being retained in regimental hospitals instead of being evacuated to Scutari,'[130] though the extent of provision for the well proved more variable.[131] The regimental facilities were supported by the provision of

---

129 For a comprehensive account of this hospital see R. Huntsman, M. Bruin, and D. Holttum, 'The Naval Hospital at Therapia', *Journal of the Royal Naval Medical Service*, 88:1 (2002),.pp.5–27.
130 Shepherd, *Crimean Doctors*, 1, p.295.
131 Supplies Commission Report, pp.38 & 284–8.

divisional or brigade hospitals managed by medical staff officers (Figure 3.11). With time the number of available beds in the regimental and divisional hospitals, and the various general hospitals in the Crimea, increased to 2,000–2,500, and as medical admissions declined during 1855 the number of available beds increased and there was capacity to cope with nearly all eventualities.[132]

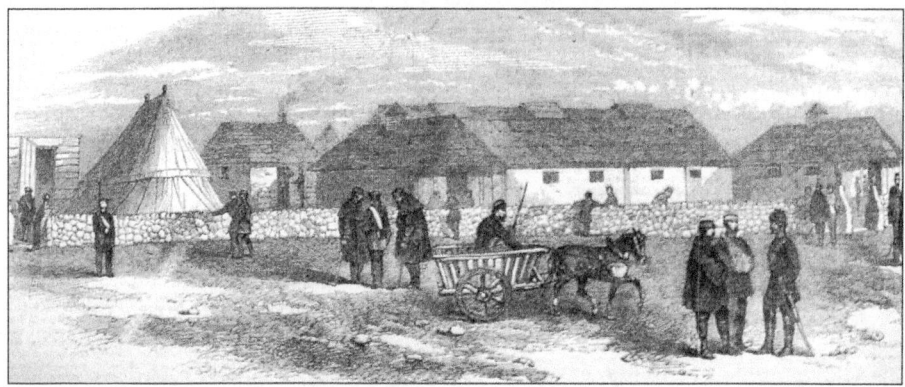

Figure 3.11 Brigade hospital of the Light Division. (From a sketch by Julian Portch, *Illustrated Times*, 12 July 1856, p.4)

Convalescing in camp: When in Bulgaria the PMO of the 1st Division recommended that following discharge from hospital patients could be treated as out-patients or do light duty in camp, and it is probable that this practical policy was adopted by other divisions.[133] For example, in the Coldstream Guards camp 'One tent per company was apportioned [in January 1855] for the use of convalescents [...] usually men recently dismissed from hospital with trivial affections (*sic*: afflictions) [...] it was often thought desirable to afford such men [...] a few days rest from the unceasing toil [...]'[134]

When the railway became operational it was used to convey convalescents from Balaklava to the camps while there are other references to convalescents working in hospitals and even some on constructional work, although some of those 'attending at stables' in hot weather often 're-appeared on the sick list.'[135]

3.3.3 Provision for battlefield casualties

Spencer Wells reported that medical officers together with an orderly who 'carried such instruments and necessaries as may be immediately required' were on duty in

---

132 Shepherd, *Crimean Doctors*, 2, pp.469–70.
133 Memorandum, 2 August 854; Royal Commission Report, Appendix LXXIX, p.154.
134 *Medical and Surgical History*, 1, p.113.
135 AG to Sir Colin Campbell, 3 April 1855; TNA: WO 28/108 and *Medical and Surgical History*, 2, p.136.

the trenches for up to 24 hours. In each 'battery in the first parallel, a sort of hut, in a tolerably sheltered spot, is used as a surgery.' The men are then transferred to the rear once any emergency first aid has been completed, a distance of at least a mile. The French, on the other hand, had advance field hospitals where primary operations could be performed and he commented that most 'medical men seemed to think this plan better than ours.'[136]

In anticipation of the assault on Sevastopol on the 18 June 1855 Hall issued a Medical Department Memorandum outlining plans for the care of the wounded in advanced dressing stations, or 'Temporary Field Hospital,'[137] the Camp General Hospital and Regimental hospitals, viz:

> (1) Regimental hospitals should be in a perfect state of readiness for the reception of wounded; (2) A medical officer of each regiment engaged will follow the column and staff surgeon of Division should be present to give directions. [...] They will see that prompt aid is afforded to the wounded when, required, and get them carried off by the Croats and Ambulance to the hospitals in rear as soon as possible. All the medical officers of the Divisions will be on duty; and as many as can be spared from the Cavalry Division and Balaklava, will repair to the front; (3) Superintending officers will make arrangements for forming temporary field-hospitals in the ravines, as near to the scene of action as safety will admit. Here those cases that require immediate operation will be attended to, and then sent either to their own regimental hospitals, or to the general hospital in the rear of the Third Division. [...] care must be taken that there is an ample supply of water, stimulants, and surgical appliances.[138]

On the day before the second assault on Sevastopol, Hall issued a Medical Department Order that required the medical officers of all Divisions to be on duty while one medical officer of each regiment engaged was to follow the men into the trenches and a staff surgeon was to take direction of the right and left attack. Advanced dressing stations for the wounded were provided in piquet house ravine and the ravine in front of the 4th Division where those requiring immediate treatment could be attended to while 'ambulance wagons and mules carrying litters and chairs performed the service of transporting those who could not walk with wonderful rapidity' to the divisional and regimental hospitals in camp. These had a capacity of 1,294 beds. In addition, there were three fully equipped hospital transports located in the harbour, viz. the *Severn* (120 berths), *Poietiers* (100) and *Imperador* (120).[139]

---

136 *Medical Times and Gazette*, 30 June 1855, pp.648–50.
137 See Shepherd, *Crimean Doctors*, 2, pp.470–1 for the experiences of Assistant Surgeon J. Cowan, 55th Regiment, in a 'Temporary Field Hospital' on 8 September 1855.
138 Reproduced in *The Lancet*, 28 July 1855.
139 Shepherd, *Crimean Doctors*, 2, p.471 and Smith, *Précis of Letters*, 2, p.108 & Appendix 8, p.588.

3.3.4 Preparations for the second winter

Some weeks before the second assault on Sevastopol Hall reported to the Smith that: (1) with the exception of the Cavalry Division at Kadikoi, which is close to Balaklava, each Division has a reserve store of medicines, materials and medical comforts; (2) there has been no want of water and there is nothing to apprehend in that there has been some rain; (3) application has been made to repair all present huts, viz. 170 hospital huts, 122 store huts, and 80 officers' huts; (4) every precaution has been made to provide for the approaching winter. Several regiments have their medicine chests with them in camp; (5) hospitals have covered kitchens, mostly built of stone. Latrines with paved pathways are in the course of erection and every precaution is being made to provide for the approaching winter; (6) the regimental hospitals have the appearance of hospitals in fixed quarters with iron bedsteads, bedding etc. These would be difficult to move if this had to be done in a hurry.[140]

Towards the end of November 1855 the GOC, Light Division, stressed: 'the necessity of giving every assistance possible to ensure the immediate repairs necessary for rendering the regimental hospitals as complete as circumstances will admit; he expects no exertions will be spared to secure this object before the rigour of winter sets in. Lord William Paulet will occasionally make an inspection of the regimental hospitals.'[141]

3.4 Mediterranean ports

The British Army maintained a number of garrisons in the Mediterranean and these provided scope for accommodating convalescents. Malta was an obvious place for this and also for disembarking invalids too ill to proceed to England, for example, patients with sloughing wounds on *Talavera* and *Sultana*.[142]

The medical facilities on the island were poorly developed in the summer of 1854 as there were only 120–150 beds for the sick;[143] and they probably remained in a rudimentary state during the campaign since Captain Galton and Dr Sutherland reported in 1861 that there was no single good military hospital on the island.[144] Nevertheless, by October, Hall felt able to 'apply officially for lighter cases of disease to be sent to Malta, rather then England', although the proposal had to be 'put [...] in official shape

---

140 Hall to Smith, 7 September 1855; RAMC: 397/F/CO/1/2/3091 and Smith, *Précis of Letters*.
141 TNA: WO 28/90.
142 PMO, Malta to Smith, 9 January 1855; Smith, *Précis of Letters*. Sloughing is the shedding of dead tissue.
143 PMO, Malta to Smith, 26 July 1854; Smith, *Précis of Letters* and Hall, *Observations*.
144 HCPP 1863 (3207) XIII.475: *Report of the Barrack and Hospital Improvement Commission on the Sanitary Condition and Improvement of Mediterranean Stations*, p.21.

for the naval authorities to act.'[145] A few weeks later Hall told the PMO, Scutari that Raglan was anxious that invalids should be sent to England and convalescents to Malta as expeditiously as you can manage,'[146] thus releasing space at Scutari for more casualties.[147]

A month later the GOC, Malta reported ample accommodation for convalescents on the island, and inevitably the increased number of both invalids and healthy troops prompted a request for 'additional medical officers' together with 'a purveyor, a steward, and wardmasters.'[148] By April 1855, however, the 'want of accommodation' necessitated Raglan suspending sending sick to Malta,[149] although by this time plans were afoot for developing a convalescent hospital or depot on Gozo.

It was planned to send a draft of the 'not very sick' from Scutari to Corfu in *Dunbar* in January 1855,[150] though some patients were wounded and others were in a 'disgraceful state [...] suffering from dysentery, debility after fever, chest complaints and rheumatism.'[151] Not surprisingly their arrival prompted a request for additional medical staff.[152] The returns for these 463 invalids prepared during February to November 1855 indicated that over two thirds probably returned to their regiments although after four months some patients were not sufficiently fit to be repatriated to England.[153]

Panmure's plan to establish a depot there for invalids was abandoned in favour of a hospital for 500–1,000 men at Gozo,[154] possibly because it was on the direct route to the Black Sea, unlike Corfu. Smith was also against the plan because 'during the hot season fever of a severe type often appears, and invalids would be less able to resist than healthy troops.'[155]

In March 1855 Panmure instructed the GOC, Malta to 'take measures for the establishment of a convalescent depot for a 1,000 men on Gozo' but it is possible their letters crossed as earlier in the month he informed Panmure of difficulties encountered

---

145 Hall to Smith, 27 October 1854; Smith, *Précis of Letters* and Royal Commission Report, Appendix LXXIX, p.103. For example, a disembarkation return in TNA: WO 25/1187 indicated that HMS *Arethusa* left Scutari for Malta on 9 November with 146 convalescents arriving there on 20 November 1854. The health of the invalids was 'tolerably good under the circumstances' and there were no deaths. Similarly, *Jura* sailed from Scutari on 15 December with 283 invalids arriving at Malta on 21 December 1854.
146 Hall to Cumming, 10 November 1854; RAMC: 397/F/CO/1/1/892.
147 Cumming to Smith, 10 November 1854; Smith, *Précis of Letters*.
148 Hall to Cumming, 27 November 1854; RAMC: 397/F/CO/1/1/961; Smith informed the PMO, Malta on 9 January 1855 to expect 10,000 men to be quartered on the island; Smith, *Précis of Letters*; and PMO, Malta to Smith, 9 January 1855; Smith, *Précis of Letters*.
149 PMO, Malta, to Smith, 18 April 1855; Smith, *Précis of Letters*.
150 Paulet to AG, 8 & 14 January 1855; TNA: WO 28/186.
151 PMO, Corfu to Smith, 3 February 1855; Smith, *Précis of Letters*.
152 Smith to Deputy Secretary, 2 February 1855; Smith, *Précis of Letters*.
153 TNO: WO 28/185 and AG to QMG, 15 June 1855; TNA: WO 28/197.
154 Undersecretary to Smith, 10 April 1855; Smith, *Précis of Letters*.
155 Smith to Military Undersecretary, 13 March 1855; Smith, *Précis of Letters*.

in obtaining accommodation for the Army as relationships between the military and civil authorities and private property owners was ill defined, though Fort Chambray, on Gozo, was in the process of being refurbished as a hospital or convalescent depot, and it would be ready in about five weeks.[156]

Smith was apparently not consulted officially about the plan,[157] though he had 'no doubt that [Gozo] would prove a most eligible locality.'[158] He took matters forward by requesting the appointment of staff for a 300-bed hospital,[159] only to be informed that the plan was for 500 convalescents,[160] later increased to 1,000–1,500. The barrack could accommodate 500[161] and hence the Commissary-General was instructed to provide 40 huts for 25 men, although Panmure favoured tents rather than new buildings.[162] The huts provided by Messrs Weikersheim of Vienna[163] proved unsatisfactory and the cost of rendering them habitable was £3,580. The sum was subsequently authorized by Panmure.[164]

Smith suggested 15 medical officers of various grades for 500–1000 men[165] and shortly afterwards his request for passage to Gozo for three medical officers was confirmed,[166] while 14 wardmasters and orderlies passed the Isle of Wight en route for Gozo on 17 August 1855.[167] In the first instance it was planned to obtain hospital stores from Marseilles[168] and Vienna.[169] These arrived on *Earl of Mulgrave* on 15 May,[170] while equipment prepared in England by early May[171] was not dispatched until over two months later.[172] In the mean time, Panmure ordered that any stores duplicating those supplied by Weikersheim should be forwarded to other hospitals.[173]

---

156 Panmure to GOC, Malta, 12 March and GOC, Malta to Panmure, 7 March 1855; TNA: WO 6/70 & TNA: WO 1/513.
157 Referred to in Deputy Secretary to Smith, 10 April 1855; Smith, *Précis of Letters*.
158 Staff Surgeon Armstrong to Smith, 6 March 1855; Smith, *Précis of Letters* and Smith to Armstrong, 13 March 1955; Smith, *Précis of Letters*.
159 Smith to Military Undersecretary, 30 March 1855; Smith, *Précis of Letters*.
160 Undersecretary to Smith, 7 April 1855; Smith, *Précis of Letters*.
161 PMO, Malta to Smith, 18 April 1855; Smith, *Précis of Letters*.
162 Panmure to GOC, Malta, 24 April 1855; TNA: WO 6/70.
163 Following the loss of *Prince* the ambassador in Vienna – Earl of Westmorland – arranged a contract with Weikersheim to supply warm clothing; *Morning Post*, 10 January 1855.
164 Panmure to General Pennefather, 29 October 1855; TNA: WO 6/71.
165 Smith to Military Secretary, 18 April 1855; Smith, *Précis of Letters*.
166 Smith to Military Secretary, 30 April 1855; Smith, *Précis of Letters* and Smith to DIGH Gibson, 9 May 1855; Smith, *Précis of Letters*.
167 *The Times*, 20 August 1855.
168 Deputy Secretary to Smith, 19 April 1855; Smith, *Précis of Letters*.
169 Military Secretary to Smith, 8 May 1988; Smith, *Précis of Letters*.
170 PMO, Gozo to Smith, 18 May 1855; Smith, *Précis of Letters*.
171 Smith to PMO, Malta and Undersecretary, 1 & 9 May 1855; Smith, *Précis of Letters*.
172 Director of Transport Service to Smith, 21 July 1855; Smith, *Précis of Letters*.
173 Military Undersecretary to Smith, 9 June 1855; Smith, *Précis of Letters*, p.646.

Panmure informed Simpson and Paulet on 18 July that the GOC, Malta would notify them when Gozo was ready, viz. 500 beds in Fort Chambray and 500 in huts.[174] In August the hospital could accommodate 250–300 and the medical staff comprised 1 DIGH (Dr J.B. Gibson), four surgeons, and 16 assistant surgeons.[175] There are no records of this hospital in the *Medical and Surgical History*,[176] though Smith recommended its use when he counselled against repatriating patients to England during the winter,[177] while during the evacuation of the Crimea invalids and convalescents from the 'late seat of war' were quartered there. The 31st Regiment landed on Gozo on 16 June 1855;[178] and lost several men from cholera during the weeks that followed.[179]

Panmure informed Paulet that he could 'avail' himself of accommodation for 400 convalescents in Gibraltar 'for relieving the hospitals in the East.'[180] However, Hall, who had lived there for four years, considered it unsuitable for convalescents during the summer and recommended they should be sent to England;[181] an opinion reinforced by a board of Medical Officers.[182] Authority was, however, given for transports returning to England to embark any invalids from regiments serving in the Crimea if required.[183]

Paulet was subsequently instructed not to send patients there in summer,[184] though some invalids unfit to proceed to England were landed at Gibraltar and attached to a regiment in the garrison while under treatment.[185] They then continued to England following the approval of a Medical Board.[186]

---

174 TNA: WO 6/71.
175 <maltaRAMC.com> consulted on 15 September 2015.
176 The monthly reports of the AG in Malta recorded a total of only 280 deaths during the 27 month period, April 1854–June 1856; TNA: WO 17/2160-2.
177 Smith to Undersecretary, 5 November 1855; Smith, *Précis of Letters* and Royal Commission Report, Appendix LXXIX, p.77.
178 *The Times*, 12 June 1856 and TNA: WO 25/1188.
179 Malta Family History website entry for Fort Chambray, Gozo. There are no entries in the register for invalids evacuated to there from the Crimea.
180 Panmure to Paulet, 2 April & 6 May 1855; TNA: WO 6/70.
181 Hall to QMG, 12 May 1855; RAMC: 397/F/CO/1/1/2974.
182 Smith to the Undersecretary, 20 June 1855; Smith, *Précis of Letters*.
183 Newcastle to GOC, Malta, 24 January 1855; TNA: WO 6/70.
184 Military Undersecretary to Smith, 5 July 1855; Smith, *Précis of Letters* and Panmure to Paulet, 7 July 1855; TNA: WO 6/71.
185 For example, Gibraltar Garrison Orders, 6 March, 10 June, 11 July, 9 August, 25 September, & 24 October, 1855 & 14 January & 7 July 1856; TNA: WO 284/71 & 72.
186 Gibraltar Garrison Orders, 1 January ; TNA: WO 284/71 and *The Times*, 12 January 1855

3.5 Other locations considered

Newcastle suggested to Raglan during November 1854 that Rhodes might prove suitable for convalescents and HM's consul was making enquiries,[187] while Stratford confirmed that the Porte had agreed to the establishment of a sanatorium there.[188] Early in January Herbert, noted that he had heard that 'Rhodes is best for climate and buildings' but it would be difficult to supply as it is 'without much trade or market,'[189] and this, coupled with a lack of suitable public buildings,[190] meant that Smyrna was considered a better option, although Nightingale preferred Rhodes.[191]

Panmure instructed Paulet on 16 February to ascertain whether Mitylene would make a suitable venue for a hospital though it proved 'ineligible' on inspection.[192] Finally, a Dr J.B. Thompson suggested to the military authorities that Sueida (now Samnadağ) at the mouth of the Orontes as a location for a convalescent station but it was 'quite out of the question; as it was too far away and there were no suitable port facilities.'[193]

Smith recommended that Prince's Islands in the Sea of Marmora would prove a convenient location for convalescents rather than erecting temporary hospital accommodation at Scutari, and Panmure instructed Paulet to make the necessary enquiries.[194] Smith planned to provide sufficient marquees to permit the formation of a 'breezy and salubrious camping ground' which could be moved if the 'site became objectionable.'[195] Smith also considered Proti as an alternative venue, but nothing

---

187 Newcastle to Raglan 23 November 1855; TNA: WO 6/70/155.
188 Stratford to Clarendon, 9 & 14 December 1854; TNA: FO 78/1006 & 1007.
189 Herbert to Cumming, 5 January 1855; Wiltshire and Swindon History Centre: 2057/F8/III/C/15.
190 Stratford to Paulet, 1 February 1855 in response to a request for information by Paulet, 27 January 1855; TNA: FO 78/1072, FO 195/452, and FO 352/41A/4. Incidentally, Hall informed the Military Secretary on 25 January that, though he had no report on Rhodes, he thought it should prove a suitable location for convalescents, and he could provide medical staff if requited; TNA: FO 30/91.
191 Nightingale to Herbert, 26 March 1855; McDonald, *Florence Nightingale*, p.171.
192 Panmure to Paulet, 16 February & 19 April 1855; TNA: WO 6/70 and Sir Dominic Ellis Colnaghi papers; British Library: Add Ms 59502, ff.142 & 197.
193 Hall to Raglan, 20 April; Smith, *Précis of Letters*, 1, Appendix 15 and Hall to Smith, 21 April 1855; RAMC: 397/F/CO/1/2/1872; and Smith, *Précis of Letters*. Dr Thompson, MD, was 'well known in connection with the proposed overland route to India via Snediah and valley of the Orontes.' He died of fever at Constantinople on 5 August 1855; *Gentleman's Magazine*, October 1855, p.441.
194 Smith to Undersecretary, 1 March 1855; Smith, *Précis of Letters* and Royal Commission Report, Appendix LXXIX, p.38, and Panmure to Paulet, 5 & 12 March 1855; TNA: WO 6/70.
195 Smith to Cumming, 9 May 1855; Smith, *Précis of Letters* and Royal Commission Report, Appendix LXXIX, pp.40–1.

came of either initiative.[196] Paulet was informed that permission had been obtained from the Turkish authorities to build a 'wooden hospital' to the north of Scutari at Selvi Bournou (Cypress Cape), but, again, this proposal was not put into effect.[197]

Sinope: In the spring of 1855 Hall informed the QMG that if there was the need for another hospital away from the Crimea he would recommend Sinope (now Sinop), and this opinion was echoed by PMO, Scutari who considered it 'would answer well enough.'[198] The Sanitary Commissioners subsequently reported that Sinope was 'as good a place for a large hospital as could be desired' although temporary buildings were required, and further expense would be incurred in providing storage for water.[199] Hall accepted that a deficiency of water would render the location 'ineligible,'[200] and no further action was taken. After the war Hall opined that the 'the want of water could not have been a well-founded objection, from the number of animals belonging to the Commissariat and LTC that were subsequently collected and kept there.'[201] A reasonable conclusion given there were 3,994 mules, 1,215 camels, 948 horses, and 105 donkeys there in January 1856,[202] and equidae can consume 5–20 gallons a day depending on the weather, their size, diet, and workload.[203]

3.6 Comparison of hospitals

The assessment of a hospital's performance is a vexatious topic and it emerged as an issue following the publication of reviews of Nightingale's *'Notes on Hospitals'*[204] in the *Medical Times and Gazette*[205] and *The Lancet*.[206] These notices, together with letters

---

196 Smith to Dr Bryce, 11 December 1855; Smith, *Précis of Letters* and Royal Commission Report, Appendix LXXIX, p.82. Proti, an island in the Sea of Marmora, was used to accommodate Russian prisoners.
197 Odo Russell to Paulet, 26 April 1855; TNA: FO 352/41A
198 Hall to QMG, 23 March 1855; RAMC: 397/F/CO/1/1/1684 and Royal Commission Report, Appendix LXXIX, p.118 and Cumming to Hall, 10 April 1855; National Army Museum: 007-07-16-19.
199 Sanitary Commissioners to Raglan, 19 June 1855; TNA: WO 33/1/49/55/Inclosure 14.
200 Hall to Military Secretary, 23 June 1855; RAMC: 397/F/CO/1/1/2448, TNA: WO 28/176; and Royal Commission Report, Appendix LXXIX, p.125.
201 Hall, *Observations*.
202 Commandant, Sinope to HQ, 31 January 1856; TNA: WO 28/193.
203 M. Hinton, 'On the Watering of Horses', *Equine Veterinary Journal*, 10 (1978), pp.27–31.
204 F. Nightingale, *Notes on Hospitals*, (3rd edition) (London: Longman, Green, Longman, Roberts, and Green, 1863).
205 *Medical Times and Gazette*, January 1864, pp.129–30, with further correspondence on pp.186–9, 211, 242–3, & 491–2.
206 *The Lancet*, 27 February 1864, pp.248–50, with further correspondence on pp.338–9, 365–6, 420–2, & 451–2.

from others, criticized the method used by Dr W. Farr[207] of judging a hospital on mortality rates alone, as this ignored the case load, number of doctors employed and their experience, nature of the cases admitted, ratio of medical to surgical cases, and age and gender of patients. More specifically, Nightingale was criticized for making a comparison of 'the great mortality of the large Scutari hospital' with 'the well-ventilated detached huts of the Balaclava Castle Hospital.'[208] Clearly this statement is misleading because the problems in Scutari occurred principally during the winter of 1854–55, a few months before the Castle Hospital opened during March 1855 as a convalescent hospital for surgical cases, and when conditions had begun to improve both in the Crimea and at Scutari.

An overall conclusion to be drawn from these discussions is the need to compare like with like; and this is only possible for general hospitals in operation at the same time, as illustrated in Table 3.2 The two examples that follow illustrate clearly how the differences in mortality rates can be explained simply by taking account of the use to which the hospitals were put. .

Table 3.2 Admissions to and death from wounds and injuries in the general hospitals in the Crimea

Hospital	Operational dates	All admissions	Admissions for W&I (% of all admissions)	Deaths from W&I (% of admissions for W&I)
General	1 Oct. 54–30 June 56	5,686	315 (5.5)	14 (4.5)
Castle	3 Mar. 55–30 June 56	2,554	1,834 (72)	83 (4.5)
Camp	1 Apr. 55–30 Apr. 56	1,083	740 (68.5)	184 (25)
Monastery	21 July 55–17 June 56	911	18 (2)	0

* W&I = Wounds and injuries.

(Summarized from the *Medical and Surgical History*, 2, General Hospital Returns III, IV, V, and VI)

Varna: Two hospitals were utilized during the occupation of Bulgaria, viz. a General Hospital (June–November 1854) and an Invalid Depot (August 1854–January 1855). Both were open between August and November and during this time they admitted 894 and 577 patients respectively of whom 208 (23 percent) and 35 (six percent) died, thereby confirming that the Depot was utilized principally for men who were convalescent.

Crimean general hospitals: During the period April–December 1855 men suffering from gunshot wounds (*Vulnus sclopitorum*) were treated principally in two hospitals, the

207 Farr was an epidemiologist and statistician employed in the General Register Office, London.
208 *The Lancet*, 27 February 1864.

Camp General Hospital which was close to the front and which received men shortly after injury, and the Castle Hospital which was opened specifically for men recovering from their wounds. In this time 730 and 1782 patients were admitted to the two hospitals respectively with 184 (25 percent) and 82 (4.5 percent) deaths. By comparisons, there were only 17 admissions for gunshot wounds to the General Hospital in Balaklava out of 1,767 cases, with one death. Incidentally, as mentioned previously a policy was adopted in the spring of 1855 not to send seriously wounded men to the Bosphorus and clearly this policy was effective as there were only twelve (two percent) deaths among 701 evacuees in this category and only eleven (two percent) deaths amongst 723 patients with gun shot wounds that were treated at Scutari during the same period.

3.7 Concluding remarks

MacMunn was of the decided opinion that (1) the 'scandal' at Scutari was entirely due to Herbert's failure to organize hospitals behind the front, presumably in advance of any action with the enemy; (2) Scutari was beyond the power of Lord Raglan and his staff or his principle medical officer to control; and in a foot note to the paragraph he stressed that no one would have thought of making Sir Ian Hamilton responsible for establishing hospitals to which the sick and wounded from Gallipoli were to be evacuated. That was the duty of other authorities in communication with the War Office; and (3) Hardinge should: 'have insisted in the formation of ancillary services for war, having many months to do so, and further should have so forcibly reminded Herbert of his responsibility *in re* hospitals that there should have been no need of the hurried Nightingale mission or *The Times* Relief Fund.[209] Maxwell, on the other hand was more conciliatory as he considered that once the problems became known in London both Newcastle and Herbert did what they could to ameliorate the situation.[210]

The provision of hospital facilities in Bulgaria and the Crimea, both regimental and general, proved inadequate until the early part of 1855. This was due in large measure to the absence of suitable buildings that could be readily adapted for hospital use; the considerable increase in the number of patients with disease, particularly cholera, diarrhoea, and dysentery; and the need to cater for those wounded during action with the enemy.

As the siege progressed stationary regimental hospitals became available and these became the preferred location for providing primary health care and treating men wounded in action. General hospitals catering for different categories of patients were also developed and overall this resulted in a reduction in the need to evacuate seriously ill patients to Turkey from the end of January 1855.

209 MacMunn, *Crimea in Perspective*, pp.244, 261, & 241.
210 See Anon [Maxwell], *Whom Shall We Hang?*, pp.208–22.

4

Transportation and evacuation of invalids

4.1 Initial planning and further developments

As early as 18 February 1854 Smith intimated to the War Office the need for an Ambulance Corps (AC), staffed by fit men and not pensioners, given his experience of invaliding 20,000 men when at Chatham.[1] In contrast, Raglan's Military Secretary (Lieutenant Colonel Steele) asked the Deputy Secretary on 30 March to enlist pensioners for an AC.[2] The next month Smith proposed 800 able-bodied men should be recruited to serve as ambulance drivers, stretcher-bearers, and hospital orderlies thus relieving bandsmen and fighting men from these duties, but the Commander-in Chief (Hardinge) was not prepared to reduce the strength of regiments and Smith's advice was ignored.[3]

A scheme to form a corps in Bulgaria employing locally recruited personnel came to nothing and a unit of about 370 pensioners was subsequently raised along the lines suggested in Steele's letter. The men arrived in Bulgaria in July 1854 but proved unsatisfactory from the start because the corps was ill-equipped and the men were inexperienced in the duties required and most were considered too old and unfit for heavy work. In addition, disease, particularly cholera, soon thinned their ranks.[4]

---

1   Select Committee, 2nd Report, pp.411–2. The AC was referred to as the Hospital Conveyance Corps in other documents.
2   Presumably based on advice given by Tulloch, 30 March 1854; Supplies Commission Report, p.194.
3   Cantlie, *A History*, pp.33–4 and Shepherd, *Crimean Doctors*, 1, pp.37–8 & 79. The Hospital Commissioners subsequently recommended the Corps should comprise 'carefully selected men in the prime of life' and […] should include 'wheelwrights, farriers, harness-makers, and other artisans;' Hospital Commission Report, p.5.
4   For summaries on the development and performance of the Ambulance Corps see a memorandum by Tulloch in the Supplies Commission Report, pp.194–6 and DIGH Longmore, *A Treatise on the Transport of Sick and Wounded Troops* (London: HMSO, 1869), pp.36–40.

Before the invasion Hall recommended to Raglan that each infantry regiment should have one spring ambulance waggon and 32 bearers [stretchers] (Figures 4.1 and 4.2); the Cavalry Division four waggons and 48 bearers; and the Artillery four waggons (one per battery) and 48 bearers.[5] These requirements were not met, and the Army landed without a single functional ambulance waggon,[6] an omission that had serious consequences during the first weeks thereafter.

Raglan subsequently admitted that the 'Ambulance Corps, hastily raised on a limited scale, had proved a failure,'[7] while the Roebuck Committee acknowledged that Smith's recommendations for its constitution had been ignored, and concluded that the 'entire failure of this corps and the consequent sufferings of the army are abundantly proved.'[8]

The design of the ambulance waggons used initially proved unsatisfactory and the conveyance of invalids continued a serious problem throughout the first winter, especially as the deterioration of the roads from November precluded the use of wheeled transport. In mid-January Dr G. Lawson noted that the roads were still in a 'very bad condition, almost impossible to anything but baggage animals [though] the French are making roads for us, macadamizing them with the stone [...] but it is a very long job'.[9] Matters certainly improved when the railway came into use during April 1855, and eventually better equipment was supplied, including lighter sprung waggons and cacolets.[10]

There was no provision for a field ambulance section in the Medical Staff Corps (see Section 2.2.5), much to Smith's disappointment.[11] Plans to reorganize Corps were formulated during 1855 and it was finally integrated into the Land Transport Corps as an Ambulance Service on 31 December,[12] with a proportion of the ambulance waggons forming part of the transport allocated to Divisions.[13]

---

5   For the text see *The Times*, 20 September1854; Hospital Commission Report, pp.55–7; and Cantlie, *A History*, 2, pp.37–42 & 46–67.
6   An army staff officer ordered the vehicles etc. to be disembarked to make room for troops; Royal Commission Report, p.xlviii and *Medical and Surgical History*, 2, p.253
7   Raglan to Panmure, 30 January 1855; TNA: WO 33/1/17/55.
8   Select Committee, 5th Report, p.18.
9   Bonham-Carter and Lawson, *Surgeon in the Crimea*, p.150.
10 Cacolets comprise two chairs attached on each side of a pack saddle fitted for a horse or mule and could be used to convey patients across rough terrain. See *Illustrated London News*, 27 January 1855.
11 Smith pointed out to the Military Undersecretary on 16 March 1855 that 'many of the wounded are carried off the field by bandsman and drummers' and that this 'arrangement has proved woefully deficient;' Smith, *Précis of Letters*.
12 General Order, 28 December 1855.
13 For discussion see Cantlie, *A History*, 2, pp.71–2 & 146–7 and Shepherd, *Crimean Doctors*, 1, p.79

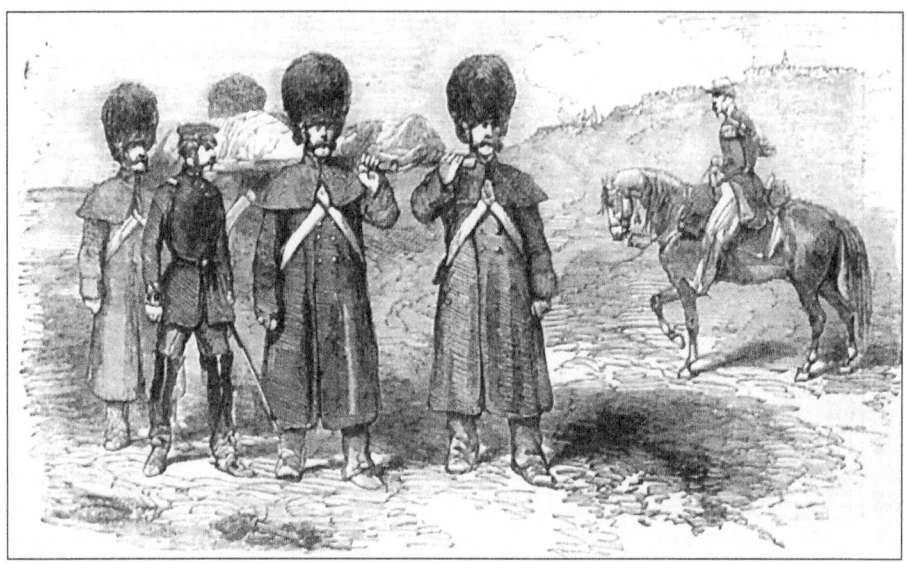

Figure 4.1 The Guards carrying a wounded officer from Inkerman. (*Illustrated London News*, 3 February 1855, p.116)

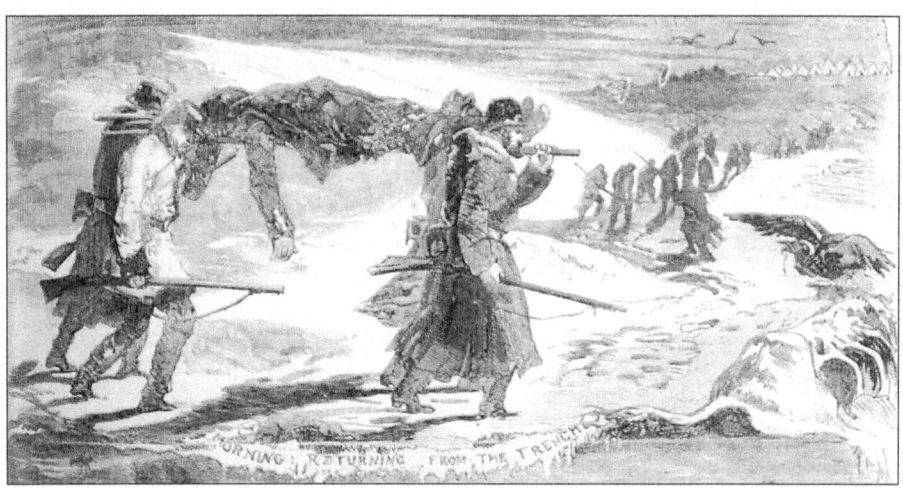

Figure 4.2 Morning: returning from the trenches. (*Illustrated Times*, 14 July 1855, p.89)

Smith also appreciated the need for hospital transport ships and on 10 February 1854,[14] and again on 4 April 1854, he proposed formally to the Military Secretary that:

---

14 Smith to Military Secretary, 10 February 1854; Smith, *Précis of Letters*.

The welfare of sufferers and of the Army will require those disabled by wounds or sickness should be removed from the vicinity of the conflicting forces. Ships, therefore, should be liberally provided, some for carrying to England, or elsewhere, men not likely to be soon available for further service; others in use in harbour, as floating hospitals. The ships [...] should be commodious steamers, high between decks, thoroughly ventilated, and having fixed berths.[15]

Smith wrote again to the Military Secretary on the same topic on 11 May,[16] but received no reply,[17] although Newcastle did forward a copy of the letter to Raglan, but not until 13 July, with the suggestion that he should confer with Admiral Boxer on the subject.[18] It is probable that Smith's initial request was not passed to the Admiralty. The Roebuck Committee was informed on 27 April 1855 that no requisition had been received from the military authorities, but if it had been, 'steps would have been taken to have had hospital ships fitted up.'[19] Cantlie suggested that fault on this occasion must have resided with the Military Secretary, Hardinge, or Newcastle.[20] Newcastle, however, claimed that he knew nothing of Smith's letters of 4 April and 11 May,[21] while Smith later received support from Kinglake:

When as early as the 11th May 1854 the Director General submitted to Horse Guards in writing a well considered plan for removing sick and wounded by appropriating beforehand due means of sea transport, and showed need of stationing in convenient ports ships prepared for reception of patients, his appeals were unanswered and apparently provoked no attention.[22]

The need for hospital ships was appreciated by the Royal Navy and HMS *Belleisle* was equipped for service with the Baltic Fleet at the beginning of March 1854 (Figure 4.3).[23] In view of this initiative it is surprising that the military authorities and the government failed to heed Smith's timely advice, and this inevitably contributed to the terrible problems encountered while evacuating the sick and wounded during the first months of the campaign.[24]

15 Smith to Military Secretary, 4 April 1854; RAMC: 397/F/CO2/7 (Manuscript); and RAMC: 524/14/2 (Typescript).
16 Smith, *Précis of letters*. Full text in Select Committee, 2nd Report, pp.415–6 and *The Lancet*, 28 July 1855. The annotation 'pressing' was included by *The Lancet*, but not in the official report.
17 Select Committee, 2nd Report, p.416.
18 TNA: WO 6/69–118–9.
19 Select Committee, 3rd Report, p.279.
20 Cantlie, *A History*, 2, pp.54–5.
21 Select Committee, 3rd Report, pp.136–7.
22 Kinglake, *Invasion*, p.49.
23 *The Times*, 4 March 1854 and *The Lancet*, 13 May 1854.
24 The topic was addressed by Cantlie, *A History*, 2, pp.21 & 54–5.

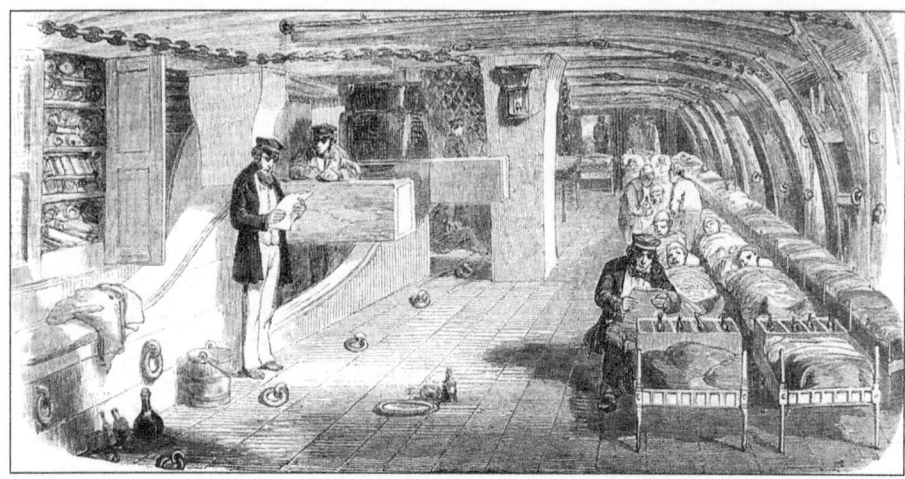

Figure 4.3 The sick-deck 'The Bellisle' hospital ship, in Faro sound. (*Illustrated London News*, 18 August 1855, p.220)

The consequences of this oversight became apparent when details of the management of the wounded after the battle of the Alma, and the voyages to Turkey involving the *Kangaroo*, *Dunbar*, *Colombo*, *Trent*, and *Avon*, were publicised by the press. Much unwarranted criticism for these catastrophes was subsequently and unreasonably laid at the door of the AMD. This obviously upset Smith, Hall, and their colleagues, and serves to illustrate a general lack of understanding of how an army on campaign functioned. However, it is clear that Martineau appreciated where the responsibility lay when she wrote after the war:

> After the first landing in the Crimea the sick seem to have been thrown upon the mercies of chance [with the surgeons] being the victims rather than the perpetrators of the mistake as the according to the rules of the Army, the medical department is dependent on other departments for ambulance and transport of sick and wounded. [...] The QMG and naval commanders, one would think would consult with the chief medical officer present and [the embarkation of] the serious sick and wounded, how to provide for them on board the ships, and where to take them. [But] nothing of the sort was done [after the battle of the Alma.]'[25]

The dilemma is simply explained. The AMD had no executive authority and hence it was dependent on cooperation from the military authorities and the Royal Navy to transport patients on land and to evacuate then from the peninsula by sea. Initially

---

25   Martineau, *England and Her Soldiers*, p.93.

vessels were 'told off' for this purpose by the naval authorities on an ad hoc basis until mid-December 1854. Steamers were then selected to provide a shuttle service across the Black Sea, a policy which remained in place until the end of the campaign.

4.2 The Black Sea theatre

4.2.1 Evacuation from Bulgaria

When the allied armies landed in Bulgaria during June the troops were reasonably healthy but as the sick list lengthened Raglan requested that the hospital accommodation ashore should be supplemented by the use of *Monarchy* that could accommodate 90 men in comfort, while the evacuation of the sick to Scutari commenced at about this time, for example on *Teignmouth*.[26] The increasing numbers reporting sick necessitated an urgent request to the Royal Navy by the QMG [Airey] on 30 August for 'sufficient boats to convey 300 sick on board [...] *Bombay*[27] and *Cornwall*,' while a few days later Hall informed the PMO, Scutari that '*Bombay* and *Mercia* will bring 400 and 250 convalescents.'[28] He continued by emphasizing that: 'We have had an enormous number of sick thrown on our hands all at once, and have been much pressed to provide for them in any way' and pointed out that 'it is Lord Raglan's wish to gradually get the sick away from this and they will be sent down when they become convalescent, and opportunities for transport present.'[29]

In all about 1,250 patients were admitted to the Hospitals on the Bosphorus in the period June–August 1854. The problem, which ceased to be an issue in Bulgaria when the army sailed for the Crimea, was resolved when the general hospitals were closed and the remaining patients transferred to Abydos or elsewhere (see Section 3.2.2).

4.2.2 Invasion of the Crimea

During early August 1854, Hall had recommended to Raglan the need to set three ships apart for the sick and wounded[30] and on the 26 August he was notified by Sir George Brown that *Andes* and *Cambria* had been selected,[31] though neither was avail-

---

26 Major Wellesley, AQMG, to Captain Rawstone, RN, 30 July 1854; TNA: WO 28/196 and RAMC: 397/F/CO/5. The employment of *Monarchy* in this capacity proved a temporary measure.
27 A fine Indiaman of upwards 1,300 tons burthen; *The Times*, 21 September1854.
28 Lord de Ros, QMG, to Admiral Lyons, 30 August 1854; TNA: WO 28/196 and Hall to Smith, 4 September1854; Smith, *Précis of Letters*. Incidentaly, *Mercia* was substituted for *Cornwall* and Hall estimated about 2,000 sick were left behind in Bulgaria.
29 Hall to Menzies, 2 September1854; RAMC: 397/F/CO/1/1/682. Incidentally, Cantlie, *A History*, 2, p.42 implied that Hall ordered these vessels to Scutari. This is incorrect as the Royal Navy controlled the movement of all transport vessels.
30 Hall to Smith, 5 August 1854; Smith, *Précis of Letters* and Mitra, *Life and Letters*, p.315.
31 RAMC: 397/F/CO/10/1. Hall informed the PMO, Scutari, and Smith of this development on 26 & 29 August respectively, RAMC: 397/F/CO/1/1/642 & 665.

able until after the invasion as they were 'filled and overcrowded with troops by the authorities.'[32] Hall, who considered that neither vessel was very desirable,[33] found *Andes* very dirty and badly ventilated,[34] and the captain a 'drunken ill-conditioned man.'[35]

Hall's preparation for the invasion was severely compromised because he was not informed of the plans in advance, though he suggested to the QMG on 11 August that it would be convenient if medical stores and equipment could be shipped on vessels to be employed as hospital ships.[36] Needless to say the request went unheeded.

Hall was only told officially on the 26 August that the fleet was due to sail on 1 September and this short notice led him to complain formally about his exclusion from the planning process in his evidence to the Hospital Commission and the Royal Commission on 16 January 1855 and 19 June 1857 respectively;[37] while in his draft memoirs he wrote:

> No intimation was given to me by the QMG of the precise date, and order of embarkation of the Army from Varna; and the consequence was that some ships had several medical officers on board, others none, some had medicines and stores, others none, and every effort to remedy these defects during the few hours the vessels remained in the bay after the men were embarked was unsatisfactory and ineffectual.[38]

Incidentally, Hall was not alone in making this point. For example, on 4 September 1854 Lieutenant Colonel A.H. Gordon told his father, the Prime Minister, that 'Lord Raglan very wisely keeps his plans very close and few people really know what he intends to do.'[39]

Prior to the invasion Hall issued a memorandum for the guidance of medical officers and this was well received by Russell who wrote: 'Great care has been taken by the medical authorities to make the department as efficient as possible, and Hall has issued a circular containing directions and suggestions as to surgical practice, which is highly spoken of.'[40] It did not contain specific advice on the evacuation of invalids though it was obviously going to be necessary to remove as many as possible so the

---

32   RAMC: 397/F/RT/1/1. *Andes* and *Cambria* transported part the 33rd and 50th Regiments to the Crimea; *The Times*, 21 September1854.
33   Hall, on *John Masterman*, to Smith, 15 September1854; RAMC: 397/F/CO/1/1/695.
34   Hall, diary entry, 15 September1854; RAMC: 397/PC/1/6.
35   RAMC: 397/F/RT/1/1.
36   RAMC: 397/F/CO/1/1/533. The text is reproduced in Hospital Commission Report, p.57, and was referred to by Mitra, *Life and Letters*, pp.316–7.
37   Hospital Commission Report, p.339 and Royal Commission Report, p.178.
38   RAMC: 397/F/RT/2.
39   British Library: Add. Ms 43225.
40   *The Times*, 21 September1854 and other newspapers. For a version printed locally see RAMC: 397/F/CO/6/13.

advance towards Sevastopol was not hindered. The matter had not been overlooked entirely, however, as evinced by a memorandum issued to each Division:

> When the troops disembark all soldiers [...] unfit to land will be left on board. [...] A steamer will [...] collect all these [...] and convey them to Scutari. Medical Officers will be placed on board [...] A return of the probable number of non-efficient men is to be sent as soon as possible to the Principal Medical Officer on board the 'Tyrone' [...] Orderlies in proportion of one man for every 12 sick men are to be selected to accompany the sick.[41]

Hall was aware of this memorandum, but he received no information on the numbers involved from the divisional commanders.[42] On the 15 September the Royal Navy's Agent of Transports (AoT) instructed that 'all sick troops and sick women remaining on board the transports be sent by tomorrow noon to the *Kangaroo*.'[43] The net result was the vessel was overwhelmed and chaos ensued. A second vessel, *Dunbar*, was employed to carry some of the sick and both vessels arrived at Scutari on 22 September. The British public was made aware of the '*Kangaroo* affair' when reports were published in *The Times* on 2 and 9 October 1854. The first was from Russell, who was with the Army, and the second from Thomas Chenery, who was based in Turkey. They were dated 16 and 25 September respectively and there is little doubt that though both exaggerated the conditions on both transports they must have been horrendous, but for reasons that were outwith the direct control of the AMD.

Cantlie provided a brief description of the incident and concluded that despite Hall's denials 'the transports were most inadequately staffed, and it is a distressing fact that the conditions on *Kangaroo* were the precursors of those on many similar voyages.' He considered that neither Hall nor Dumbreck had attempted 'to provide the sick with [the palliases] on board *John Masterman*, or to supply soldiers as orderlies.'[44] Cantlie's points may have been well intended but in Hall's defence it may have proved impractical to obtain bedding if it had been stowed under other items of equipment or the Navy was unable or unwilling to arrange the transfer between the ships. In addition, the prospect of an imminent engagement with the enemy would have reduced the opportunity for detailing medical officers for service afloat while Hall could take no responsibility for the provision of orderlies as this rested solely with the military authorities.

---

41 QMG to GOC, Divisions, 10 September 1854; TNA: WO 18/199/2.
42 Hall, *Observations*.
43 Cantlie, *A History*, 2, p.48.
44 Cantlie, *A History*, 2, pp.48–9. It was not until the New Year that the MSC replaced some military orderlies (AG to Hall, 21 February 1854; TNA: WO 28/125) or civilians (QMG to GOC, Malta, 1 March 1855; TNA: WO 28/137).

4.2.3 Transfer of patients from camp to Balaklava

Management systems for transferring patients from the camps to Balaklava, a distance of six miles or more along poorly constructed roads, were inadequately developed during the early months. Not surprisingly things did not always run smoothly, and Raglan choose to admonish the AMD for some of the problems that arose, rather than the military authorities who rightly should have shouldered most of the blame as they were responsible for the movement of the troops (see Table 4.1).

Table 4.1 Correspondence concerning the transfer of invalids from camp to Balaklava, December 1854–August 1855

Date 1854–55	Abstract [Reference]
7 Dec.	About 600 sick will be brought by the French Ambulance tomorrow, weather permitting. […] apply for the boats to be in readiness and ensure comforts are placed on board […] and soup and some nourishment is ready for them on arrival. Application must be made tonight for orderlies. [Hall to PMO, Balaklava; RAMC: 397/F/CO/1/1/1040]
11 Dec.	There are near 785 sick men sent from [camp] but nearly 300 have yet to be embarked at three p.m.. Everything has been done to get them on board but it is almost impossible to manage satisfactorily with so large a number in one day. [with] many […] on stretchers it causes great delay, and in future I think it would be very desirable if a smaller number were sent down at the same time. It would also add much to the comfort of the sick if the orderlies […] were detailed and on board ship the previous evening. [DAQMG, Balaklava to QMG; TNA: WO 28/192]
12 Dec.	The French will lend 300 ambulance mules on the 14 December [and] steps should be taken immediately to accommodate 350 sick. [Hall to PMO, Balaklava; RAMC: 397/F/CO/1/1/1072]
21 Dec.	Today when in Balaklava I received a note at half past one from the AG to provide for the reception of 600 sick to be taken down in the morning by the French ambulance. The ships are not even appointed. How is it possible to make them comfortable? [Hall, dairy; RAMC: 524/15]
26 Dec.	In consequence of nobody knowing the sick were coming and there was a delay in embarking them before dark. [DAQMG, Balaklava to QMG; TNA: WO: 28/196]
28 Dec.	The sick did not arrive at Balaklava until half past three. It was near five until they were all embarked. There was no delay in the boats. [Balaklava report to QMG; TNA: WO 28/196]
30 Dec.	Great inconvenience from ships ready for sick not being reported, it is impossible to send sick, which is daily necessary, unless it is known that accommodation is provided for them. Inform if there is a vessel is now disposable, answer by bearer. [QMG to AoT; TNA: WO 28/137]
25 Jan.	A large number of sick came down today without warning after intimation had been given to the AG that there was no accommodation. They appear to have come down independently [having been sent by] the PMOs of Divisions. [PMO, Balaklava to Hall; Royal Commission Report, Appendix LXXIX, p.204]
14 Feb.	A great irregularity has taken place in the arrival of the sick at the General Hospital for Balaklava and […] the sick have been detained for some considerable time in the cold. [Memorandum issued by PMO, Light Division; RAMC: 1139/LP10/12]

Date 1854–55	Abstract [Reference]
15 Feb.	Great inconvenience having been felt […] at Balaklava from sick being sent down without any previous notice being given […] due notice shall be given to them when there is accommodation for their sick on board ship, they must not be sent down there being no room for them at the hospital. [AG, Memorandum to Divisions; TNA: WO 28/122]
14 Mar.	Thirty sick men from the front are now waiting at the hospital for admission into which we can receive only three. There is here a marquee but fatigue men are not to be had for its erection. (The letter was annotated at HQ that the men were sent from the 4th Division without authority and without notification and there was no ship available to receive them.) [Medical officer, General Hospital to Commandant, Balaklava; TNA: WO 28/161]
5 Apr.	Ten men of the RA were sent down for embarkation but there was no ship ready to receive them. They have been admitted to the General Hospital on a temporary basis. This is of great inconvenience as the hospital is already full and they were laid on the floors of wards already overcrowded. [Medical officer, General Hospital to PMO, Balaklava; Royal Commission Report, Appendix LXXIX, pp.190–1]
11 May.	The PMO should ascertain that there is room for patients in the Hospital before he applies for transport from camp. [AG to GOC, Cavalry Division; TNA: WO 28/109]
26 May	Wounded men are frequently sent to Balaklava without due notice being given to the Commandant consequently no parties with stretchers are ready to carry them to the hospitals causing great suffering to the patients. [AG, Memorandum to Divisions; TNA: WO 28/123]
26 May	Six wounded men were sent down to Balaklava without notice on the 24th inst to the great inconvenience of all concerned. [AG to GOC, 3rd Division; TNA: WO 28/109]
29 Aug.	The prompt removal of sick and wounded from camp to better quarters is obviously of the first important, time cannot always be given for the preparation of documents, and a delay in proper settlements will be the result. Notifications of the removals of soldiers […] are made to assist […] COs and others and it is hoped that although delay may sometimes occur in the balancing of accounts the interests of the soldiers will not ultimately suffer. [AG to GOC, 2nd Division; TNA: WO 28/110]

Shortly after the invasion Dumbreck, who was deputizing for Hall while at Scutari, was severely reprimanded by a General Order on 11 October, without any properly constituted inquiry having taken place.[45] Briefly, a verbal order from Dumbreck did not reach the PMO, Balaklava with the consequence that nothing had been prepared for invalids when they arrived during inclement weather.[46] Raglan accused the PMO of 'gross neglect', which was hardly fair given he had not received the message, and not surprisingly Dumbreck, who was enjoined to give written orders in future 'was affronted' as he argued with justice, 'that it was customary to give verbal orders in the army, even at the highest level.'[47, 48]

45 TNA: WO 28/49 and *The Times*, 28 October 1854.
46 Dr J.C.G. Tice, although he was not named in the Order.
47 Shepherd, *Crimean Doctors*, 1, pp.160–1.
48 The incident was reported in *The Times*, 28 October and this provoked a strong reaction in support of the AMD from the editor of *The Lancet*, 4 November 1854.

The decision to publish this Order was taken without consulting Hall, which was a gross breach of etiquette if nothing else, revealed that Raglan 'appeared to show scant appreciation of the transport conditions.' It was, however, erroneous of Shepherd to suggest 'there was nothing to suggest that [...] Raglan saw fit to investigate the reasons for the defects of the system'[49] since he ordered that future conveys of sick should be accompanied by both a medical officer and a DAQMG who was to ensure arrangements were made for the reception of the invalids, and that the 'ticket' that should accompany each invalid was given to the medical officer on the ship.[50]

The military authorities in Balaklava were required to inform headquarters of the accommodation available for invalids by the evening of each day. The departments of the AG and QMG, whose co-operation was crucial, could then arrange for Divisions to send down the appropriate number the next day, and for the medical officers to be selected by Hall. This system was not foolproof, however, and on occasions invalids arrived without notice, or too late in the day to be dealt with before nightfall, or when there was no ship available upon which to embark (see Table 4.1).

Panmure subsequently asked Raglan why these problems had not been addressed, and, inter alia, he held the QMG responsible for neglecting to construct a suitable road between the camp and port.[51] It is inconceivable that the AG and QMG were unaware of their responsibilities though the following an exchange of letters during July 1855 indicates that matters were not entirely resolved even by that time:

> QMG: We must come to some arrangement and notification about sick going down. Some day, if I am not before hand informed, that boats etc. are required, there will be some disaster. The boats, fatigue parties etc. are told off for duty over night. Sick coming unexpectedly down is very embarrassing.
>
> AG's response: As soon as vessels have been reported our sick may be expected daily so long as there are vessels to receive them. It is a daily business. [...] The numbers carried down by the cavalry vary certainly but not very much. 70 or 80 are the most they convey. We now know precisely how many horses the cavalry will send up. The other modes of conveyance have increased of late [...] Some 20 men per diem may be counted in by those individual exertions of divisions. In cases the cacolets for men, being extra conveyance, we always give ample notice. The daily duty of the ordinary cavalry description is one which never ceases so long as there are ships.[52]

---

49 Shepherd, *Crimean Doctors*, 1, p.160.
50 General Order, 11 October 1854 and AG to Commandant, Balaklava, 17 February 1855; TNA: WO 28/108. A General Order of 8 January 1855 instructed that patients sent to hospital should be issued with a prescribed form of admission ticket available from the Purveyors.
51 Panmure to Raglan, 12 February 1855; TNA: WO 33/1/13/55.
52 QMG to AG, 9 July 1855 and reply; TNA: WO 28/195.

The twelve ambulance waggons employed at Inkerman proved of the 'greatest use' but they were insufficient to convey the wounded to Balaklava,[53] and assistance had to be sought from the French,[54] although the numbers involved meant that the process still took some time[55] (see Figures 4.4 and 4.5 for ambulances in use early in the campaign).

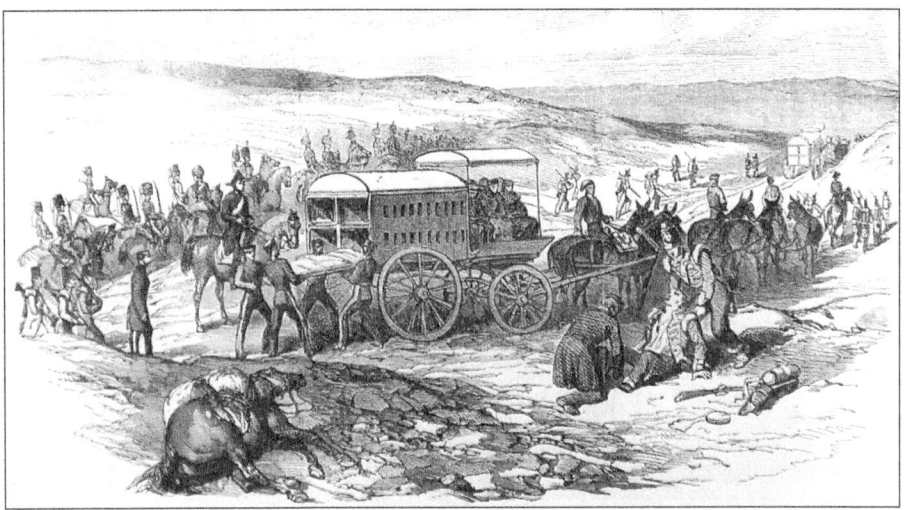

Figure 4.4 Siege of Sebastopol – Dr Smith's new hospital waggon. (*Illustrated London News*, 4 November 1854, p.448)

Clearly the AC did not come up to expectations for several reasons, one of which was that many of the men were former infantry soldiers who knew little about handling horses and driving the waggons, while the lack of smiths, farriers, and wheelwrights meant that damaged vehicles could not be repaired readily.[56] It was essential that the horses had to be of sufficient size and strength to do what was expected of them. The animals also became 'knocked up' as a consequence of the heavy work and the insufficiency of feed and forage,[57] and many perished,[58] while the theft of transport

53 Hall expressed regret of not having the forty originally brought from England; Cantlie, *A History*, 2, p.77.
54 Hall to Smith, 7 November 1855; RAMC: 397/F/CO/1/1/876; Smith, *Précis of Letters*; and Wiltshire and Swindon History Centre: 2057/F8/III/B/317 (Copy).
55 Special Correspondent, 12 November 1954; *Illustrated London News*, 9 December 1854.
56 Hospital Commission Report, p.5.
57 Hall to QMG, 19 November 1854; RAMC: 397/F/CO/1/1/934; TNA: WO 28/196; Supplies Commission Report, p.161; and Royal Commission Report, Appendix LXXIX, p.103.
58 *Medical and Surgical History*, 1, p.301.

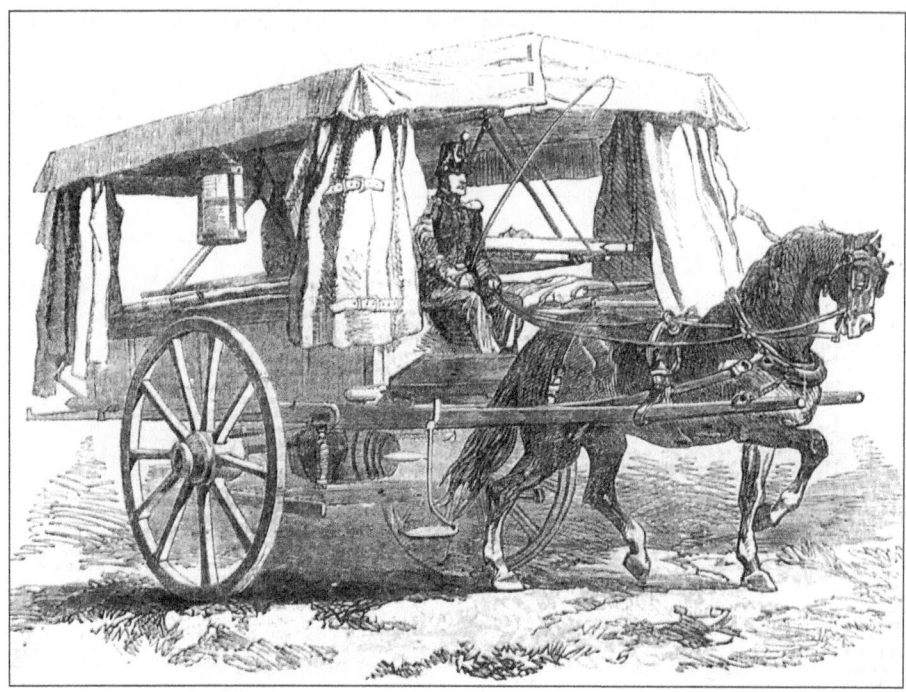

Figure 4.5 Ambulance for the wounded. (*Illustrated London News*, 30 December 1854, p.693)

cattle rendered the ambulance arabas at Headquarters inoperable as they could not be immediately replaced.[59] Surprisingly, perhaps, Hall's request to use buffaloes a few months later for a 'want of horses' was refused.[60]

After Inkerman, Hall requested that spare Commissariat waggons should be used to convey the sick,[61] and, although Raglan was in favour it proved unworkable because of the need to supply rations with the limited transport the Commissariat had available.[62] In December RA waggons and horses were employed to assist with relieving the sick list,[63] but this was not sufficient, and Hall was placed in the humiliating position

---

59 Hall to QMG, 29 November 1854; RAMC: 397/F/CO/1/4/975 and TNA: WO 28/196. Another problem in this regard was the slaughter for human consumption of bullocks used to tow the hospital wagon as recorded in a transcript in the author's procession of a letter written by Assistant Surgeon J.I.P. Williams, 1st Battalion, Rifle Brigade, on 1 October 1854. The original letters, together with Williams's medals, were sold by DNW on 27 June 2012.
60 Hall to QMG, 3 February 1855; TNA: WO 28/140 & 176.
61 Hall to QMG, 5 November 1854; RAMC: 397/F/CO/1/1/865 and TNA: WO 28/196.
62 Medical Department Memorandum, 25 November and PMO, 4th Division to Hall, 26 November 1854; Royal Commission Report, Appendix LXXIX, pp.162–3.
63 Medical Department Memorandum, 9 December 1854; RAMC: 397/F/CO/1/3.

of having to 'get a loan of the French ambulance' because he had no alternative 'as relief is now of the most vital importance [and] we shall be glad to avail ourselves of it.'[64] (Figure 4.6) And just as well perhaps, as one surgeon opined on 12 December that if it had not been for the 'French Ambulance not a single man could be moved from the camp. The famous ambulance carriages [having] long since stopped work.'[65] In addition, some sick were carried to the port by regimental bât horses, officers' chargers, and cavalry horses[66] (Figure 4.7) with the involvement of the Cavalry Division being authorized officially when early in 1855 it was ordered to 'furnish horses daily until further orders to carry sick to Balaklava.'[67]

Herbert was informed by the AG [Estcourt] that 'the two-wheeled ambulance carts sway about, and are liable to upset on rough ground and are [...] inferior to your four-wheeled ones; but all our useless now that the roads became impassable [during November.]'[68] It is then that the French cacolets proved their worth (Figure 4.8). Hall informed Smith that mules fitted with packsaddles, chairs and reclining litters, were needed,[69] and this was also recommended by the Hospital Commissioners with the additional proviso that 'light vehicles like Irish jaunting cars to transport invalids' and ambulance waggons 'lighter than those sent out' should also be provided.[70] When Smith appreciated the circumstances he placed an order for '200 litters, 200 chairs, and 210 pack saddles be sent as soon as possible,' with the caveat: 'they should be sent when half the order is filled.'[71] Hall informed the QMG when he heard of this,[72] although this equipment did not arrive until the summer.

On receipt of a request from Smith dated 22 December Hall convened a committee comprising himself and three Divisional PMOs to consider the performance of the available ambulance conveyance. They were generally in favour of the French mule cacolets, although there was a tendency for them to sway, and there was risk of the animals stumbling or falling. The wheeled waggons available were considered too heavy, especially on poor roads after rain, and they recommended the ample provision of lighter waggons drawn by horses for men reclining, and Bianconi cars for patients

---

64   Hall to PMO, Light Division, 5 December 1854; Royal Commission Report, Appendix LXXIX, pp.107 & 148.
65   J.A. Bostock, *Letters from India and the Crimea* (London: George Bell, 1897), pp.213–4.
66   Evidence to the Supplies Commissioners; Supplies Commission Report, pp.115, 145 & 383.
67   AG to GOC, Cavalry Division, 19 January 1855; TNA: WO 28/108.
68   Herbert to Smith, 24 December 1855; Select Committee, 4th Report, pp.343–4.
69   Hall to Smith, 20 December 1854; RAMC: 397/F/CO/1/1/1148; Smith, *Précis of Letters*; and Supplies Commission Report, pp.169–70.
70   Hospital Commission Report, pp.5–6.
71   A total of 122 pairs of litters, 74 pairs of chairs, and 55 cars were sent to the East in 10 vessels between 7 April and 25 August 1855; Store Department, Pall Mall to Smith, 7 September1855; Smith, *Précis of Letters*.
72   Smith to Ordnance Office, 16 January 1855; Smith, *Précis of Letters* and Hall to QMG, 5 February 1855; RAMC: 397/F/CO/1/1/1396.

146 Victory Over Disease

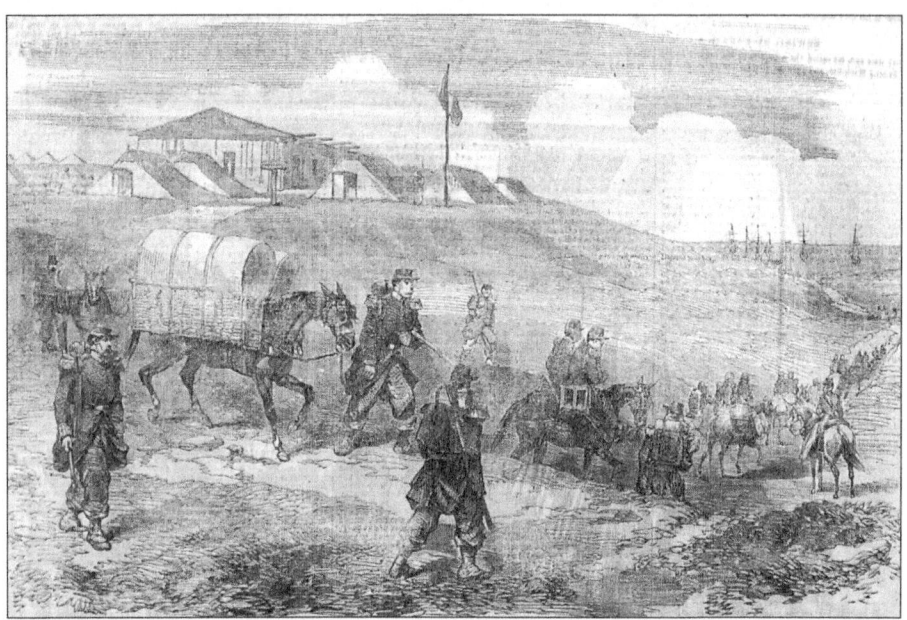

Figure 4.6 French ambulances, before Sebastopol. (*Illustrated London News*, 16 December 1854, p.625)

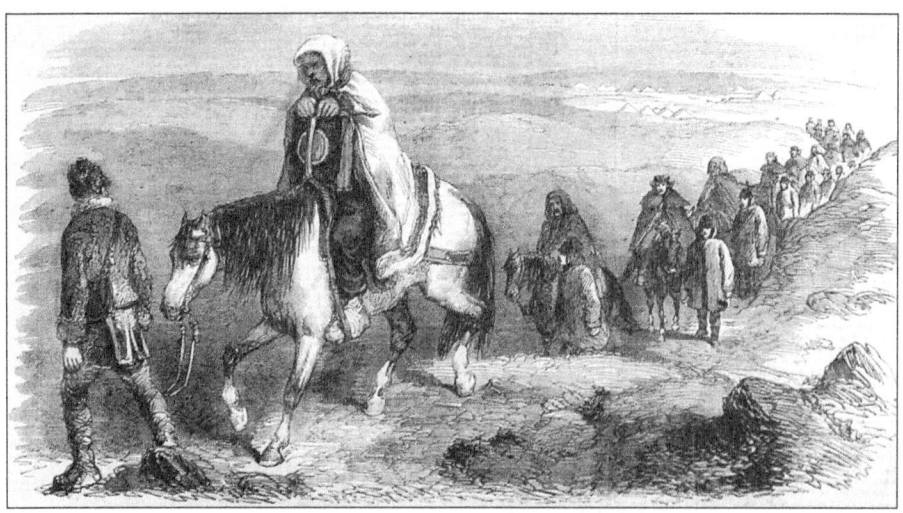

Figure 4.7 Carrying the frost bitten to Balaclava. (*Illustrated London News*, 3 March 1855, p.213)

Transportation and evacuation of invalids 147

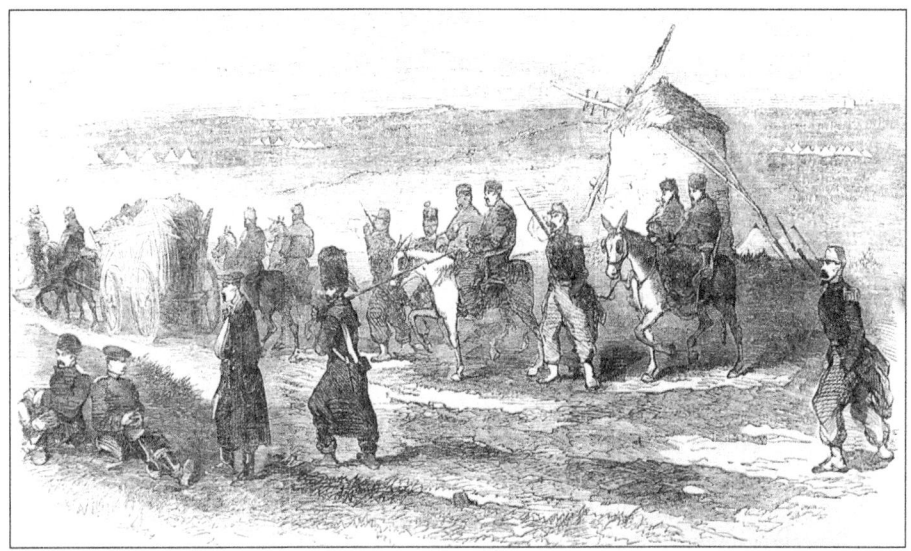

Figure 4.8 French cacolets carrying wounded before Sebastopol. (*Illustrated London News*, 27 January 1855, p.80)

who can sit.[73] They also stressed that men operating the service should have knowledge of horses as there were few effective drivers and not one who could shoe a horse or repair a damaged waggon.[74]

When military activity increased during the spring Hall found it necessary to call the QMG's attention to:

> the state of the ambulance wagons [...] In the event of an engagement with the enemy we have not a single ambulance wagon efficient, and beyond canvas bearers no means of carrying the wounded off the field, and to have them exposed at this season would seal their doom.[75]

It is understandable that Hall should have taken such a pessimistic view given that at the end of May the AC could only muster transport for 308 patients, and then only if unsuitable waggons or those out of repair were included.[76] The French Army, in contrast, provided 250 mule seats and five vans for each 10,000 men.[77]

---

73 The passengers were seated on benches arranged along the side of the carriage with them looking outwards.
74 Hall to Smith, 20 January 1855; RAMC: 397/F/CO/1/1/1350 and TNA: WO 1/374/313 (Copy).
75 Hall to QMG, 11 February 1855; RAMC: 397/F/CO1/1/1424.
76 TNA: WO 1/374/313/No. 2, 24 May & No. 3, 31 May 1855.
77 *North Wales Chronicle*, 4 November 1854, quoting the *Spectator*.

Following a request from Panmure[78] a Committee comprising Hall and an officer from the RA and LTC was convened and their recommendations included, inter alia, an 'extension of the mule litter and chair and Irish car conveyance' and the provision of a 'lighter [...] spring carriage on four wheels for [...] four wounded men in recumbent posture.' The Committee also concluded that 'mixed conveyance for reclining and sitting patients [was] objectionable' and that the limit for any conveyance should be four.'[79] This report, and associated documents, was forwarded to London together with a summary by Raglan: 'It is difficult to fix on the most eligible form of hospital carriage, so many different opinions existing on it. The carriage should be light with four wheels, with a canopy and curtain overhead. It should only contain four men, and there should be a space underneath for their accoutrements and packs. It should be drawn by horses abreast.'[80]

Fortunately the British forces had no further major contact with the Russian field army,[81] and just as well perhaps, because even after the fall of Sevastopol Hall concluded that the Corps was still 'imperfectly organized and would not work well if the Army was to take the field.' The AC was eventually subsumed into the LTC on 31 December 1855, and from then on it was involved essentially on garrison duty.

The AC was under the control of the QMG initially and medical officers had to apply to his staff for transport to be provided. Inevitably this layer of bureaucracy was considered unsatisfactory by Smith who considered that divisional PMOs were the best judge of an invalid's needs, and should be able to apply directly for ambulances without reference to an AQMG.[82] Panmure subsequently instructed that this policy should be adopted,[83] and when Hall heard he also stressed that 'the demands made by the Inspectors of Hospitals on the Ambulance branch [...] should be attended to without reference to any other authority.'[84] The matter was finally concluded when the AG ordered that requisitions for medical conveyance signed by a 'superior' medical officer could be sent direct to the Divisional Transport Officer without reference to the AQMG.[85]

Hall also considered that it 'would be advantageous to have a due proportion of the ambulance attached to each Division, such an arrangement will have to be made if the Army takes to the field, and perhaps it will be as well to have it carried into effect at once.'[86] The DG of the LTC agreed with this, but only when staffing levels permitted.[87]

---

78 Panmure to Raglan, 7 May 1855; TNA: WO 6/70/111.
79 Hall to AG, 25 May 1855; RAMC: 397/F/CO/1/2/2177 and TNA: WO 1/374/313 (Copy).
80 Raglan to Panmure, 4 June 1855; TNA: WO 1/374/313.
81 The British Army was not involved in the battle of the Tchernaya.
82 Smith to Military Secretary, 17 & 31 July 1855; Smith, *Précis of Letters*.
83 Panmure to Simpson, 11 August 1855; TNA: WO 6/71/88.
84 Hall to Military Secretary, 26 August 1855; RAMC: 397/F/CO/1/2/3000.
85 AG, Memorandum, 3 September1855; TNA: WO 28/175.
86 Hall to Military Secretary, 26 August 1855; RAMC: 397/F/CO/1/2/3000.
87 Memorandum prepared by the DG, LTC, 31 August 1855; TNA: WO 28/175.

The evacuees: It was the responsibility of regimental surgeons to ensure that 'no men unable to bear removal are sent away,'[88] while Raglan desired 'great care be taken that the whole of this service be well performed.'[89] The PMOs were enjoined to ascertain that there was room for patients in the hospital before applying for transport from camp,[90] while the Commandant at Balaklava made the important, and seemingly obvious request: 'Unless a distinction is made [...] between the sick and wounded it is impossible to make the necessary arrangements for the conveyance of the wounded to the sanatorium, each wounded man requiring five men to carry him up to the hospital.'[91]

The ever practical Hall ordered that the men should have breakfast before departure and take their blanket and great coat with them. The accompanying medical officer was to carry restoratives (spirits and wine) and a small cup,[92] while the AG specified that three fatigue men were required to place a man on a mule, one to hold the opposite side of the litter, and two to lift the sick man.[93] Incidentally, some months later a medical officer commented on his role in this duty:

> Our [...] wounded [are sent] to Balaclava in [...] ambulance carts [with] an assistant surgeon [...] We rather like the job as it saves us trench duty. [...] It is drawn by four mules and the surgeon rides alongside clears the road of Turkish donkey carts and uses his authority in monopolising the whole road.[94]

Towards the end of 1854 the men evacuated to Scutari were 'ragged and destitute of clothing' despite there being 'a quantity of warm clothing in Balaklava.'[95] This was confirmed by the Commandant there who noted that the patients were 'lousy and naked.'[96] In order to rectify this problem the AG instructed that the sick should take their knapsacks with them, and if they lacked warm clothing it should be issued.[97] A few weeks later Brigadier Paulet [Commandant on the Bosphorus] reported that though the 'sick came down better than they did' there was still room for improvement

---

88 PMO, 4th Division to Regimental Surgeons; Royal Commission Report, Appendix LXXIX, p.170.
89 AG to Sir J. Campbell, 13 December 1854; Royal Commission Report, Appendix LXXIX, p.166.
90 AG to OC, Cavalry Division, 11 May 1855; TNA: WO 28/109
91 Commandant, Balaklava to AG, 10 April 1855; TNA: WO 28/194.
92 Medical Department Memorandum, 10 December 1854; RAMC: 397/F/CO/1/3 and Royal Commission Report, Appendix LXXIX. pp.108 & 165.
93 AG's Memorandum, 10 December 1854; TNA: WO 28/122 and Royal Commission Report, Appendix LXXIX, p.165.
94 Assistant Surgeon D. Greig, letter, 15 June 1855; Hill, *Letters from the Crimea*, p.93.
95 Nightingale to Raglan, 29 December 1854; National Army Museum: 1968-07-293-9.
96 Paulet to Romaine, 7 January 1855; Robins, *Romaine's Crimean War*, p.66.
97 AG's Memorandum, 3 January 1855; TNA: WO 28/122.

as some still were without clothing,[98] a situation that was confirmed by Nightingale.[99] The subsequent arrival of sufficient clothes for the troops favoured a resolution of the problem and the QMG was informed that clothing in Balaklava had been sent to Scutari for the benefit of men who had already been evacuated.[100]

The railway: The first use of the railway for invalids was recorded by Russell on 2 April 1855: 'The first human cargo [...] was sent down to Balaklava to-day [...] in less than half an hour. The men were propped up on their knapsacks, and seemed very comfortable. What a change from the ghastly processions [...] some weeks ago, formed of dead or dying men, hanging from half-starved horses, or dangling about on French mule-litters!'[101]

The railway was used regularly up to twice a day for this purpose if ships were in harbour,[102] while it was also used to convey convalescents from Balaklava back to camp.[103] There is no evidence that waggons were adapted as ambulances though this was probably unnecessary as the opening of the Camp General Hospital in April 1855 and improvements in the regimental hospitals meant seriously injured patients could be treated in camp and not transferred to Balaklava and beyond.

Incidentally, Hall was also pleased that it meant that more malt liquor could be delivered to the camp, and this 'would be better for the men than spirits,'[104] while conversely McMurdo noted that the conveyance of the sick retarded the transport of ammunition to the front,[105] though if this became a pressing issue road transport could be used so that the turn round of the trucks was not delayed by the loading and unloading of patients.[106]

4.2.4 Preparation of vessels as hospital transports
Hospital ships were a source of considerable vexation for Hall during the first four months of the campaign,[107] presumably as most were employed on an ad hoc basis. The time between their selection by the AoT and sailing was frequently too short for them to be suitably modified. A problem compounded by the inadequate resources in Balaklava given that the Roebuck Committee was informed that it took 10–14 days

---

98 Paulet to Raglan, 20 January 1855; National Army Museum: 1968-07-393-8.
99 Raglan to QMG, 14 February 1855; TNA: WO 28/192.
100 DAQMG, Balaklava to QMG, 14 February 1855; TNA: WO 28/192.
101 *The Times*, 18 April 1855.
102 DAQMG to QMG, 8 June 1855; TNA: WO 28/192.
103 For example AG, Balaklava to GOC, Balaklava defences, 3 April 1855; TNA: WO 28/108.
104 Hall to AG, 21 March 1855; RAMC: 397/F/CO/1/1/1672.
105 DG, LTC to QMG, 10 June 1855; TNA: WO 28/175.
106 See for example DG, LTC to QMG, 10 June 1855, with an annotation by Raglan; TNA: WO 28/175.
107 Mitra, *Life and Letters*, p.349. Mitra continued 'for in Dr Hall's diary repeated mention is made of his fruitless applications for the speedy fitting up of such vessels.'

to fit a ship with standing berths or cots.[108] In addition, supplying transports placed a strain on AMD's limited supplies,[109] especially if bedding and other equipment was not returned to Balaklava.[110]

The QMG requested the AoT to nominate the hospital ships as the need arose. He also asked that at least 24 hours notice be given of the intended departure time.[111] Conversely, the AoT stressed the desirability of the early appointment of medical officers, with the required medicines, comforts, etc.[112]

Early in December Hall stressed once again the absolute necessity of having large and commodious steamers' to 'run regularly between Balaklava and Scutari.'[113] The issue was obviously appreciated at HQ since the AG privately informed the AG in London that:

> We must have two or three vessels fitted up, steamers as hospital ships, on board which should be officers, purveyors, and orderlies always living. [...] We are continually sending sick men to Scutari. Work as hard as they will the Medical Officers cannot keep things decent, much less clean as they ought to be. The sick are laid on the deck [...] often without a bed. [In addition there is a need for] a corps of orderlies at a rate of one to 10, the regulation rate [...] and surgeons.[114]

Fortunately Raglan agreed, and after negotiations with the AoT Hall was requested to nominate permanent medical officers to serve on *Australian*, *Brandon*, *Melbourne*, and *Sydney*.[115] The vessels were fitted up in Constantinople, including provision of standing beds and a surgery.[116] Three were ready by 12 February,[117] while *Severn* was also adapted for hospital use in England.[118] Nearly a month later Russell noted that there were more patients requiring evacuation than these vessels could carry, despite

---

108 Select Committee, 3rd Report, pp.303–5.
109 Hall to Smith, 23 February 1855; RAMC: 397/F/CO/1/1/1519.
110 Dumbreck to PMO, Scutari, 22 October 1854; RAMC: 397/F/CO/1/1/802.
111 QMG to AoT, 4 December 1854; TNA: WO 28/137.
112 AoT to QMG, 7 October 1854; TNA: WO 28/196.
113 Hall to QMQ, 4 December 1854, RAMC: 397/F/CO/1/1/1017; TNA: WO 28/196; and Royal Commission Report, Appendix LXXIX, pp.107–8. Incidentally, on 1 December Paulet recommended to Raglan that 'it would be advisable to fit up and provide with bedding three or four ships and retain them solely for moving the sick and taking back those fit for duty; National Army Museum: 1968–07–293–8.
114 Estcourt to AG, Horse Guards, 3 December 1854; National Army Museum: 1962–10–95.
115 QMG to Hall, 23 December and Hall to QMG, 24 December 1854; TNA: WO 28/137 and RAMC: 397/F/CO/1/1166.
116 AoT to QMG. 21 December 1854; TNA: WO 28/196 and Boxer to QMG, 27 February 1855; TNA: WO 28/183.
117 Russell, 12 February; *The Times*, 24 February 1855.
118 *The Times*, 21 January 1855. The Admiralty informed Admiral Lyons on 19 March that *Severn* had been 'fitted up' and that ship's surgeon was to be paid £100 p.a. to assist with the medical care of the patients; ADM 2/1317.

about 1,200 being transported in the previous three weeks, but things must have eased thereafter as only 725 were evacuated during the next three weeks.[119]

Soon after the invasion, written instructions were issued to medical officers employed on hospital ships.[120] While it appeared that the PMO at Balaklava was solely responsible for inspecting vessels for invalids until 12 December 1854, when a General Order directed that inspections were to be undertaken by a Board comprising the Commandant of Balaklava, the DAQMG and PMO doing duty there, an Assistant Commissary General, and the Transport Agent or his deputy. With the exception of the last mentioned, 'this Board is constituted in conformity with the regulations of the service.'[121] The Board was required to obtain the following information during an inspection, viz. the number of invalids and medical officers, and their rank; the state of the bedding and accommodation of the sick; conveniences for the sick, including utensils, drinking cups, mess tins, etc.; cooking facilities; the number of WCs, and their state of repair; ventilation; and the supply of medical stores and comforts, groceries etc. and any other points which might be relevant.[122]

It is possible that the General Order of 12 December was issued when HQ appreciated that the Queen's Regulations had been overlooked for several months,[123] although this did not inhibit Raglan from unfairly admonishing Hall and Dr R. Lawson, the PMO at Balaklava, in a General Order of the 13 December (see the summary of the *Avon* affair below), or from informing Paulet of these developments thus: 'The state of the *Avon* was too shocking and here I had a Court of Enquiry upon it. The report [...] rendered it necessary for me to give a strong order for the examination of them [before] being used [...] for the sick and [so] ensure the poor sufferers being more comfortable in future on their passage across the Black Sea.'[124]

The General Order of the 12 December was supplemented by a more specific Medical Department Order which enjoined medical officers on hospital transports to:

> pay [...] attention to the cleanliness, ventilation and fumigation [...] see the sick are as comfortably accommodated as circumstances will permit [...] the food is of good quality and properly cooked [...] the men [should] receive any medical comforts used [...] make out a nominal roll of men embarked with details of disease etc. which will be handed over to the principal medical officer at Scutari. [...] The orderlies should be divided into three watches.[125]

---

119 Russell, 19 March; *The Times*, 3 April 1855 and *Medical and Surgical History*, 2, pp.470–1.
120 Dumbreck to Tice, 19 October 1854; RAMC: 397/F/CO/1/1/795. (The text was not reproduced.)
121 Hospital Commission Report, pp.16 & 335. The requirement for a Commissary Officer was rescinded in a General Order of 18 October 1855.
122 QMG to Major Mackenzie, 7 December 1854; TNA: WO 28/196
123 *Queen's Regulations* (1844), p.325.
124 Raglan to Paulet, 15 December 1854; National Army Museum: 6807/393/8.
125 RAMC: 397/F/CO/1/3.

Problems encountered on hospital ships included insufficient notice being given to the AMD;[126] a change in the vessel after embarkation had commenced which resulted in 'added discomfort for the sick as it [was] almost impossible to fit up [alternative] ships at a few hours notice;'[127] a shortage of available medical officers; insufficient orderlies and sea sickness or illness amongst them while en route; a lack of cooperation from the civilian crew, for example, drawing of water or assistance with the invalids;[128] and delays in the vessels return from Scutari because of difficulties in obtaining coal and water.[129]

4.2.5 Embarkation of patients at Balaklava

When Dumbreck forwarded his reaction to the General Order of 14 October 1854 to Smith he pointed out that embarking patients in a poorly equipped and cramped harbour was a 'vexatious [task] that has brought considerable obloquy on the department, deservedly, or not,'[130] and he was not alone in finding the task 'a most troublesome business.'[131]

The extremely unsatisfactory state in the port and town of Balaklava was described graphically by Mrs Henry Duberly on 28 November and 3 December,[132] and *The Times* correspondent on 1 December.[133] At this time Lawson informed Hall that the increased number of vessels in the harbour made it difficult to embark the sick from the place then in use, and suggested developing a location on the West side that would allow the patients to be embarked directly if a small jetty was built and the approach roads were improved.[134] He also requested that notice should be given at least the evening before of the expected arrival of patients so that arrangements can be made for their reception, and that they should be despatched to arrive before sunset. Hall subsequently ordered that 'Sick [...] must not be sent off until Dr Lawson [...] has been warned [...] for the number is too great for any ordinary means to meet.'[135] The difficulty in embarking patients under these circumstances was also outlined by the Hospital Commissioners:

---

126 Hall to Smith, 16 December 1854; RAMC: 397/F/CO/1/1/1095 and Smith, *Précis of Letters*.
127 Hall to QMG, 29 January 1855; RAMC: 397/F/CO/1/1/1358.
128 Medical officers evidence to the Hospital Commissioners, 8 & 12 December 1854; Hospital Commission Report, pp.302 & 201.
129 Despatch, 12 October; *The Times*, 26 October 1854.
130 Dumbreck to Smith, 12 October 1854; RAMC: 397/F/CO/1/1/753 and Smith, *Précis of Letters*.
131 Assistant Surgeon Taylor, letter, 11 December 1854; *Journal of the Royal Services Institution* (1957), pp.234–5.
132 C. Kelly (ed.), *Mrs Duberly's War* (Oxford: University Press, 2007), pp.109–10 & 118.
133 *The Times*, 18 December 1854.
134 Lawson to Hall, 27 November 1854; TNA: WO 28/196. Hall referred this to the QMG who did not object to the proposal; RAMC: 397/F/CO/1/1/947 and TNA: WO 28/975.
135 Hall to PMO, Cavalry Division, 1 December 1854; RAMC: 397/F/CO/1/1/989.

> The sick and wounded [are] taken to the wharf, where a medical officer [sees] to their embarkation, and to afford medical assistance when necessary. The men are embarked in boats, under the orders of a naval officer, and put on board the vessels [...] Except in [one] instance (involving Dr Tice), we did not hear of any delay having arisen, beyond that incidental to the necessarily slow process of embarking a large number of helpless men in a limited number of open boats, and transhipping them to larger vessels.[136]

William Simpson's water colour of the embarkation of invalids directly from the beach at Balaklava has resulted in the assumption by some commentators that the procedure was always thus. However, the port facilities were improved gradually and by the end of January 'a pier had been constructed for the embarkation of the sick and wounded,'[137] 'planks were set across the road [...] so patients and orderlies did not have to walk through mud,' and an application was made for a hut on the wharf for the accommodation of the sick,[138] a very necessary development in the view of Russell and the PMO, Balaklava:

> Russell: There they lie just as they were let gently down on the ground by [...] their comrades, who brought them on their backs from camp with the greatest tenderness, but who are not allowed to remain with them. The sick appear to be tended by the sick, and the dying by the dying.[139]

> PMO: [...] a little more comfort to the sick [who are] brought down [on] mules, from which they are very hurriedly dismounted [and the] poor creatures are left sitting either in the mud or on any convenient plank. The tent on the other side of the road is much too far off [...] and I [...] suggest the immediate erection of one or two wooden huts close to the wharf, to be provided with benches, stove, etc. so that the more exhausted might have shelter, till they could be conveyed on board ship.[140]

Improvements obviously continued to be made and by the time the Sanitary Commissioners arrived at the beginning of April 1855 they found:

> there was a jetty [which was] nearly on the same level as the side of the boat into which the sick were placed [and this] was always done with great care. [...] the

---

136 Hospital Commission Report, p.16. It would appear that the Commissioners may have been misinformed on this point.
137 Elphinstone, *Journal*, pp.79–81.
138 AG to Commandant, Balaklava, 25 January 1855; TNA: WO 28/108 and Hall to QMG, 3 February 1855; RAMC: 397/F/CO/1/1/1379.
139 Despatch, 1 December; *The Times*, 18 December 1855.
140 PMO, Balaklava to Commandant, 23 January 1855; Supplies Commission Report, p.203.

boat was rowed [to] the 'sick ship'. [...] The sick who were able [...] walked up the ladder [while] those on stretchers were lifted on board by a simple contrivance, [which was] hoisted [...] by means of a pulley, and kept in a horizontal position. [...] the stretcher was carried below, by two men, and the patient transferred to a swing cot. [...] this method [could be] simplified by bringing the ambulances down to the shore under the stern of the 'sick ship', and by having, a brow constructed by which the sick might be carried directly on board. [Raglan] authorized the construction of the works on the 21st April, 1855, but the pressure of the siege operations [meant it was not completed until] the end of the year. During the whole period the Commissioners had every reason to be satisfied with the careful and considerate manner with which the duty of embarking the sick was performed by the officer in charge.[141]

4.2.6 Employment of hospital transports

The *Medical and Surgical History* included a return of 187 voyages made by 66 vessels in which the sick and wounded were evacuated from the Crimea to Turkey following the landing of the allied armies on 14 September 1854.[142] All were merchant ships except HMS *Vulcan*[143] and the details provided for each voyage included the vessel's name and tonnage; the number of officers and men who embarked and died during the voyage; the dates of departure and arrival; and the names of the medical officers on board. No distinction was made between sick and wounded patients until the 92nd voyage departing on 31 March 1855 while, the time taken for disembarkation was not provided for all voyages until much the same time. Each hospital transport was required to carry a regulation number of orderlies, usually under the command of a sergeant.[144] The number comprising this detail was given regularly from the 6 March (83rd departure).

The first vessels (*Kangaroo* towing *Dunbar*)[145] left the Crimea on 17 September while the last departed on 4 June 1856. The majority of patients were disembarked

---

141 Sanitary Commission Report, pp.145–7.
142 *Medical and Surgical History*, 2, pp.465–477. Pages 478–80 provide details of vessels transporting patients to Abydos (5 voyages), Smyrna (10) and Renkioi (10). Twenty of the 25 were from the Crimea and were included within the listings on pp.469–477. The other five departed from Varna (1) or Turkey (4) have been omitted from the foregoing analyses.
143 Shepherd, *Crimean Doctors*, 1, p.137 pointed out that HMS *Vulcan*, being a naval vessel, would have been better stocked with stores and medical equipment than the civilian transports.
144 The ratio one orderly to 25 patients was set by the military authorities; AG to Lieutenant Colonel Daveney, 15 December 1855; RAMC: 397/F/CO/6/17 and TNA: WO 28/122.
145 A report from Scutari recorded *Kangaroo* and *Dunbar* had 600 and 500 sick on board respectively; *The Times*, 9 October 1854. The official numbers given in the *Medical and Surgical History*, 2, p.465 were 452 and 357 respectively with 23 (5.1 percent) and 22 (6.2 percent) men dying during the voyage.

at Scutari, though from December 1854 until February 1885 hospitals at Abydos and Smyrna were utilized respectively with the hospital at Renkioi receiving patients from October 1855. In all 887 officers and 28,904 NCOs and men were evacuated on sailing vessels (44 voyages) and steamers (143), and of these 12 (1.5 percent) and 1,292 (4.5 percent) respectively died during the voyage.[146]

Expressing the results on a monthly basis takes no account of military situation and accordingly further analyses will consider the voyages in the following categories: Phase I: after landing in the Crimea (3 voyages); Phase II: after the battle of the Alma (8); Phase III: before Sevastopol, October 1854 (2); Phase IV: after the battle of Balaklava (7); Phase V: after the battle of Inkerman (6); Phase VI: winter Period 1, mid-November to mid-December when the formal survey of hospital transports was ordered (9); Phase VII: winter Period 2, mid-December to the mid-February 1855 when a General Order authorized the issuing of lime juice to all troops (34);[147] Phase VIII: spring and summer campaign, February to 17 September 1855 (84); and Phase IX: occupation of Sevastopol until the final evacuation (34).

Of the 187 voyages 143 (76 percent) were made by 41 steamers and 44 (24 percent) by 25 sailing vessels. Up until mid-December sailing vessels and steamers were used almost equally (19 and 16 respectively) but thereafter steamers predominated, and thus provided a more reliable service. Only one sailing vessel (*Gomelza*) departed between 13 January and 13 June 1855, while none were used after 3 December 1855, presumably because bad weather could be expected.

New vessels were engaged during all phases of the campaign with 23 (92 percent) of the 25 sailing vessels and 32 (78 percent) of the 41 steamers being employed for the first time by the end of Phase VII in mid-February. Fifty-five (83 percent) of the 66 hospital vessels had been engaged by the end of phase VII although only 77 (41 percent) of the 187 voyages had been completed. Conversely, only eleven new vessels were employed during the remaining 16 months, presumably to replace those in need of repair or whose contract had terminated.

Almost half (93 of 187) of the voyages involved vessels used only once or twice, while nearly a third (57 of 187) were made in those making six trips or more, with a maximum of 22.

A total of 39 (59 percent) and 13 (20 percent) of the 66 ships were used only once or twice respectively with 44 (85 percent) of vessels in these categories having sailed by mid-February 1855 (Phase VII) with five of the remainder being engaged after the siege was over. Only three of the 25 sailing vessels completed more than three voyages while nine (22 percent) of the 41 steamers were employed between six and 22 times.

---

146 The total mortality among those embarked would be higher than this figure as those dying after arrival would have been included in the hospital returns.
147 It is not implied that lime juice caused the reduced mortality, rather it provides evidence that the standard of living of the troops had definitely improved by that time and worst of the privations of the winter were over.

Officers went on board ship for the 'recruitment of the health' but it was not until the summer of 1855 that Panmure desired 'that arrangements should be made with the naval authorities that [...] accommodation may be prepared on board ship [...] as floating hospitals for 500 to 600 men.' The Port Admiral was requested to 'name vessels for this service,' and to take care there was sufficient room allowed between cots for medical officers to attend the patients. Several vessels were fitted up within a few days despite a shortage of carpenters, and provided for 921 patients, together with 426 additional beds in the hospitals.[148] It has not been established how much use was made of these vessels though some were later employed on the shuttle service to Turkey.

4.2.7 Mortality among evacuees

Mortality during the voyage was high after the Alma (13 percent of 2,582 evacuees). This is not surprising given that the transfer of the wounded to the shore was undertaken with considerable difficulty and unnecessary suffering as the British position was several miles from the coast, and there were no ambulance waggons. Personnel from the Royal Navy assisted with the task[149] and superintended the embarkation of the wounded,[150] and hence Hall, who would have been fully employed on the battlefield, concluded that 'it was the Naval Authorities' fault that the vessels were overcrowded.'

The mortality was much reduced to four percent in the weeks up until the battle of Inkerman (Phases III-V); it then increased during the first part of the winter when the health of the Army had deteriorated considerably (Phase VI: 14.9 percent of 1,527 evacuees). However, mortality was lower during the second winter period at six percent (Phase VII) despite the rate increasing among the troops in camp until January, which suggests that, inter alia, there had been selection for less critically ill patients coupled with improved conditions on the ships following the issuing of the General Order of 12 December.

Overall, nearly a third of 1,292 ship-board deaths occurred on thirteen vessels departing before mid-October 1854 (Phases I-III) while the evacuation of invalids following the battles of the Alma, Balaklava, and Inkerman was completed by 11 November 1854 (26th voyage). By that time 6,597 (23 percent) of the invalids had been evacuated with nearly half (3,200, 48 percent) being conveyed in sailing vessels, compared to 13.5 percent (3,047) for the remainder of the campaign. All but about

---

148 QMG to Admiral Lyons, 30 March, QMG to Boxer, 30 March & 1 April, DAQMG to QMG, 4 April, and AQMG to QMG, 10 April 1855; TNA: WO 28/192. The vessels included *Ottawa* (100 evacuees), *Severn* (140), *Australian* (100 if not full of platforms), *St Hilda* (91), *Wm Jackson* (110), *Orient* (110), *Robert Lowe* (100), *Poieties* (100), HMS *Leander* (50), HMS *Wasp* (20), and *Ottawa* (100).
149 Dr J. Rea to Dundas, 8 November 1854; Wiltshire and Swindon History Centre: 2057/F8/IV/D/1h: The naval personnel sent ashore comprised 30 medical officers and 1,000 seamen and marines.
150 Hall to Spence, 10 November 1854; Smith, *Précis of Letters*, 1, Appendix 2, pp.689–701.

five percent of deaths had been recorded by the end of January, viz. the end of Phase VII, although by that time only 77 (42 percent) of voyages had been completed and 7,826 (55.2 percent) of the patients had been evacuated (calculated from Table 4.2).

Table 4.2 Number of hospital ships departing from the Crimea during different phases of the campaign, September 1854–June 1856

Phase of the campaign		No. of departures			No. of men			
					evacuated		dying (% of evacuees)	
Event	Dates	Sail	Steam	Total	Sail	Steam	Sail	Steam
I After landing	17–20 Sept. 1854	1	2	3	350	744	22 (6.3)	48 (6.5)
II After the Alma	21–30 Sept.	5	3	8	1,388	1,194	278 (20.0)	63 (5.3)
III Before Sevastopol	1–13 Oct.	2	0	2	462	0	14 (3.0)	0
IV After Balaklava	14–31 Oct.	4	3	7	588	524	45 (7.7)	18 (3.4)
V After Inkerman	1–11 Nov.	2	4	6	412	905	14 (3.4)	26 (2.9)
VI Winter Period 1*	12 Nov.–11 Dec.	5	4	9	650	887	126 (19.4)	102 (11.5)
VII Winter Period 2†	12 Dec.–16 Feb. 1855	8	34	42	1,105	6,721	182 (16.5)	301 (4.5)
VIII Spring and summer campaign	17 Feb.–17 Sep.	13	63	76	1,076	8,086	14 (1.3.)	27 (0.3)
IX After the siege	18 Sep.–4 June 1856	4	30	34	217	3,575	3 (1.4)	9 (0.25)
Whole campaign		44	143	187	6,248	22,656	698	594

* Up until a General Order of 12 December 1854 regulated inspection of hospital transports.
† Up until a General Order of 16 February 1855 authorized the issued of lime juice to all troops. (This date was chosen arbitrarily as evidence that conditions for the troops were improving in the Crimea; clearly the issuing of lime juice would not in itself have been responsible for reducing the mortality on the hospital ships.) There were no departures between 13–26 October, 1–6 November 1854, and 18–26 September 1855 respectively.

(Summarized from the *Medical and Surgical History*, 2, pp.465–77)

At least one medical officer was present on board each transport, with two, and 3–5 respectively, being employed on 95 (51 percent) and 20 (11 percent) of the 187 voyages. For the majority of voyages the names of the medical officers are listed although on 19 voyages from April 1855 the second member of the medical team was either a hospital dresser or a dispenser, viz. *Brandon* (seven voyages), *Imperador* (five), *Severn* (three), *Clifton* (one), and *Melbourne* (three). The sick and wounded were entered separately in the returns from 31 March 1855. Of 11,113 men evacuated thereafter only 719 (6.5 percent) were wounded, and it is likely they were not in a critical condition as only one died (0.14 percent), thus providing evidence that the policy from that time was to treat the most seriously wounded men in the Crimea.

Evacuees from infantry regiments: The numbers of men in the infantry regiments who died in general hospitals or on board ship tended to decrease as the time that the regiments spent on active service, although there was considerable variation in the various categories specified in Table 4.3. A similar pattern was also noted for the numbers of these patients who were invalided home.

Table 4.3 **The number of NCO and men in fifty-two infantry regiments who died in general hospitals and on board ship, and who were invalided home according to the month of arrival in the East**

Month of arrival (1854–55)	Number of regiments	Median (range) number of men dying in general hospitals or on board ship	Median (range) number men invalided home
April–June	25	150 (100–370)	262 (112–415)
July–September	6	159 (83–273)	203 (184–261)
October–December	9	81 (37–230)	186 (152–265)
January–March	3	34 (14–41)	106 (62–160)
April–June	6	10 (4–17)	118 (69–152)
July–September	3	4 (1–8)	65 (14–936)

(Column 3: *Medical and Surgical History*, 1, Regimental histories; Column 4: Sayer, *Despatches*, endpaper)

4.2.8 Disembarkation of patients at Scutari

The port facilities at Scutari were rudimentary initially and could only be used in calm weather as the comparatively shallow water precluded ships mooring along side the pier, and open boats and small steamers had to be employed to convey patients ashore.[151]

In addition to stormy weather delays in disembarkation were caused by swell and heavy seas resulting in waves breaking over the landing place; strong currents; late arrival in the day or after dark; the unavailability or late arrival of vessels for transferring patients to the shore;[152] and the want of hospital accommodation owing to overcrowding. The Hospital Commissioners were clearly sufficiently concerned to recommend that alternate hospital accommodation should be sought where 'embarkation and disembarkation [...] can at all times be effected without difficulty or danger;'[153] while the Hon. the Revd S.G. Osborne summarized the problems encountered at the pier head:

---

151 Hospital Commission Report, p.23.
152 The Admiralty informed the Under Secretary at the War Department on 26 February 1855 that 'active steps were being taken for despatching tugs to the Bosphorus' for 'landing the sick and wounded;' ADM 2/137.
153 Hospital Commission Report, p.51.

The nearest entrance to the Barrack Hospital is [about] a quarter of a mile from the so called pier [...] Passing [...] down a broad paved road for all passengers [...] for the stores [...] for the sick and wounded, in short for everything [...] so utterly inconvenient, and inadequate [...] If the wind blew [the surf] made landing next to impossible; in the ordinary breezes [...] the approach in anything but a large boat was dangerous [...] I have seen the bodies of the dead, stores for the living, munitions of war, sick men staggering from weakness, wounded men helpless on stretchers, invalid orderlies waiting to act as bearers, oxen yoked in arabas, officials [crowded] on this narrow inconvenient pier, exposed to drenching rain, and so bewildered [...] that the transaction of any one duty, was quite out of the question.[154]

Once ashore there is an uphill climb up to the Barrack, though Menzies the PMO considered the distance trifling,[155] with the stretcher cases being carried by fatigue parties or Turkish labourers.[156]

The pier at Scutari was extended by early December 1854.[157] Paulet was authorized by the government to further lengthen the pier to enable landing in nearly all weathers,[158] and that boats must be purchased and retained, with proper crews, for the use of the hospital.[159] The improvements, which involved the sinking of 9ft wooded piles to give a depth of water of 14ft[160] and the construction of a jetty of wood and stones,[161] meant that when they arrived the Sanitary Commissioners appeared generally satisfied with the care with which the invalids were disembarked.[162]

The pier nearest to the General Hospital was a little more sheltered but the route to the hospital was longer and steeper while the Kuleli hospital was the best served as it was on the shore of the Bosphorus and larger vessel could moor along side (see Figure 3.2).

4.2.9 Causes célèbre

The problems encountered on the voyages of several hospital ships received more prominence than others, and a summary involving three of them follows:

Colombo: The vessel sailed for Scutari on 22 September 1854 with one staff surgeon and three assistant naval surgeons to attend 27 officers and 453 men and,[163] though

---

154 Osborne, *Scutari*, p.7. Osborne referred to the unsatisfactory condition of the pier in his evidence to the Roebuck Committee; Select Committee, 2nd Report, pp.387–8.
155 Hospital Commission Report, p.303.
156 The barrack was 130ft above sea level.
157 Own Correspondent, 5 December; *The Times*, 21 December 1855.
158 For a plan see TNA: MPH 1/1133.
159 Newcastle to Paulet (Cabinet paper), 5 January 1855; TNA: WO 33/1/8/55; Wiltshire and Swindon History Centre: 2057/F8/III/C/65; and TNA: WO 6/70.
160 Elphinstone, *Journal*, p.292.
161 TNA: MPH 1/1133.
162 Sanitary Commission Report, pp.26–7.
163 *Medical and Surgical History*, 2, p.465.

conditions on board were extremely harrowing, the reports in the English newspapers were an exaggeration.[164] When Hall heard of these accounts he asked the surgeons for details and reported to Raglan on 11 November that: 'the medical officers [...] in charge of wounded [on *Colombo*] repudiate with indignation and scorn the statement in *The Times* of their inhumanity to the unfortunate people on board, and the story of maggots crawling about contaminating their food is pure fiction.'[165]

On 21 November, Hall received a further report from a naval surgeon which seemingly provided an account of the voyage, somewhere between the apparent overstatements in the press, and terse response that Hall made to Raglan:

> The scene on board [was] terrible. The [...] suffering [...] scarcely exaggerated. Such a lamentable state is [...] attributed mainly to the following perhaps unavoidable circumstances: (1) the ship being over crowded and the wounded kept a long time on board; (2) [insufficient] medical men [...] and (3) the want of medical stores. [...] The wounds having 'bred maggots' was owing [...] to the wounded having being exposed to the burning sun [and] the wounds not having been attended to for many hours [...] it was impossible from the paucity of assistance that [proper] attention could have been bestowed on each. There are some errors in the newspaper statement [...] there were a total of 591 souls, 30 of whom died. It is therefore absurd the state that 'the surgeons had to pick their way through the heaps of dying and dead.'[...] I consider the article [was written] to call the public attention to the system of conveying the wounded and the want of adequate surgical assistance in such an emergency than to throw aspersions on our characters individually.[166]

Hall was, nevertheless, sufficiently impressed with the ship's company in these circumstances that he subsequently informed Raglan that: 'It is a justice I owe to Dr Bourne, Captain Methuen, the officers and crew of the *Colombo* to bring under the notice of the Field Marshal the uniform kindness and attention shown to all sick and wounded soldiers.'[167]

Trent: Raglan admonished Hall in an 'angry memorandum' in which he inferred that the AMD 'cared little [of] what became of [the invalids]' because the *Trent* sailed for

---

164 For example, despatches dated 27 & 28 September; *Daily News* and *The Times*, 10 & 13 October 1854.
165 RAMC: 397/F/CO/1/1/901 and Wiltshire and Swindon History Centre: 2057/F8/III/B/324 (copy).
166 A.S. Wright, HMS *Leander*, to Hall, 21 November 1854; RAMC: 397/F/CO10/4.
167 Hall to Military Secretary, 11 February 1855; RAMC: 397/F/CO1/1/1423. Incidentally, there is a snuff box in the London Museum presented by Colonel Frederick Horn and officers of the 20th Regiment to James Smith of *Colombo* in appreciation of his services during the voyage to the East.

Scutari on 25 November 1854 with only two assistant surgeons on board and no staff surgeon. Hall subsequently pointed out that *Trent* was well founded and that the two 'intelligent and talented young men' were quite capable of 'taking medical charge' but owing to a shortage of medical officers 'not sending [a staff surgeon] was a matter of necessity, not choice on the part of Dr Lawson' and 'it would be desirable if this [deficiency in staffing] could be remedied.'[168]

Avon: Raglan received a complaint about the condition of a soldier in board *Avon* on 28 November 1854 and he instructed the AG and Hall to investigate. A committee of enquiry then placed the blame on Lawson, the PMO at Balaklava, although he had not been on trial, merely being called as a witness. Raglan then issued a General Order on 13 December, in which Lawson and Hall were castigated. They were never granted the right to reply to the allegations although Hall was later able to refute the suggestion that the vessel had not been properly equipped.

Lawson was replaced and transferred to Scutari by a General Order on 15 January 1855, but he was never brought to trial or allowed to see a copy of the proceedings by which he was condemned.[169] No reason for this was given for but it may have been that Raglan let the matter drop when he realized that the headquarters staff had disregarded the Queen's Regulation which stipulated that any ship used to transport troops should be inspected by both a staff officer and a medical officer.[170] The issue was regularized by a General Order dated 12 December and to which reference has been made.

4.2.10 Return to duty
It was imperative that convalescents should return to duty as soon as possible and shortly after the invasion men were returned to the Crimea in surprisingly large numbers. For example, *Himalaya* and HMS *Valorous* sailed from Scutari to Balaklava with 600 and 530 men on 16 October and 9 November 1854,[171] while Hall, who sailed on *Himalaya*, reported that about 1,700 had already rejoined since the beginning of the month.[172] Similarly, Stratford informed Clarendon that Boxer 'had sent up about [1,000 men] with the expectation of adding five or six hundred in two or three days,'[173] with a further 150 sailing on *Medina* the next month.[174]

168 Hall, diary, 17 December 1854; RAMC: 524/15/6.
169 Several commentators have suggested that Hall appointed Lawson to this post. However, this is incorrect as the move was confirmed by a General Order and thus had Raglan's approval.
170 *Queen's Regulations* (1844), p.325
171 TNA: ADM 7/576.
172 Hall to Smith, 20 Oct; Smith, *Précis of Letters* and Hall to Raglan, 27 October 1854; RAMC: 397/F/CO/1/1/819.
173 Stratford to Clarendon, 25 October 1854; TNA: FO 78/1004.
174 Paulet to AG, 8 & 14 January 1855; TNA: WO 28/186.

When the regular shuttle service to Scutari was instituted it was agreed with the naval authorities that the hospital ships should return empty to the Crimea. However, on occasions they were employed to convey healthy troops, an unsatisfactory policy as Hall sensibly pointed out:

> If duty men are embarked on board ships that have conveyed sick, the vessels should be well cleaned and fumigated before they go on board, and on no account should they be permitted to use the same equipment as the sick. This would detain the vessel two or more days at Constantinople and it would require as many at Balaklava before she would be in a fit state [to] embark sick again.'[175]

4.2.11 Concluding remarks

Many of the problems associated with the transport of the sick and wounded, either on land or at sea, resulted from the failure of the government and the military authorities to develop a comprehensive plan for this crucial activity.[176] In consequence, no advanced provision was made for either a suitably equipped and manned Ambulance Corps[177] or dedicated ships for use as hospital transports or floating hospitals.

The transfer of patients from camp to Balaklava took place almost daily and on occasions the lack of suitable transport caused considerable difficulties for the AMD who had to rely on assistance from the French.[178] Inevitably there were some local failures in communications which resulted in hardship for the patients. Matters improved during the spring of 1855 with improvements in the regimental hospitals, the opening of the railway, and the repairing of the roads.

Vessels employed for evacuating patients were selected on an ad hoc basis during the first three months of the campaign and inevitably many would have been unsatisfactory in terms of on-board facilities, equipment, and personnel. The service became more regular from mid-December when dedicated steamers began to provide a shuttle service across the Black Sea. This arrangement proved generally satisfactory as there was little adverse comment, apart from occasional problems associated with either embarkation or disembarkation.

Mortality on the voyage to Turkey was greatest during the first weeks following the invasion when many of the invalids were either severely wounded or suffering from cholera, or both. The death rate started to decrease after the turn of the year suggesting improvements in the management of patients on shore and afloat, and the need to send patients with a poor prognosis to Scutari becoming less pressing. From mid-February 1855 until the end of the campaign there were only 53 (0.4 percent)

---

175 QMG to Military Secretary, with a comment by Hall, 13 April 1855; TNA: WO 28/192.
176 For a discussion see Shepherd, *Crimean Doctors*, 2, pp.386–7.
177 It was near the end of 1855 before the Ambulance Corps was fully equipped with vehicles etc.; see Shepherd, *Crimean Doctors*, 2, p.463.
178 Hall to PMO, Scutari, 9 & 12 December 1854; RAMC: 397/F/CO/1/1/1040 & 1072.

deaths among the 11,905 patients evacuated thus confirming that during this time most of those evacuated would have been convalescents.

4.3 Repatriation to England

Invalids were repatriated prior to the invasion using several vessels, viz, HMS *Simoom, Niagara, Tonning,* HMS *Vulcan, Orinoco, Harbinger, Mangerton, Palmyra*,[179] and *Golden Fleece*[180] but this would have been more for convenience than necessity, and it was not until the departure of *Libertas* from Scutari on 16 October 1854[181] that matters became more pressing and hospital transports from the East began to arrive regularly in English ports, principally Portsmouth, from the beginning of 1855.[182] These events were reported in *The Times* and other newspapers and varied from one liners to accounts giving details of the voyage, the passengers, particularly officers,[183] and the various hospitals to which the invalids were distributed.

In February 1855 Smith suggested to the War Office that the sick and wounded should only be brought back to England in 'streamers with appropriate fittings' and they could not be transported at that time of year 'without risk of serious suffering from inclement or severe weather.'[184] The need to repatriate invalids during the second winter was less urgent though he advised once again that it would 'not be expedient to transport the sick and wounded back to this country [...] from the beginning of December to the following April,' and they should be treated at Scutari, Gozo, and Gibraltar.[185] Initially Panmure was 'unwilling to accede to this request as he wished they should return to England as usual,' although he subsequently changed his mind.[186]

The electric telegraph became available during the campaign, and although there is no evidence it was employed routinely by the AMD, its use allowed advanced warning if invalids needed hospitalization on arrival. For example, Smith informed the PMO,

---

179 *The Times*, 17 April, 5 & 30 May, 5 & 23 June, 2 & 9 August, and 6 October 1854. Incidentally, invalids brought home on HMS *Vulcan* and *Tonning* travelled to Dublin from Portsmouth in *Ajax*; *Isle of Wight Observer*, 17 June 1854. A disembarkation return in TNA: WO 25/1187 recorded the arrival of *Mangerton* at Gravesend from Malta on 14 September with 63 NCOs and men from 12 regiments together with 82 women and 127 children.
180 *Morning Post*, 20 July 1854.
181 TNA: ADM 7/576.
182 For additional details see M.J. Hoad and A.T. Patterson, 'Portsmouth and the Crimean War', *The Portsmouth Papers*, No. 19 (1973).
183 The names of officers leaving the Crimea with a medical certificate for Turkey, England, or elsewhere were published in General Orders.
184 Smith to Military Undersecretary, 27 February 1855; Royal Commission Report, p.469.
185 Smith to Undersecretary, 5 November 1855 Smith, *Précis of Letters* and Royal Commission Report, Appendix LXXIX, p.77
186 Military Undersecretary to Smith, 9 November 1855; Smith, *Précis of Letters*.

Plymouth that four ships from Scutari would touch there and that he should disembark up to 150 before they proceeded to Portsmouth,[187] while Codrington telegraphed that 60 of 244 invalids embarked on *Thames* on 17 June 1856 would require medical treatment,[188] and these were sent to Chichester on arrival.[189]

4.3.1 Provision of hospital transports

Smith addressed the problem of evacuation the sick and wounded 'from the vicinity of conflict' in May 1854 and he emphasized the need for 'a liberal supply of ships, some to convey periodically to England men never likely to become available for further service.' This advice was not heeded and in the following January he found it necessary to recommend that two good steamers would prove sufficient for transporting medical stores to the East and that the public would be 'ensured against any unnecessary loss' if they were used to carry home invalids when returning.[190] Similarly, Dr H. Mapleton, sometime Raglan's physician, advocated the employment of dedicated vessels for the purpose, especially during the summer as the heat in Turkey and Malta 'would impair recovery.' He calculated that four steamers of 2,000 tons could convey 2–3,000 men every six weeks. These ships would require a permanent staff of medical officers, orderlies, cooks, washermen, etc. but despite this outlay the policy would obviate the vast expense of setting up hospitals in Smyrna, Abydos, etc., places which would also prove unsuitable in the summer owing to the hot weather expected.[191]

Panmure informed the House of Lords that: 'As soon as we can obtain [...] transports it is [intended] to establish a communication every week to 10 days direct between Scutari and England [...] steamers fitted up as hospital ships, which will bring home [...] 300 or 400, or perhaps 500 [...] who will be far sooner restored to health [...] in this country, than [...] where they now are.'[192]

He then told Paulet that he was hoping to secure the services of six steamers not required by the Navy to provide a weekly service between Scutari and England,[193] and, though Palmerston informed MPs on 19 February 1855 that the War Department intended to make arrangements for a 'periodical service' between Constantinople and England for 'bringing home such invalids as [can] be transported by sea,'[194] nothing come of it, and two sailing transports, the *Great Tasmania* and *Saldanha*, were engaged instead on 29 March.

187 Smith to PMO, Plymouth, 28 April 1856; Smith, *Précis of Letters*.
188 Undersecretary to Smith, 24 June 1856; Smith, *Précis of Letters*. A later message reported 24 French nurses were on board.
189 PMO, Portsmouth to Smith, 9 July 1856; Smith, *Précis of Letters*.
190 Smith to Deputy Secretary, 23 January 1855; *The Lancet*, 28 July 1855.
191 Report by Mapleton, 5 February 1855; HCPP 1857–58 (425) XXXVII.105: *A Report* [...] *Relative to the Sanitary Condition of the Army of the East* [...] *by Dr Mapleton*. See also Royal Commission Report, Appendix LXXIX, p.196–7.
192 *The Times*, 17 February 1855 and referred to in Lorne, *Viscount Palmerston*, p.142.
193 Panmure to Paulet, 9 March 1855; TNA: WO 6/70.
194 *The Times*, 20 February 1855

Mapleton was sent to Liverpool to superintend their modification,[195] but found them being fitted for troops in health and not invalids. The number of berths was then reduced, the bunks widened from 22 to 26 ins., and additional patent air tubes installed to improve ventilation.[196] Smith was requested to advise on dietary matters as the owners were to victual for the troops both out and home,[197] and then to nominate medical officers.[198] Smith's suggestion to appoint permanent medical staff[199] was approved,[200] as was the appointment of two hospital sergeants and one steward to each vessel, while the orderlies, in the ratio of 1:20 sick,[201] were to be volunteers from line regiments.[202]

Two sets of apparatus for hoisting the wounded on board were ordered,[203] and on 19 April the vessels were ready for sea.[204] Mapleton also recommended that the boxes for the horses should be cleared away before the return journey as they were a source of filth and an obstruction to ventilation.[205] Only twelve sick officers should be evacuated so that each had a separate cabin; and that every mess should be answerable for all equipment to prevent its illegal disposal as this would leave the vessel under equipped for the return voyage.[206]

In September Smith and Dr J. Forrest inspected *Great Tasmania*, *Saldanha*, the three-decker *Britannia*, and the General Military Hospital in the Portsmouth Garrison. They expressed their satisfaction in the state of the ships for invalids, the condition of the hospital, and the treatment and progress of the patients.[207]

---

195 Smith to Mapleton, 31 March 1855; Smith, *Précis of Letters*.
196 Mapleton to Smith. 2 April 1855; Smith, *Précis* For details of the fittings see *Morning Chronicle*, 27 April 1855. Following their return to England it was decided to install rotary ventilation machines and Smith suggested that a person acquainted with the apparatus should travel with the vessels; Smith to Undersecretary, 14 September 1855; Smith, *Précis of Letters*.
197 Director of Transport Services to Smith, 23 March 1855; Smith, *Précis of Letters*.
198 AG to Smith, 9 April 1855; Smith, *Précis of Letters*.
199 Smith to Undersecretary, 13 April 1855; Smith, *Précis* and Royal Commission Report, Appendix LXXIX, p.47.
200 Military Undersecretary to Smith, 17 April 1855; Smith, *Précis of Letters*.
201 Military Undersecretary to Smith, 25 April 1855; Smith, *Précis of Letters*. See also Memorandum No. 942, 2 May 1855; TNA: WO 123/151.
202 Military Secretary to Smith, 1 May 1855; Smith, *Précis of Letters*. Smith issued a list of 15 regulations for display on the vessels; Smith to Undersecretary, 8 May 1855; Smith, *Précis* and Royal Commission Report, Appendix LXXIX.
203 Smith to Director of Transport Services, 14 April 1855; Smith, *Précis of Letters*.
204 Mapleton to Smith, 19 April 1855; Smith, *Précis of Letters*.
205 The horse stalls were removed before departure. PMO, Portsmouth to Smith, 5 May 1855; Smith, *Précis of Letters*.
206 Smith to Undersecretary, forwarding Mapleton's letter, 20 April 1855; Smith, *Précis of Letters*.
207 *The Times*, 19 September 1855. *Saldanha* and *Great Tasmania* arrived in Portsmouth on 5 August and by 1 September respectively.

Smith hoped that the two vessels would convey invalids from the Crimea to England without calling at the hospitals of the Bosphorus,[208] while he suggested that the vessels should be towed by a steamer when 'calmness prevailed.'[209] The naval authorities in Gibraltar, Malta and Turkey were requested to assist in this regard,[210] and *Assistance*, *Charity* and *Prompt* were used for this purpose.[211] *Great Tasmania* and *Saldanha* only completed two round trips and were paid off 22 March and 7 April 1856 respectively.[212]

Several steamers equipped as permanent hospital transports operated a shuttle service between Balaklava and the Bosphorus from January 1855 but none was told off permanently for the voyage to England, and judging by the number of different vessels employed during the campaign, their selection must have been frequently on an ad hoc basis.[213] The military authorities had no official role in the selection of these vessels, as this was the responsibility, of the Royal Navy but to minimize the risk of adverse criticism Smith enjoined Hall to ensure that all transports conveying sick to England should be minutely examined and that all the specifications for provisions, medical comforts, etc. should be exact.[214]

No comprehensive list of the transports involved in this service was published. A survey of the dates of arrival in British waters of 160 voyages involving 115 vessels reported in *The Times* and elsewhere has revealed that 38 (33 percent) were sailing vessels, which undertook a quarter of the voyages; 61 (53 percent) were screw steamers; and 16 (14 percent) paddle wheel steamers. These were utilized for 87 (54 percent) and 32 (20 percent) of the voyages respectively.

There are several reports in *The Times* of quarantine regulations being imposed at Corfu, Gibraltar and Malta, particularly with respect to cholera or smallpox, while more specifically, the need for allied transports and civilian trading vessels to obtain Turkish Bills of Health became the topic of a correspondence between the British consul at Smyrna, J.W. Brant, Stratford and Clarendon following the opening of

---

208 Smith to Military Undersecretary, 16 June 1855; Smith, *Précis of Letters*.
209 Smith to Military Undersecretary, 31 July 1855; Smith, *Précis* and Royal Commission Report, Appendix LXXIX, p.70.
210 Military Undersecretary to Smith, 10 August 1855; Smith, *Précis* and Smith to Undersecretary, 10 September 1855; Smith, *Précis* and Royal Commission Report, Appendix LXXIX, p.74.
211 HCPP 1856 (345) XLI.341: *Return of all ships engaged as regular transports, with the names (stating whether steam or sailing), from Jan 1st, 1855, to Apr 1st, 1856; the date of the engagement, with a list of ships in the service at the latter date, their registered tonnage, rates of freight, and mulcts or deductions for the same, and why made; in steam ships, the horse power, the time occupied in their passages, and where information has been received, the quantity of coals or fuel consumed per hour*. See also *The Times* 22 February & 8 March 1856.
212 HCPP 1856 (345) XLI.341.
213 Conache, *Britain and the Crimea*, p.81 implied incorrectly that a regular transport service to England was established.
214 Smith to Hall, 30 November 1855; Smith, *Précis of Letters*.

the hospital at Smyrna. Brant thought that vessels involved in the war effort were exempted from quarantine and that it would be reasonable for other traders to be similarly privileged. However, it transpired that the Turkish authorities had not relaxed the regulations and Stratford considered there was no chance of the official policy being changed.[215] Clarendon responded to this robustly by stating that HM's government was surprised that:

> The Turkish authorities are not only not disposed to relax [...] quarantine as regards merchant vessels, but [...] impose it against transports engaged in the service of the Sultan's allies. The importance of avoiding the delays [...] of quarantine systems, as regards vessels employed in the service of the Allied forces, is so evident, that [...] that the Porte will [...] see the necessity [...] for the exemption of all transports from the quarantine regulations.[216]

It has not been established if this matter was resolved but sympathy for the Turkish authorities should be entertained since many invalids arriving at Smyrna during the first four months suffered from infectious disease; with fevers, diarrhoea, and dysentery accounting for 689 (53 percent) of the 1,311 patients.

4.3.2 Voyage to England

Smith reminded Hall that all transports conveying sick to England should be inspected to ensure that 'all the specifications for provisions, medical comforts, etc. should be exact.'[217] Hall subsequently issued a Medical Department Order on the subject on 11 December 1855.[218] The Queen's Regulations also required that vessels should be appropriately inspected before departure, although, in view of the many employed to transport invalids it is probable that the facilities on board were not always ideal. For example, Hall considered *Libertas* was 'not well calculated for the purpose.'[219] His misgivings were confirmed by Staff Surgeon Baxter who travelled on the ship.[220] Raglan sanctioned that the *Emeu* could transport 'ineffective men to Malta'[221] and, though Dr Tice reported that she was 'too filthy' to receive invalids

---

215 Brant to Stratford, 4 October and Stratford to Clarendon, 2 October 1855; TNA: FO 78/1090.
216 Clarendon to Stratford, 16 November 1855; TNA: FO 78/1068.
217 Smith to Hall, 30 November 1855; Smith, *Précis of Letters*.
218 RAMC: 397/F/CO/1/3.
219 Hall, *Diary*, 7 October 1854; RAMC: 397/PC1/6–8. *Libertas*, which also conveyed naval invalids, arrived at Devonport on 24 December, where some invalids were disembarked, before sailing on to Chatham; *Hampshire Telegraph and Sussex Chronicle*, 30 December 1854.
220 Smith to Military Secretary, 2 January 1855 Smith, *Précis of Letters*.
221 Hall to Smith, 2 November 1854; RAMC: 397/F/CO/1/1/855 and Smith, *Précis of Letters*.

while at Balaklava,[222] she subsequently sailed from Scutari for England with about 400 invalids, together with 'perhaps 100 women', so relieving 'the barracks and hospital very much.'[223]

When *Himalaya* arrived at Portsmouth early in 1855 she was 'not very cleanly [...] on the lower deck where the troops and the women and children were berthed next to 8–10 horses with the result the stench was almost sickening'[224] (Figure 4.9) Smith complained officially only to be informed by the Admiralty, via the Military Secretary, that although fitted for horses she had been used for invalids at the urgent request of the military authorities in Malta.[225] Some months later the PMO, Portsmouth reported that when *Lady Eglington* arrived she appeared 'short-handed and not very clean.'[226]

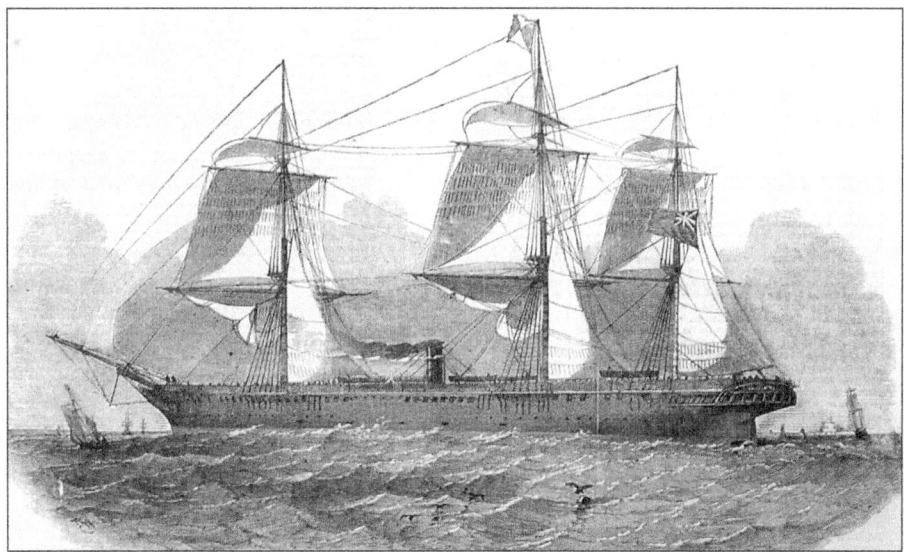

Figure 4.9 "The Himalaya" steamship. (*Illustrated London News*, 21 January 1854, p.48)

222 AoT to QMG, 3 November, with an annotation by Hall, 4 November 1854; TNA: WO 28/196.
223 Commandant, Scutari, to AG, 9 November; TNA: WO 28/186 and PMO, Scutari to Smith, 14 November 1854; Smith, *Précis of Letters*. A return in TNA: WO 25/1187 recorded that *Emeu* left Scutari 11 November and disembarked 115 wounded convalescents and others at Malta on 17 November.
224 *The Times*, 3 & 4 January and *Hampshire Telegraph and Sussex Chronicle*, 6 January 1855.
225 Smith to Military Secretary 8 January and his reply of 24 January 1855; Smith, *Précis of Letters*.
226 PMO, Portsmouth to Smith, 17 May 1855; Smith, *Précis of Letters*.

Mapleton considered that the health of patients would 'tend to improve on the voyage especially as they knew they are going home,'[227] and this was indeed the case on *Arabia, Croesus, Julia, Lord Raglan, Hydaspes, Alma, Orinoco, Niagara*, and *Robert Lowe*,[228] while some men on *Great Britain, Great Tasmania, Arabia*, and *Niagara* were fit enough to be granted furlough on arrival.[229]

The manner in which the invalids were catered for on *Orinoco* and *Sultana* attracted praise,[230] while Staff Surgeon Saunders reported that invalids on *Arabia* enjoyed 'every possible comfort' when on voyage from Malta.[231] Letters of appreciation addressed to the medical officer and the master and crew on HMS *Neptune, Orinoco, Sultana, Great Britain, Imperatriz*, and *Euxine* were published.[232]

On occasions military priorities influenced the management of transports conveying invalids. Passengers on *Ripon* were disembarked at Malta as the vessel was required to transport French troops.[233] *Cambria* then conveyed the invalids to Liverpool where some were retained in the parish hospital until convalescent.[234] The remainder travelled to Strood by train via Coventry and London,[235] despite Smith considering it preferable to send them to Chatham by sea as they would remain 'lodged in comparative comfort, in a splendid roomy vessel [and] would be sheltered from [...] the weather,' rather than be transported overland by rail; a journey 'too long for men in delicate health to sit in an erect posture' and during which time they may have up to twelve 'removals [...] into and out of vehicles.'[236] The Admiralty agreed with this suggestion but Horse Guards 'desired that the men might be landed at once,' an instruction that was followed such that only nine men were sent to the Royal Infirmary and 187 to Chatham by train.[237]

---

227 Report by Mapleton, 5 February 1855; HCPP 1857–58 (425) XXXVII.105. See also Royal Commission Report, Appendix LXXIX.
228 *The Times*, 5 & 8 March, 16 May, 5 & 21 July, 12, 15, & 29 October, and 12 November 1855.
229 *The Times*, 13 August, 3 & 13 September & 2 November 1855
230 *The Times*, 12 and 28 February 1855.
231 *Medical Times and Gazette*, 15 March 1856.
232 *The Times*, 12 & 28 February and 20 August 1855; *Medical Times and Gazette*, 6 October 1855 and *The Times*, 14 May 1856.
233 *Hampshire Telegraph and Sussex Chronicle*, 13 January 1855. Disembarkation return in TNA: WO 28/1187: *Ripon* left Scutari on 25 December with 132 NCOs and men who were wounded convalescents in whom bowel complaints were prevalent. Two died on the voyage and she arrived at Malta on 31 December 1954.
234 Disembarkation return in TNA: WO 25/1187: *Cambria* left Malta on 3 January and arrived at Liverpool on 15 January with 139 invalids from 15 regiments together with 24 women and two children. There was one death.
235 *The Times*, 20 January 1855.
236 Memorandum from Smith to Secretary at War, 20 January 1855; Royal Commission Report, Appendix LXXIX, p.29.
237 The QMG informed Smith on 24 January that Hardinge appreciated the 'measures so handsomely adopted by the authorities in Liverpool' but he was 'desirous not to trench

The weather and sea conditions also influenced the progress of vessels. Embarkation on *Great Tasmania* was delayed at Balaklava because of bad weather,[238] and she made three unsuccessful attempts to pass through the Straits of Gibraltar.[239] Gales or contrary winds slowed the progress of HMS *Arethusa, Harbinger,* HMS *Malacca*, which was unable to make headway with her steam, HMS *Bellerophon, Dunbar, Golden Fleece, Germania, Hope, Alma,* and *Cape of Good Hope*.[240] The invalids on *Talavera* 'suffered much' during severe weather on the voyage before she became 'wind bound' in Plymouth Sound for some days; *Ripon* put into Corunna to the 'great relief of the invalids [and] officers and crew who were much exhausted'; while disembarkation from HMS *Arethusa* and *Thames* was delayed due to the weather.[241] A low tide delayed *Candia*'s progress from Southampton to Portsmouth,[242] and the tide presumably affected other vessels from time to time, although, being a common occurrence, this would rarely merit comment.

Equipment failures and navigational errors caused delays on occasions. Newspaper reports noted the voyages of the *Golden Fleece* and *Himalaya* were prolonged due mechanical failure; the speed of *Simla* was reduced to six or seven knots when her screw broke about 100 miles from Ushant; both hawsers parted in a heavy gale when *Thames* was towing *Columba* about 30 miles off Cape Finisterre; *Drawback* (sic: *Drobak*) broke adrift from *Severn* off Cape Bon; *Adelaide* experienced 'a heavy gale [and] the sick suffered severely […] and several temporary berths […] on the troop deck […] were broken;' and HMS *Highflier* had to return to Malta to repair the expansion valve.[243] *Perseverance* ran aground on Isola Point after leaving Corradino, Malta with 410 invalids. The 'united power' of *Dragon, Magicienne, Shearwater,* and *Argo* failed to extricate her and all men, together with cargo and ballast, had to be disembarked before she was re-floated.[244] *Gibraltar*, the last hospital ship to leave Balaklava, broke down in the Sea of Marmora and was towed to Gallipoli by *Cumberland*, and then to Spithead by HMS *Urgent*, where she arrived on 16 August.[245]

When evacuation of the Crimea became imminent instructions which required the inspection of vessels carrying troops by a medical officer and an army and naval

---

upon their hospitality longer the necessary;' Smith, *Précis of Letters*.
238 AG to GOC Divisions, 14 January 1856; TNA: WO 28/124.
239 *The Times*, 1 March 1856.
240 *The Times*, 4 January, 8 February, 28 March, 2 & 11 April, 24 May, 6 June, 20 September, and 12 October 1855.
241 *The Times*, 7 & 12 February 1855 and 21 January 1856; PMO, Chatham to Smith, 25 February 1855, Smith, *Précis of Letters*; PMO, Portsmouth to Smith, 6 July 1856; Smith, *Précis of Letters*.
242 *Daily News*, 8 January 1855.
243 *Morning Post*, 20 July 1854 and *The Times*, 3 January, 18 April, 14 May, 15 September 1855, and 26 May and 3 July 1856.
244 *The Times*, 29 July 1856.
245 *The Times* and *Caledonian Mercury*, 18 & 19 August 1856.

officer were reissued.[246] The whole operation was effected in a relatively short time and between 1 May and 1 August 1856 125 vessels disembarked 2,183 officers, 57,888 men and 3,931 horses at Portsmouth. These numbers are exclusive of those conveyed to Liverpool, Plymouth, Woolwich, and destinations overseas, but presumably included invalids who travelled with their regiments although no information on the point was published.

The scale of this operation had implications for the hospitals at home and in this context the Invalid Depot at St Mary's Barrack, Chatham was informed in early May 1856 that 3,500 invalids were en route from the East, thus prompting preparations for their arrival, including the provision of 450 extra beds.[247]

Severn left Balaklava on 12 June with 350 invalids while '*Thames* will embark 234 more today.'[248] *Severn* towed the Norwegian bark *Drobak* with invalids from Scutari,[249] and following her arrival at Devonport some invalids were admitted to the military hospital while others were sent to their depots in Ireland, with the remainder being transferred to *Britannia*, located at Spithead from 4 July.[250] The last hospital ship to leave Balaklava was *Gibraltar* (see above), the sick having been placed on board on 11 July, the day before the final evacuation.[251]

4.3.3 Arrival in England

In January 1855 instructions were issued requiring a return of invalids admitted to hospital, or otherwise disposed of, being sent to the Invalid Depot at Chatham,[252] while from February 1855 ships touched at Plymouth to ascertain what accommodation was available at Chatham and elsewhere, and to disembark patients if it was insufficient.[253] Officers in charge of invalids were required to report to the AQMG on arrival, and following landing the invalids were to be inspected medically in order to decide on their future destination.[254]

Himalaya was the first steamer to arrive in Portsmouth with 'wounded and invalided officers from both services [and] men [...] from 42 different regiments [and with

---

246 QMG to the Commandant and AQMG, Balaklava, 14 April 1856; TNA: WO 28/134.
247 *The Times*, 3 May 1856.
248 Hall to Smith, 5 July 1856; Smith, *Précis of Letters*. *Severn* also transported soldiers' wives not allowed to embark with their husbands and a large proportion of the female nursing establishment.
249 Several men with ophthalmia joined *Drobek* at Gibraltar on 10 July 1856; TNA: WO 284/72.
250 PMO, Devonport to Smith, 3 July; Smith, *Précis* and *The Times*, 5 July; *Hampshire Telegraph and Sussex Chronicle*, 5 July, in which the vessel is named *Drawback*; and *Isle of Wight Observer*, 12 July 1856.
251 PMO, Balaklava to Smith; 11 July 1856; Smith, *Précis*
252 Simpson, AAG, to GOC, Portsmouth, 26 January 1855; TNA: WO 3/117.
253 See Smith, *Précis*, I, pp. 371, 380, & 393.
254 Circular issued by the AG, 15 October 1855; TNA: WO 123/151 & WO 28/193, and reproduced in *The Times*, 1 November 1855.

others] a total of 845 souls.' She had been ordered from Malta by Admiral Stewart when seemingly unfit for sea and mechanical failures prolonged her voyage, while bad weather 'caused a great deal of discomfort to the invalids' although 'everything that could be done to make them as comfortable as the circumstances would admit.' Some invalids were brought ashore aboard a tug while disembarkation was delayed owing to a want of 'organization' due to the presence of 'small officials' but no 'head'. There were no ambulances, or men at hand to assist those who 'were wholly or partially footless, legless, armless, or eye-less', although the severely wounded were subsequently carried to hospital in Portsea on stretchers or went by omnibus, while those in a fit state were sent to Chatham by rail. A further problem was the ransacking of luggage 'on the open jetty, before a single officer or man was allowed to leave for home or hospital.' This 'disgraceful exhibition' was 'as painful to the few Custom house officers [...] compelled to perform the duty as it was to a bystander to witness.'[255]

Smith requested the PMO, Portsmouth for a full account of events in order to 'exonerate' the medical officers from blame,[256] and fortunately procedures had improved by the time *Candia* arrived a week later. The 'unprotected gang board [...] to the jetty' was replaced by 'well-stepped and substantial double-railed landing stages' made 'quite secure' by carpenters,[257] while the regulations requiring 'rigid examination' of baggage by customs officials, and which had resulted in 'great dissatisfaction', were relaxed to cover only 'doubtful cases'.[258]

When Hardinge heard of these events the GOC at Portsmouth was informed that the Purveyor should supply 'such articles as are considered essential for the comfort and cleanliness' of the 'gallant soldiers.' The expenditure incurred was subsequently approved by the Deputy Secretary.[259]

When HMS *Retribution* docked on 24 January 1855 'Admiral Cochrane himself was present on the jetty' and 'nothing could exceed the careful attention paid to the landing of the stretcher cases, the more urgent of whom were taken to the garrison hospital and the rest to a new auxiliary hospital [...] established near the Milldam.' Some 'cases walked ashore' while others were 'helped by blue jackets to a waiting omnibus.'[260] (Figure 4.10) Similarly, the report of the arrival of *Mauritius* noted that 'since the first unfortunate cargo [of the *Himalaya*]' the sick have 'received a progressive amount of attention and consideration from all the government authorities.'[261] Several subsequent reports also contained additional comments and these are summarized in Table 4.4.

---

255 *The Times*, 4–6 January 1855 and *Hampshire Telegraph and Sussex Chronicle*, 6 January 1855.
256 Smith to PMO, Portsmouth, 9 January 1855; Smith, *Précis of Letters*.
257 *The Times*, 9 January 1855.
258 *The Times*, 20 January 1855.
259 AG, Horse Guards to General Smith, 25 January 1855; TNA: WO 3/117.
260 Hoad & Patterson (1973) and *The Times*, 26 January 1855.
261 *The Times*, 5 February 1855.

Table 4.4 Press reports published following the arrival in British waters of ships conveying invalids

Vessel	Abstract	The Times (all 1855)
Avon	Dense fog found the authorities unprepared for her arrival, although matters were soon rectified. 'Dr. Robinson [...] superintended the removal of the worst cases' although the 'the bulk will not be disembarked until the morning' allowing suitable arrangements to be made while 'Mr. Hoddes, the collector of Customs at Portsmouth, with an efficient staff, was promptly on board [...] to see that no unnecessary delay, or overhauling took place with the baggage.'	13 January
Avon	The *Avon* shared in the destructive effects of the great hurricane [...] In other respects she is in good condition and order, and being much cleaner than the *Himalaya* [...]	*Daily News*, 13 January
Cork steamer	On 15 January invalids arrived at Gravesend on the Cork steamer from Plymouth. 'The whole were in a very sickly state; they were very cold, complained that they had nothing to eat since Sunday evening, and they had to stand on the deck during the passage. [...] Ten men were admitted into hospital and 68 sent to the Invalid Depot for further examination.'	16 January
Harbinger	These cases were all doing well [...] and will leave for Chatham this morning without being disturbed. But why could not the ship have been despatched from Malta to Chatham direct, instead of first going to Southampton on Monday, waiting there all night, then going to Portsmouth yesterday, and staying there all night, finally leaving for Chatham this the third day after their arrival in England? Disembarkation return in WO/25/1187: Left Scutari on 10 January and arrived at Chatham on 12 February with 81 invalids from 34 regiments; their health was indifferent, but there was only one death.	7 February
Arabia	No medical officer or other official was sent off to the *Arabia* while at Spithead to see what was the nature of the cases and which the most urgent to be got to hospital.	5 March
Dunbar	Anchored at eight a.m. off Portsmouth, but up to 6 o'clock at night no military authority [...] had been off to her [although] Major-General Breton [...] asserted that 'as soon as a vessel is notified Surgeon Odell and Major Dalgetty [went to] make the necessary arrangements for landing the men.' (In the event *Dunbar* sailed on to Chatham)	11 April
Medway	[...] not taken into harbour yesterday – upwards of 50 hours after reporting herself. The captain could get no one to authorize their coming in on Saturday morning. The Port-Admiral had gone [...] with a squadron of honour for the Emperor of the French; the Admiral-Superintendent of the Dockyard [...] was sitting as president of the court-martial [...] and he does not appear to have deputed anybody to do the duties of the port [...]	16 April
Victoria	'two days and a-half having lapsed since her arrival! The poor fellows [...] complained of the unnecessary confinement to which they had been subjected. The delay [...] is another of the many flagrant cases which have at various times been recorded. [...] no blame can be attached to the Admiralty officials at Southampton, for [her arrival] was forwarded by telegraph to London. [...] and it was not until too late on Monday night to send the passengers ashore that any knowledge existed of the wishes at head-quarters.'	2 May

Vessel	Abstract	The Times (all 1855)
Cornwall	'went into Portsmouth harbour yesterday to land invalid soldiers [...] but no arrangements were made for their removal until 11 o'clock. Thus the invalids lost the train by which such unfortunates are usually forwarded to Chatham invalid depot (8.30 a.m.), and will not be landed until this morning. [...] there was no general commanding the garrison or any staff surgeon to see to the landing and removal of these poor fellows.'	10 May
Germania	'arrived at Spithead yesterday [...]The [invalids] will not be disembarked until this day, there being no accommodation for them in barrack quarters.'	6 June
Ripon	'arrived at Southampton yesterday [...] The distressed British seamen, however, remained on board the transport during the night, and will be despatched to their various destinations by the Admiralty department at Southampton this day.'	6 November

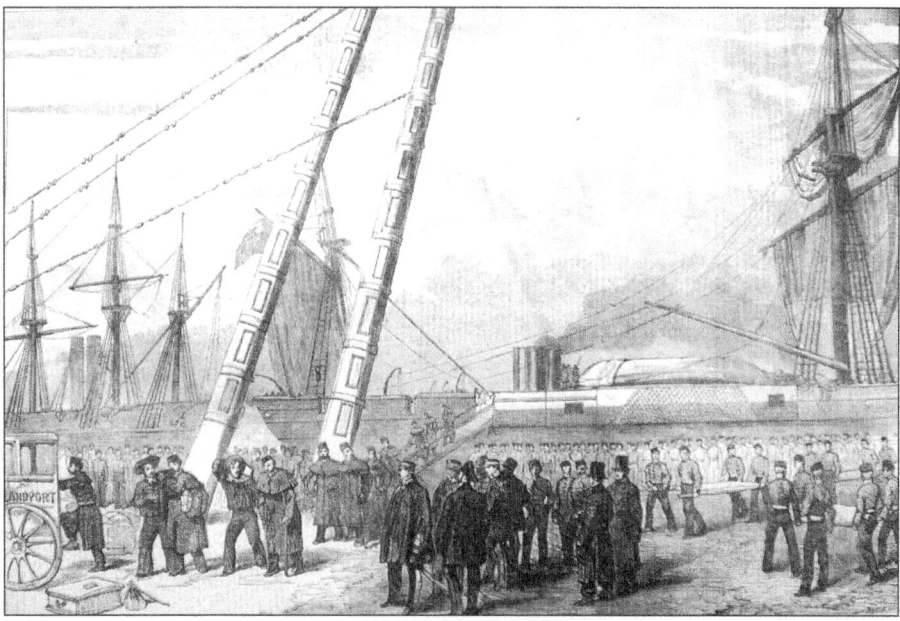

Figure 4.10 Landing the wounded from 'HMS Retribution', at Portsmouth. (*Illustrated London News*, 17 February 1855, p.153)

Himalaya hoisted a yellow (Q) flag on arrival at Spithead indicating illness on board, although she soon obtained *pratique* (a licence to enter port), while the troopship *Conrad* was quarantined in Plymouth Sound, because of 'an informality about her bill of health,' as was HMS *Cressy* on arrival at Spithead from the Baltic, although no reason was recorded.²⁶² On the other hand, there was no specific mention of quarantine when *Black Prince*,²⁶³ HMS *Resolute*,²⁶⁴ *Emeu*,²⁶⁵ and HMS *Firebrand*²⁶⁶ arrived with cases of cholera on board.

In some cases tugs or tenders landed the sick when disembarkation was delayed, although this was not without risk or discomfort. For example, 'one Guardsman died of exposure while being transferred in a open boat [from *Libertas*] to the hospital in Stoke during inclement weather; a tragedy that would have been avoided if arrangements had been made for disembarkation at Plymouth,²⁶⁷ while invalids landed in *Sprightly* from HMS *Neptune* had to be wrapped in blankets to shield them from the cold, being all on deck.²⁶⁸

Sprightly also assisted disembarkation from *Himalaya* as did *Pygmy* from HMS *Neptune*, an unnamed tug from *Victoria*, *Comet* from *Camperdown* and *Lancashire*, and *Echo* from *Gibraltar*.²⁶⁹ Similarly, *Confeance* landed invalids from *War Cloud* at Devonport while a few who had 'lost their passage on *Australian*' at Gibraltar were taken ashore by boat from HMS *Centaur* following her arrival at Spithead.²⁷⁰

Charitable initiatives: Examples of kindness shown to the invalids were acknowledged by the press (Table 4.5), although on one occasion this was considered excessive and banned by the military authorities, except under the direction of the medical officer.²⁷¹ Incidentally, the plight of the troops at the front resulted in a number of important organized charitable initiatives. See Section 10.4 for a brief summary.

Women and children: A large number of women and children were sent home during the course of war. A War Office Memorandum issued before the war set out the expenses which legally married women and legitimate children aged 14 and under could claim when returning home.²⁷² They would be transported by steam vessel or railway, if available, and when walking the women and children would receive 1½d

---

262 *The Times*, 18 September 1854 & 28 July 1856.
263 *The Times*, 13 June 1855
264 Military Secretary to Smith, 17 July and Staff Surgeon Teevan to Smith, 19 July 1855; Smith, *Précis of Letters*.
265 PMO, Portsmouth, to Smith, 11 September; Smith, *Précis of Letters* and *The Times*, 15 September 1855
266 Admiralty to Smith, 17 July 1855; Smith, *Précis of Letters*.
267 *The Times*, 27 December 1854.
268 *Isle of Wight Observer*, 17 February 1855.
269 *The Times*, 12 Feb, 2 & 9 May, 20 August 1855, and 26 May & 16 July 1856 and
270 *Hampshire Telegraph and Sussex Chronicle*, 3 March and *The Times*, 5 & 6 June 1855. A General Order issued in Gibraltar on 25 May named two serjeants, one corporal and five privates assigned to the 66th Regiment until their passage home was arranged; TNA: WO 284/71.
271 *Medical Times and Gazette*, 14 April 1855.
272 Memorandum No. 1155, 12 March 1855; TNA: WO 123/181. (1d was worth approximately 31p at today's prices.)

Table 4.5 Generosity extended to invalids following their arrival in England

Vessel/ donor	Abstract	Reference (all 1855)
Himalaya	The Relief Association 'expended a considerable sum […] assisting the poor women and children' brought home on the vessel.	*HT&SC*, 6 January
Candia	Refreshments of all kinds were spontaneously tendered to [the invalids] […] but the commanding officer declined to accept it.'	*ILN*, 17 January
Candia	Messrs J. and G. Cokesby, merchants of Southampton, with great kindness and consideration, sent porter as a present to the invalided soldiers […] The wounded men spoke in the highest terms of the treatment received at Scutari.	*Daily News*, 8 January
Sir Frederick Smith	Major-General Sir Frederick Smith, RE […] has been constant in his visits to the poor sick and wounded soldiers […] and they were on Thursday also visited by Lady Smith who distributed among the suffers comforts and delicacies in the shape of jellies, blancmange etc. […] Mr Emmanuel and several other townsmen have collected newspapers and other things, and forwarded them for the use of the gallant patients.	*IoWO*, 10 February
Sir Frederick Smith	Sir Frederick Smith reported that he had 'received nearly 100 volumes of books of interesting biography, etc., which I intend depositing in the hospital […] in a book case I am having made for them […]' Pocket handkerchiefs, neck comforters, muffatees, etc., were added to the confections dispensed by Lady Smith on Tuesday, the muffatees principally of her own and her friends' knitting.	*IoWO*, 24 February
Talavera	'The report that the soldiers were in a personal state of uncleanliness is without foundation' but they were 'unprepared for the prevailing inclement weather, especially as they would have to encounter a cold passage [to] Chatham' and 'General Eden […] sent warm clothing from his private store to some of the poor fellows, a large portion of whom left Scutari with a single suit.' […] 'Earl of Mount Edgecumbe has afforded them constant supplies of vegetables from his own gardens' and before departure of the men expressed themselves in most grateful terms for the warm clothing, fruit, etc, sent off to the ship by the Mayor and other inhabitants of Plymouth.'	*The Times*, 12 February
Neptune	Quartermaster Paton was indefatigable in seeing to their evening meal and breakfast on Saturday morning. Their rations being drawn, Mr Chamney, purveyor to the Queen, gratuitously, though late at night, undertook to cook the gallant sufferers' provisions at his bakery. Mr Paton was at his post next morning to see each man get his allowance before leaving for Chatham invalid depot. [The men] expressed their warmest gratitude to Lord Methuen, commanding the Wilts Militia, his officers and men, whom they loudly cheered on leaving.	*The Times*, 14 February
Arabia	[…] the bounty of the Princess Mary of Cambridge was manifested towards these poor invalids by the distribution of warm and comforting clothing, such a flannels, etc., for which they appeared heartily grateful.	*The Times*, 6 March
HMS *Malacca*	The invalids […] shared the bounties distributed by Major General and Lady Smith […] consisting of clothing, personal comforts, and nourishing confections. Major General and Mrs Bentinck have also forwarded a quantity of similar good things […] to distribute among the sick.	*The Times*, 28 March
The Queen	Her Majesty has [sent to the General Hospital, Portsmouth] silk pocket and neck handkerchief and neck ties, hemmed by herself and ladies of the Court, together with arm-slings, etc.	*IoWO*, 28 July

and 1d a mile, plus 2d and 1d subsistence for every eight miles travelled. An allowance was also paid if they were delayed waiting at port for transportation.

Mutinous crews: The transports chartered by the government were manned by civilians not subjected to martial law and there were reports of mutinous behaviour on arrival, seemingly on account of disagreements of over conditions of employment. For example, by the crews of *Avon*,[273] *Mauritius*,[274] *Harbinger*,[275] and *Arabia*.[276]

4.3.4 Transportation from the port to other destinations
The arrival of large numbers of incapacitated invalids posed logistical problems as bearers would be required for stretcher cases and wheeled transport for longer journeys.[277] Smith considered that properly fitted wagons were preferable to omnibuses,[278] if they could be 'hired and rendered available at one hour's notice, [279] and, although he voiced no objection to omnibuses if men could be moved 'quickly and with without risk of injury,'[280] there was one adverse report of their use for 'those wounded in the legs, or suffering from diarrhoea.'[281]

Pressure on space meant that only 'bad' cases could be hospitalized in Portsmouth[282] with the others being sent to several destinations following disembarkation. For example, of 109 patients arriving in March 1856 seventeen were admitted to hospital, 44 were ordered to Chatham or Chichester, and 37 to their depots,[283] while, of those landing in the next month 40 remained in hospital in Portsmouth, with the remainder going to Chichester (38) Chatham (37), depots (20), London (15), and Woolwich (14).[284]

There are reports that the men received a hearty breakfast before departure for Chatham and were given cooked rations for the journey,[285] although there were 'grave

---

273 *The Times*, 15 January 1855.
274 *The Times*, 5, 6, 10, 13, & 17 February 1855.
275 *The Times*, 12 February 1855.
276 *The Times*, 6 March 1855.
277 Deputy Secretary to Smith, 5 May 1955; Smith, *Précis of Letters*.
278 Smith to Deputy Secretary, 5 May 1855; Smith, *Précis of Letters*.
279 Smith to Military Secretary, 11 January 1855; Smith, *Précis of Letters*.
280 Smith to Surgeon Gibb, 6 June 1856; Smith, *Précis of Letters*.
281 *Medical Times and Gazette*, 6 October 1855, p.356.
282 Smith to Military Secretary and PMO, Portsmouth, 21 & 30 April 1855; Smith, *Précis of Letters*. For example, 50–60 of 200 invalids on HMS *Neptune* and 33 of 242 on *Arabia* required 'immediate care'; PMO, Portsmouth, 8 March & 4 April 1855; Smith, *Précis of Letters*.
283 PMO, Portsmouth to Smith, 30 March 1856; Smith, *Précis of Letters*.
284 PMO, Portsmouth to Smith, 18 April 1856; Smith, *Précis of Letters*.
285 For example, men from *Mauritius, Neptune, Orinoco, Sultana,* and *Arabia*; *The Times*, 5, 12 & 28 February & 6 March 1855.

medical objections in sending patients [to Chatham] by rail during winter'[286] as they 'suffered much discomfort from the cold and the state of their wounds deteriorated thereby',[287] particularly 'unhealed stumps and gunshot wounds.'[288] A partial solution was to issue each man with 'two blankets or rugs to wrap round their legs as they acquire no advantage from their great coats.'[289] This advice was not always heeded, however, as invalids were moved to other locations without blankets,[290] and Smith found it necessary to reiterate that 'cases of phthisis and bowel complaint' should not be moved to Chatham 'unless the journey can be made without inconvenience or suffering.,' although he was anxious men who were fit enough for discharge should be sent to Chatham for disposal.[291]

Some patients that landed at Plymouth travelled to Chatham by train and on one occasion during March 1855 Hardinge asked the Mayor of Bath if the town could accommodate 136 wounded men overnight as it was a two day journey. This was achieved by housing them in the United Hospital, General Hospital and Guildhall Banqueting Room, while eight women and fifteen children travelling with them stayed in the Council Chamber. A collection was made locally and each man was given half a guinea with the balance defraying the cost of the Crimean Memorial in Bath Abbey Cemetery which was dedicated on 29 May 1856.[292]

4.3.5 Hospital facilities in England
Several hospitals in England treated invalids from the East but unlike the nine general hospitals in the Crimea and Turkey no details about their performance were included in the *Medial and Surgical History*, although general tables giving the reasons for repatriation and the causes of death were published.[293]

Many of the barracks in 46 towns in England and Wales had hospitals,[294] and, although several were located near a major port, it was only those at Chatham, Devonport, and Portsmouth that were used on a regular basis, while those at Dover and Walmer were not utilized as the Admiralty considered it 'inexpedient to land invalids eastwards of Portsmouth.'[295] Not surprisingly Smith enquired of the Military

---

286 Smith to Military Secretary, 16 February 1855; Smith, *Précis of Letters*. Incidentally, Smith proffered similar advice to the PMO, Portsmouth on 14 January 1856; Smith, *Précis of Letters*. The journey necessitated a journey via London and then by road from Strood to Chatham as the railway line did not then cross the Medway.
287 PMO, Fort Pitt, to Smith, 13 February 1855; Smith, *Précis of Letters*.
288 PMO, Fort Pitt, to Smith, 21 December 1855; Smith, *Précis of Letters*.
289 Smith to Undersecretary, 15 November 1855; Smith, *Précis* and Royal Commission Report, Appendix LXXIX, p.78.
290 PMO, Portsmouth to Smith, 21 January 1856; Smith, *Précis of Letters*.
291 Smith to PMOs at Portsmouth and Chichester, 23 August 1856; Smith, *Précis of Letters*.
292 W. Hanna, 'Bath and the Crimean War, 1854–1856', *Bath History*, 8 (2000), pp.148–71.
293 *Medical and Surgical History*, 2, pp.229–30 & 290.
294 Royal Commission Report, pp.440–1.
295 QMG to Smith, 1 March 1855; Smith, *Précis of Letters*.

Secretary how it was proposed to supply further accommodation, as, if 'the influx may be so great', the hospitals at Chatham, Plymouth and Portsmouth would prove inadequate,[296] and at the same time suggested that the Admiralty be asked to assist with the provision of accommodation at Haslar and Chatham if required.[297] In addition to developments at Chatham additional rooms were fitted up in Plymouth and Portsmouth for 226 and 80 respectively, with those at Portsmouth being ready at 'an hours notice.'[298] Further developments at Plymouth and Portsmouth, the modification of barracks at Chichester and the adaptation of two naval ships for hospital use eventually resulted in there being 1,300 beds available in all locations by the end of July 1855.[299] From the 21 February until the end of the campaign the average number of vacant beds in any week was never less than 650.[300]

The barracks at Deptford and Woolwich, and the Liverpool area were considered for possible use, but nothing came of these initiatives, although invalids from the RA and RS&M were sent to the Ordnance Hospital at Woolwich.[301]

Chatham: Fort Pitt was built as a defensive stronghold on the high ground overlooking Chatham and the Medway. The original barracks had been converted into hospital wards, offices, etc.[302] and was the only general hospital used for invalids returning from overseas, and had accommodation for only 170 invalids at the end of October 1854.[303] Resources at Chatham were increased by utilizing the Brompton (from February 1855) and St Mary's Barracks for accommodating invalids, and building new hospital accommodation behind Fort Pitt.[304, 305] (Figures 4.11 and 4.12)

Newspaper reports confirmed the pressure on space, particularly at Fort Pitt, and on occasions this could be exacerbated by the arrival of invalids from other places,[306] although the situation was ameliorated somewhat when a lunatic asylum opened at Fort Pitt in the spring of 1856.[307]

---

296 Smith to Military Secretary, 31 October 1855; Smith, *Précis of Letters*.
297 The Melville hospital at Chatham served the Royal Navy. The muster book for 1854 is TNA: ADM/102157.
298 Smith to PMO Portsmouth and Military Secretary, 24 & 31 October 1854; Smith, *Précis of Letters*.
299 Smith to Undersecretary, 28 July 1855; Smith, *Précis of Letters*.
300 *Medical and Surgical History*, 1, Appendix VII, p.511.
301 Smith to Military Secretary, 16 January 1855; Smith, *Précis of Letters* and Military Undersecretary to Smith, 7 March 1855; Smith, *Précis of Letters*.
302 Miles, *Accidental Birth*, p.85.
303 PMO, Chatham to Smith, 25 October 1854; Smith, *Précis of Letters*.
304 *The Times*, 22 March 1855.
305 For a commentary on the facilities at Chatham see G. Fisher, 'Treatment of the Crimean Wounded', *The War Correspondent*, 28:3 (2010), pp.33–44.
306 *The Times*, 17 July 1855.
307 *The Times*, 16 November 1855 and 18 January, 5 & 25 March and 17 May 1856.

Transportation and evacuation of invalids 181

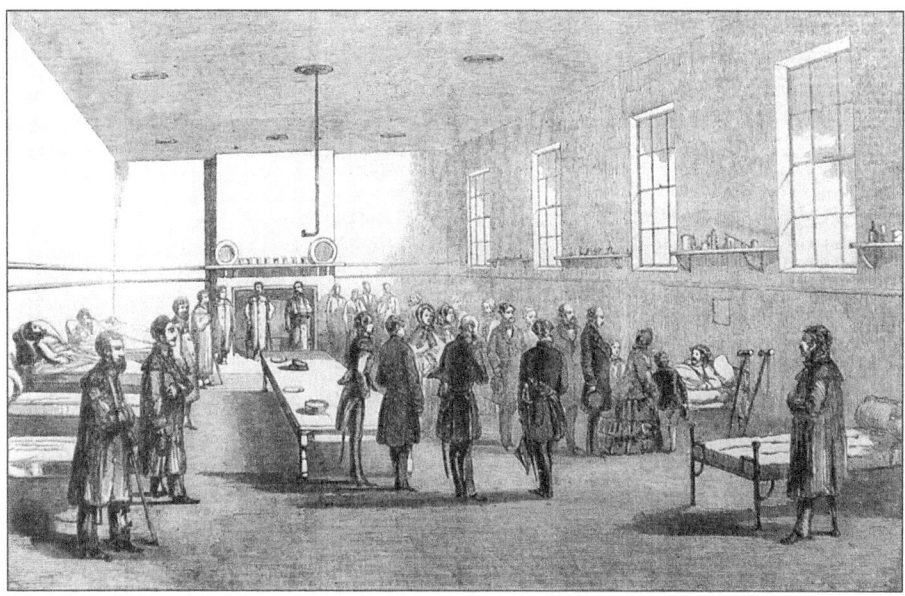

Figure 4.11 Her Majesty inspecting the wounded troops, at Fort Pitt hospital, Chatham. (*Illustrated London News*, 10 March 1855, p.236)

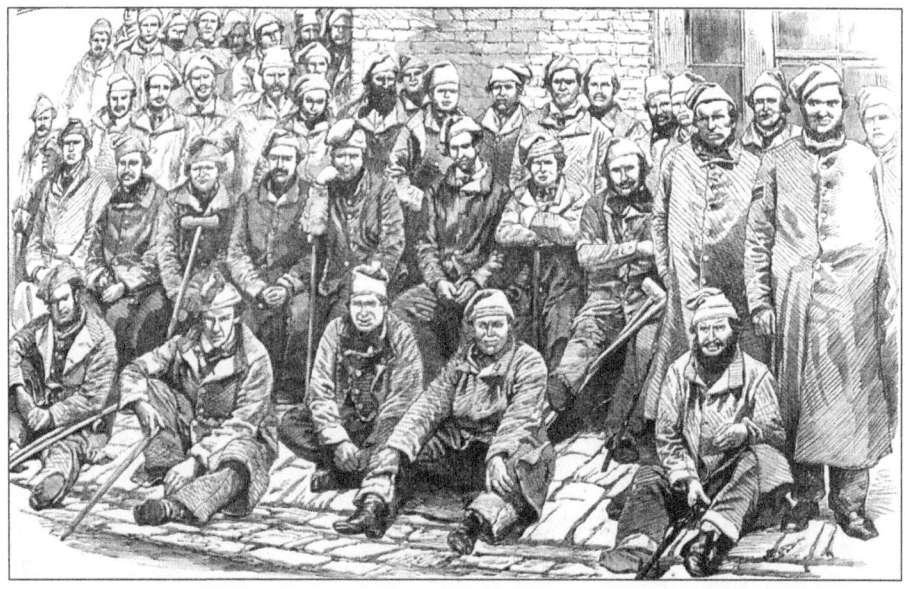

Figure 4.12 Invalided soldiers before the hospital barracks, at Brompton. (*Illustrated London News*, 21 July 1855, p.69)

Palmerston subsequently informed MPs that arrangements would be made to treat invalids 'in proper and suitable hospitals'[308] but despite this assurance the facilities at Chatham were generally considered both inadequate and antiquated, and this occasioned the publication of a number of critical comments. For example, the barracks at St Mary's, housing men awaiting discharge, was considered a 'dungeon' by a 'medical officer',[309] while the Garrison Hospital was still regarded as inadequate in 1856 and Fort Pitt had to be used to accommodate the sick.[310] The generally unsatisfactory state of the facilities was confirmed by the reminiscences of DIGH G.R. Dartnell who noted that:

> The Queen and party walked across to see the Casemate Barracks [...] She went into one or two of the upper rooms and was quite horrified at them. 'Are these really the barrack rooms of these invalids?' she said to me: I said, 'Yes indeed they are your Majesty' and Prince Albert, looking over towards the splendid Convict Prison recently built [completed 1850] said 'Well it seems very extraordinary that there should be no difficulty in obtaining money to erect a magnificent building like this for convicts, and that it should be impossible to find the means of building a commonly comfortable Barrack for convalescent soldiers.'[311]

The Queen was obviously content about the medical treatment men received but she was concerned about the conditions on the buildings. On 5 March 1855 she wrote to Panmure:

> The wards more like prisons than hospitals, with windows so high nobody can look out of them; and the generality of the wards are small rooms, with hardly space for you to walk between the beds. There is no dining-room or hall, so the poor men must have their dinners in the same room in which they sleep, and in which some may be dying, and at any rate suffering, while others are at their meals.[312]

An outbreak of erysipelas resulted in the postponement of the Queen's third visit (see below) and this prompted the editor of the *Medical Times and Gazette* to state his views in no uncertain terms:

> We hope that this measure [to build a new military hospital at Netley] is taken in order to supersede the necessity of retaining the present Military Hospital at Fort Pitt, an establishment which [...] is a disgrace to a great nation. Originally intended only for barracks, this building is wholly unsuited for the reception of sick and wounded troops, its wards are low, close, and ill-ventilated; the beds,

308 *The Times*, 20 February 1855.
309 *The Times*, 11 August 1855.
310 *The Times*, 18 January 1856.
311 *Journal of the Royal Army Medical Corps* (1904), 3, p.92.
312 Raymond, *Queen Victoria's Early Letters*, pp.209–10.

owing to deficiency of space, are too close together; the accommodation for convalescents is wholly inadequate.[313]

The first patients from the East were admitted on 4 January 1855. A few vessels sailed directly to the Thames; for example, *Culloden*, *Libertas*, *Sultana*, and *Dunbar*.[314] The majority of invalids were landed at Portsmouth and travelled by train via London to Strood were they were assisted by a fatigue party to waiting ambulances, spring vans, or omnibuses for the journey across the Medway to Chatham. Following a medical examination, the men were sent to either the supplemental hospital at Brompton Barracks for further treatment, the Casemate Barracks, the invalid depot at St Mary's Barracks, to await discharge, or, if deemed insane, to Fort Pitt.[315]

It was reported that on arrival at Chatham the patients were given gratis from the government: two shirts, two pairs of socks, two towels, one belt, one pair of boots, two brushes, one pot of blacking, one kerchief, one shell jacket, one pair of trousers, one forage cap, one knife, fork, and spoon. Two flannel guernseys and two pairs of flannel drawers used to be issued but this was stopped as many of the soldiers sold them to slop dealers when discharged.[316]

Medical officers were given authority to requisition for clothing if it was 'absolutely necessary [for] the securing [an invalid's] health and comfort whilst under treatment or when about to leave hospital.'[317] The general appearance of convalescents can be judged from an engraving of the reading room at St Mary's, while a group photograph of patients at the Brompton Barracks in hospital denim coats was reproduced in the *Illustrated London News*.[318] A diagram based on the photograph identifying several of the men by Dartnell is preserved in the Royal Archives at Windsor.[319]

Smith informed the Deputy Secretary on 28 February 1855 that he had no objection to tobacco being issued to invalids if regulated by the medical officers. The Secretary of War sanctioned its issue 'when considered desirable by the medical officer, to the extent of two ounces per week per patient' on 19 April and the PMO, Chatham instructed staff surgeons to record its issue in the diet rolls.[320]

There was a library at St Mary's while a coffee shop was established there early in 1856 although at the time offices in the Invalid Depot were found too damp and unfit for use.[321]

313 *Medical Times and Gazette*, 9 February 1856.
314 *The Times*, 1, 3 & 10 January, 28 February, and 11 April 1855 respectively.
315 *The Times*, 20 January, 28 July, 11 & 27 August, 3, 8, 10 & 13 September, 2 November, 22 & 25 December 1855, and 3 March 1856.
316 An Assistant Surgeon, Fort Pitt, 19 May; *The Times*, 22 May 1855.
317 Smith, *Précis* and Fort Pitt General Orders Book, 31 January 1855.
318 *Illustrated London News*, 8 March 1856.
319 G. Fisher, 'Doctor Dartnell's List', *The War Correspondent*, 30:4 (2013), pp.29–42.
320 Fort Pitt General Orders Book, 24 April 1855.
321 *The Times*, 7 January 1856.

A supplementary hospital at Brompton Barracks was in operation from the beginning of 1855. In 1856 a Board recommended that buildings constructed as a temporary hospital in 1855 should be used for the sick of the garrison with a part being set aside for the RS&M, a policy subsequently confirmed when the barracks were designated their headquarters.[322]

Portsmouth: This was the principal port where invalids were landed and the numbers that arrived during the first two months of 1855 are given in Table 4.6. The sick and wounded were doing well in the new Garrison Hospital in February 1855 while 'state of the patients [there was] highly satisfactory' in February 1856, though there is great room for improvement in the details of supervision and the system of dieting the patients.[323] The hospital in Portsea was located close to the docks in the Milldam Barracks[324] (Figure 4.13) and the following summer the PMO reported that there was 'a most poisonous miasma still emanating from the rampart ditch and milldam pond' and it was 'a great pity these reservoirs cannot be entirely filled up, they are frightful sources of malignant disease.'[325]

Table 4.6 Number of passengers, including invalids, landed at Portsmouth during January and February 1855

Vessel	Passengers listed in *The Times*, 21 February 1855	Total	Reported date of arrival
Himalaya	2 field officers, 3 captains; 2 subalterns, 2 staff, 18 sergeants, 1 trumpeter, 122 privates; 177 soldiers' wives, 229 soldiers' children	549 (*sic*)	3 January
Candia	1 captain, 1 staff, 14 sergeants, 181 privates, 8 soldiers' wives	205	9 January
Avon	1 staff, 20 sergeants, 1 trumpeter; 180 privates	202	12 January
HMS *Retribution*	4 sergeants; 44 privates	48	26 January
Mauritius	1 captain, 1 staff, 8 sergeants, 123 privates, 70 soldiers' wives, 93 children	296	3 February
HMS *Neptune*	10 sergeants, 1 trumpeter, 188 privates	199	9 February
Orinoco	1 subaltern, 8 sergeants, 101 privates, 9 soldiers' wives, 1 child	120	12 February
	Grand total of all passengers (and 9 horses)	1,619	

---

322 *The Times*, 21 January and 26 March 1856.
323 *Medical Times and Gazette*, 3 March 1855 and *The Times*, 21 February 1856.
324 A ward in the hospital is illustrated in *Illustrated London News*, 10 February 1855. The buildings form part of the University of Portsmouth, while Milldam House is now the Registry Office.
325 AG to Smith, 12 June 1855; Smith, *Précis of Letters*.

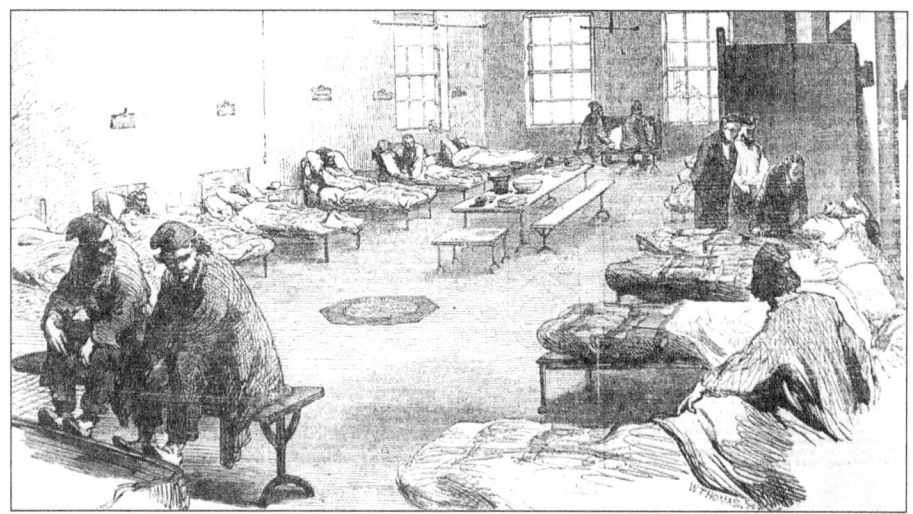

Figure 4.13 The Military hospital, Portsea. (*Illustrated London News*, 10 February 1855, p.128)

Inevitably Smith was concerned about the possibility of large numbers of invalids arriving within a short time and he recommended that only the seriously ill should be hospitalized at Portsmouth, while in November 1855 he requested additional accommodation be found so less reliance would be placed on Haslar and the hospital ship *Britannia* in cases of emergency.[326]

No detailed medical records have survived but Dr Leitch reported that 'scorbutic taint' was a complicating factor in the illnesses of many patients and that most of the 21 deaths among 34 men with phthisis pulmonaris were associated with a 'bowel complaint of a dysenteric character.'[327]

The Clarence Barracks provided temporary accommodation for invalids from *Neptune*, *Croesus*, *Indiana*, and *Niagara*,[328] and possibly *City of Norwich*, *Golden Fleece*, *Australian*, *Rockliffe*, *Hydaspes*, *Melbourne*, and *Hansa* when the name of the barrack utilized was not recorded.[329] Clarence Barracks also housed troops in transit; such as the Royal Wiltshire Militia. Commanded by Lord Methuen, they assisted with disembarkation of invalids from *Himalaya*, *Avon*, and *Neptune*, and also offered succour for women and children brought home in *Himalaya* before they departed for Ireland aboard the *Duke of Cornwall*.[330]

---

326 Smith to QMG, 6 November 1855; Smith, *Précis of Letters*.
327 *Medical and Surgical History*, 2, p.229.
328 *The Times*, 12 February, 8 March, 3 October, and 2 November 1855.
329 *The Times*, 24 May, 2 & 6 June, and 23, 27 & 30 July 1855.
330 *The Times*, 4, 12, & 13 January and 12 February, and *Daily News*, 13 January 1855.

Women and children were housed in the Camber Hospital temporarily after disembarking from *Mauritius*, as were the patients from *Arabia* in March 1855.[331] Early in 1856 militia invalids were moved there from the Garrison Hospital so that it could be reserved only for regulars.[332]

Invalids from HMS *Transit* were removed in omnibuses provided by Mr Nance, the government contractor, to quarters in the Foreshore barracks.[333] The barracks were also used by those brought home in *Brandon*.[334]

London and Woolwich: Men in the Guards arriving on *Mauritius, Talavera, Cornwall,* and *Arabia* were sent by train to London,[335] while those in the RA or RS&M on *Mauritius, Tynemouth, Canterbury, Arabia* and other vessels went into barracks in Portsmouth or Woolwich, rather than Chatham.[336] By the end of June 1855 the accommodation at the Ordnance Hospital Woolwich was proving inadequate and an additional six wards were provided in another building.[337]

Chichester: The possibility of appropriating barracks at Chichester for hospital use was discussed during February 1855.[338] Panmure authorized vacating the buildings in early April and Hardinge subsequently approved arrangements for sending invalids there from Portsmouth.[339] The barracks were in a healthy location and provided accommodation for 150 convalescents with a hospital for 60 sick and a canteen building that could be used as a surgical hospital.[340] Smith was anxious to transfer men there as soon as practicable in order to release space at Portsmouth,[341] and early in May 1855 invalids from *Chapman* and *Canterbury* were transported there from Portsmouth by train. The report continued by stating that 'nothing had been spared to render the barracks in every respect fit for the important purpose of a

---

331 *The Times*, 5 February and 7 March 1855.
332 *The Times*, 8 February 1856.
333 *The Times*, 20 October 1855.
334 *The Times*, 3 December 1855.
335 *The Times*, 5 & 12 February, 10 May, and 13 September 1855. See also Fisher, 'Treatment of the Crimean Wounded', pp.33–44.
336 *The Times*, 5 February, 7 & 14 May, 13 September 1855, and 22 January 1856.
337 *Hampshire Telegraph and Sussex Chronicle*, 30 June 1855.
338 A water colour sketch indicates that the barracks comprised a double row of buildings with a grass parade ground in front; National Army Museum: 1992-05-41.
339 Military Secretary to Smith, 9 & 24 April 1855; Smith, *Précis of Letters*.
340 Dr Forrest to Smith, 15 & 27 April 1855; Smith, *Précis of Letters*.
341 Smith to QMG, 25 April, and the reply from the Military Secretary, 3 May 1855; Smith, *Précis of Letters* and *The Times*, 14 May 1855.

hospital.'³⁴²,³⁴³ A draft of the MSC, 60-strong, joined the hospital from Chatham in May 1856.³⁴⁴

As at Portsmouth no medical records have been preserved though it was reported that invalids in a 'very bad state' were admitted as late as 6 December 1855.³⁴⁵ 'Scorbutic taint' was a common complication of other diseases, a fact that was confirmed by the beneficial effect of a 'generous diet with a liberal share of fresh succulent vegetables, and the use of malt liquor and wine.' A 'dietetic regimen, judiciously employed, [also] formed the principal feature of the treatment' in the surgical division.³⁴⁶

The hospital was still in use towards the end of 1856 as a medical staff attendant was punished by flogging and imprisonment for stealing the money (17s) of an invalid who had recently died.³⁴⁷

Stoke/Devonport: The hospital at Stoke was on the north side of Stonehouse Creek was completed in 1797 and had accommodation for 300–400 patients.³⁴⁸ However, on 25 April 1856 Smith was informed that there was accommodation for 183 at Devonport, but this could be increased by 160 with three additional medical officers.³⁴⁹ Panmure subsequently approved the proposal to occupy the vacant accommodation and Storks was requested to order the next four vessels sailing from Scutari to touch there on their voyage to England.³⁵⁰

Naval facilities: Smith was informed in early April 1855 that HMS *Britannia* and *Caledonia* were to be appropriated as hospital ships in Portsmouth and Plymouth respectively.³⁵¹ *Britannia* was ready by mid-July³⁵² and provided accommodation for 350 convalescents and a hospital for 50.³⁵³ Smith considered it would be undesirable to use her for invalids during winter if she was 'exposed to every wind that blows'³⁵⁴ and

---

342 *Hampshire Telegraph and Sussex Chronicle*, 19 May 1855
343 The Purveyor's opening stock comprised: port wine, 400 dozen; brandy, 50 dozen; stout, 200 dozen; vinegar, 18 gallons; Scotch barley 5,000 lb; sugar, 6,000 lb; tea, arrowroot, and oatmeal, 1,000 lb each; rice, 10 cwt; flesh, washing, and soft soap, five cwt each; sago, 500 lb; *Hampshire Telegraph and Sussex Chronicle*, 14 April 1855.
344 *The Times*, 14 May 1856.
345 *Hampshire Telegraph and Sussex Chronicle*, 8 December 1855.
346 *Medical and Surgical History*, 2, pp.227–8.
347 *Daily News*, 6 November 1856.
348 *Medical Times and Gazette*, 11 November 1854 and Smith and QMG, 24 July 1855; Smith, *Précis of Letters*.
349 PMO, Devonport to Smith, 25 April 1856; Smith, *Précis of Letters*.
350 Undersecretary to Smith, 30 April 1856; Smith, *Précis of Letters*.
351 Military Secretary to Smith, 4 April 1855; Smith, *Précis of Letters*.
352 Smith to Adjutant General, 13 July 1855; Smith, *Précis of Letters*.
353 PMO, Portsmouth to Smith, 9 April 1855; Smith, *Précis of Letters*.
354 Smith to QMG, 9 February 1855; Smith, *Précis* and 9 November 1855; Royal Commission Report, Appendix LXXIX, p.73.

so she was moored near the Block House Battery at the mouth of the creek leading to Haslar Hospital.[355]

Smith requested an inspection of *Caledonia* during April 1855 and by mid-July she was being fitted up at Devonport.[356] He was against augmenting the number of hospitals and asked for her to be moved to Portsmouth so that she and *Britannia* could accommodate convalescents not requiring hospitalization before being dispersed.[357] After the war *Caledonia* was towed to Greenwich where she replaced *Dreadnought* as a hospital for seamen.[358]

Major General H.W. Breton, commanding the South West District, did not favour moving severely wounded men to Chichester and suggested they should go to the naval hospital at Haslar instead.[359] Early in May 1855 Smith was informed that 100 beds could be made available there[360] and he subsequently directed that when there were 10 beds or fewer at Portsea, and transportation to Chichester was not an option, patients should be sent to Haslar together with a medical officer,[361] as the Admiralty favoured army surgeons caring for the soldiers.[362]

Smith had been unwilling to utilize hospitals at Deal and Yarmouth as they were well placed for invalids from the Baltic Fleet, and in case of emergency it might have proved difficult to relocate sick soldiers in safety.[363] However, in 1856 a formal request was made to the Admiralty to 'appropriate' 700 beds for invalids returning from the

---

355 PMO, Portsmouth to Smith, 10 June 1855; Smith, *Précis of Letters*.
356 Smith to PMO, Liverpool, 9 April 1855; Smith, *Précis of Letters and* PMO, Devonport, to Smith, 16 July 1855; Smith, *Précis of Letters*. The items required to equip *Caledonia* included bedsteads (350), blankets (700), cases, bed, hair (350), cases, bolster, hair (35), slip cases, bolster (400), slip cases, pillow (400), covers, waterproof (100), pillows, feather (350), rugs (350), sheets (1,200), spare sackings, bed (100), spare cords, bed (100), towels (200), caps (450), gowns (450), trowsers (450), waistcoats (450), slippers, pairs (450), baths, shower (400), baths, slipper (2), close stools (20), urinals (20), crutches, pairs (100), plus some domestic equipment; PMO, Devonport, to Smith, 16 July 1855; Smith, *Précis*, 2, Appendix II.
357 Smith to QMG, 24 July 1855; Smith, *Précis of Letters*. Incidentally, it would appear that *Britannia* was used for this purpose as 200 men of the 39th Regiment arriving on 21 June 1856 were transferred to her before being sent to Limerick; *Illustrated London News*, 28 June 1956.
358 *The Times*, 19 July 1856.
359 QMG to Smith, 19 April 1855; Smith, *Précis of Letters*. The Haslar Hospital was opened in 1753 and could accommodate 1,800 patients; see W. Tait, *A History of Haslar Hospital* (Portsmouth: Griffin, 1906).
360 Military Secretary to Smith, 3 May 1855; Smith, *Précis of Letters*.
361 Smith to PMO, Portsmouth, 4 May 1855; Smith, *Précis of Letters*.
362 Smith to Military Secretary, 7 March with the response on 12 March 1855; Smith, *Précis of Letters*. Incidentally, a picture of an amputee in the Haslar hospital was published in the *Illustrated London News*, 3 February 1855.
363 Smith to Military Secretary, 16 February 1855; Smith, *Précis of Letters*. Cantlie stated that the naval hospitals at Plymouth, Deal, and Yarmouth were used but he gave no reference; Cantlie, *History*, 2, p.184.

East and these were made available at Plymouth (150), Deal (200) and Yarmouth (350),[364] where 'the men will be provided with everything necessary for their care and comfort.'[365] Smith agreed to make use of Deal during the final evacuation of the Crimea and Turkey if there was insufficient space at Portsmouth or Chichester.[366]

Civilian hospitals: Suggestions were made for accommodating invalids at the Sussex Country Hospital, Brighton,[367] Norfolk Hotel, Bognor,[368] Royal Spa Bathing Infirmary, Margate,[369] Southam Infirmary,[370] and London Fever Hospital, 'apart from the fever wards.'[371] On 26 February 1855 the Undersecretary informed the House of Commons that the government would avail themselves of offers from London and other hospitals should they have occasion to do so, although at the time there was accommodation for 1,600 in military hospitals.[372] Offers were also made privately for civilian hospitals in England to be used but these were turned down, seemingly because of the administrative burden it would have imposed.[373]

Following the arrival of invalids at Liverpool on *Cambria* the Hon. Lady Cust informed Smith that 200 beds were available in the Emigrants' Home in the city.[374] Smith ordered its inspection but it proved too small and too low to be a hospital.[375] Land suitable for a new hospital was identified although this initiative was not pursued. Enmore Castle, Bridgwater was suggested for convalescent officers[376] while Appuldercombe House on the Isle of Wight was surveyed as a potential hospital for naval and army invalids,[377] but neither was apparently used.

4.3.6 Onward journeys from hospital

A General Order issued at Fort Pitt of 22 March 1855 confirmed the policy of discharging men from hospital on Tuesday and Thursday, and several reports in *The Times* during the first eight months of 1856 record that some men returned to their

---

364 Undersecretary to Smith, 14 & 19 April 1856; Smith, *Précis of Letters*.
365 DG, Naval Medical Department, to Smith, 22 April 1856; Smith, *Précis of Letters*.
366 Smith to QMG, 6 June 1856; Smith, *Précis of Letters*.
367 Military Undersecretary to Smith, 14 December 1854; Smith, *Précis of Letters*.
368 Military Undersecretary to Smith, 17 January 1855; TNA: WO 6/78.
369 Letter from the Revd J. Hodgson of St Peter's, Margate, 10 February 1855; Smith, *Précis of Letters*.
370 Letter from H.L. Smith; *Association Medical Journal*, 23 February and 9 March 1855.
371 *The Times*, 1 February 1855.
372 The number of vacant beds averaged 834 during that week in the hospitals in Portsmouth, Plymouth, Chatham and Chichester; Smith, *Précis*, 2, Appendix 45.
373 Cantlie, *History*, 2, p.136.
374 Lady Cust to Smith, 1 February 1855; Smith, *Précis of Letters*.
375 Dr Robertson to Smith, 10 & 15 March 1855; Smith, *Précis of Letters*.
376 Military Undersecretary to Smith, 15 May 1855; Smith, *Précis of Letters*.
377 *Isle of Wight Observer*, *The Lancet*, and *Medical Times and Gazette*, 23 June 1855.

depots while others were sent home with a daily pension of 6d to 2/6d together with clothing issued from the Crimean Fund in cases of need.

Several pensioners in the Ambulance Corps returning to Woolwich were sufficiently strong to proceed to their respective local districts by rail although the Quartermaster Sergeant of the Woolwich Pensioner Corps went with them to London, to see them 'safe on the train going nearest their destination.'[378] Similarly, NCOs from the depots in Chatham were selected to accompany the 'helpless sick and wounded' on their journey home,[379] although not all were so lucky. For example, invalids sent from Chatham to Dublin on *Oudine* did so as deck passengers 'in pursuance of government regulation' and 'were obliged to sleep on straw in the forehold.'[380]

Men were able to travel by train from Chatham to Gravesend by train if their onward journey involved a sea voyage[381] while the War Office entered into contracts with shipping companies for passengers travelling between ports such as London and Edinburgh and Fleetwood and Belfast.

4.3.7 *Number of invalids transported*

The reports of the vessels returning from the East occasionally included the number of invalids but an indication of the numbers that could be involved can be gauged from the passenger lists of the first six vessels that arrived at Portsmouth in 1855 (Table 4.6).

On Christmas Eve 1854 Hall noted that 650 patients were on passage to England,[382] and this increased to 2,000 by the next month.[383] In March 1855 Smith was notified that '*Indiana* is to embark 266 tomorrow; *Adelaide* 170 today or tomorrow; *Rockliffe* to go to Abydos to collect 120 for England; *Tynemouth* will leave soon with 120; *Chapman* and *Julia*, sailing vessels, are to be fitted to receive invalids,'[384] with a further 813 being evacuated from Scutari during the next month.[385]

This selection of reports made during the first few months of 1855 would suggest that the official total of 9,541 men in the cavalry, infantry, and ordnance[386] is almost certainly an underestimate as it probably does not include those sent directly to their regimental depot, or were granted leave, or travelled with their regiments when finally evacuated from the East.

378 *Morning Post*, 13 January 1855.
379 *The Times*, 17 January and 23 April 1856.
380 *Daily News*, 27 April 1855.
381 Commandant, Chatham to QMG, 3 October 1855; TNA: WO 28/192.
382 Hall to QMG, 24 December 1854; RAMC: 397/F/CO/6/43a.
383 *Isle of Wight Observer*, 20 January 1855.
384 PMO, Scutari, 22 March 1855; Smith, *Précis of Letters*.
385 Cumming to Smith, 28 April 1855; Reports on Hospitals in Turkey, p.46. The vessels employed were *Adelaide* (173 cases), *Indiana* (268), *Tynemouth* (213), *Chapman* (134), and *Julia* (184).
386 *Medical and Surgical History*, 2, p.229.

4.3.8 Post-war developments

The development of hospital facilities in England during the campaign took place on a piece meal basis and hence it became apparent there was the need for a substantial purpose built hospital which was readily accessible from the sea, as was the Royal Navy's Haslar Hospital. The foundation stone for a hospital at Netley Abbey on Southampton Water was laid by Queen Victoria on 19 May 1856,[387] too late to play a part in the war, though it proved a welcome replacement for the unsatisfactory facilities at Chatham. The Royal Victoria Hospital subsequently proved an asset during both World Wars, given its location on Southampton Water, but by the 1970s it became redundant and all but the chapel, which now houses a museum, was demolished, including the memorial to the members of the AMD who died during the Crimean campaign.[388]

A military hospital was also constructed in Sheerness, and although planned during the war, the foundation stone was not laid until July 1856. It opened the following year and was decommissioned following the closure of the dockyard in 1960.[389]

4.4 Concluding remarks

The need to repatriate large numbers of ineffective troops became apparent soon after the invasion. Four medical officers who had served in the East met in London on 8 March 1855 and concluded that the repatriation was 'most desirable, for reasons too obvious to dwell on' and that 'the beneficial effects of the voyage' and the 'escape from the crowded and polluted hospital' were 'strong arguments in favour of this measure.'[390] In addition, the spectre of a return of cholera also prompted the speedy repatriation of invalids not likely to recover.[391]

The selection of transport vessels was undertaken by the Royal Navy while the military and medical authorities were responsible for discipline and providing for the patients. There was no shuttle service of steamers to England though 10 (nine percent) of 115 vessels employed undertook 36 (22.5 percent) of 160 voyages. Two dedicated sailing transports employed from the spring of 1855 only made two round trips. Given that transports were selected on an ad hoc basis it is gratifying that there were relatively few reports of serious problems apart from the usual difficulties that may be encountered during a long sea voyage.

---

387 *Illustrated London News*, 24 May 1856.
388 For a photograph of the monument see Shepherd, *Crimean Doctors*, 2, Plate XXXVI.
389 D.T. Hughes, 'The Military Hospital at Sheerness', *Journal of Kent History*, No. 83 (2016), pp.2–5.
390 Smith to Military Undersecretary, 16 March 1855; Royal Commission Report, p.44.
391 Smith to Military Undersecretary, 16 May 1855; Royal Commission Report, Appendix LXXIX, p.54.

The military authorities made no specific plans for the management of invalids and convalescents during the run up to the campaign although several potential sites for convalescent hospitals were considered after the invasion. Gozo was seemingly the only military hospital developed specifically for this purpose although no medical records have survived.

The hospital at Smyrna was planned originally for convalescents although this was not the case for about half the time it was in use. Smyrna, like Renkioi, came into operation too late to make a significant contribution to the war effort, particularly as parts of the hospitals at Scutari and Kuleli were given over to convalescents as the campaign progressed. In addition, the Castle Hospital at Balaklava accommodated men recovering from wounds.

The hospitals at Smyrna and Renkioi were under-utilized and the staff under-employed, although this could not have been foreseen when the decisions to develop them were taken. It is not possible to determine whether the initiative was worthwhile as no comparisons can be made with the testing times of the first winter, and no official assessment of their performance was published.

There was one specific comment about providing respite in the camps in the Crimea but it is certain convalescents would have been kept in camp, especially after the fall of Sevastopol when fewer men required hospitalization.

The majority of the invalids landed at Portsmouth, rather than Chatham, which meant that vessels could be turned round quicker as the voyage was shorter. There were relatively few reports of difficulties at the port apart from some teething problems early in 1855 (Table 4.4) and hence Smith was able to inform the Roebuck Committee on 22 March 1855 that 'full provision' was being made for the reception of invalids on their arrival in England.[392] The journey to Chatham by train could prove arduous and there were complaints that some patients suffered unnecessarily, particularly during the cold weather.

Little information about the hospitals in England has survived. Provision for returning invalids was limited at the start of the campaign, but this increased with time. There was some reasonable criticism of the quality of the facilities but there was apparently no serious shortage of beds.

It was suggested after the war that the number of men repatriated was lower than expected as a proportion of those who would have been sent home under normal circumstances either died before they could be evacuated or were 'detained at the seat of war' as a consequence of the manpower shortage.[393] There were differences in the reasons for the primary admissions to the regimental hospitals and the discharge of invalids from the Army. The former being dominated by acute illness and recent wounds while the latter were for chronic disabilities; particularly those associated with

392 Select Committee, 2nd Report, p.449.
393 *Medical and Surgical History*, 2, p.227.

gunshot wounds, pulmonary tuberculosis, rheumatism, and varicose veins.[394] Further details will be presented in Chapter 8.

---

394 For the case histories on several individuals who were discharged see Fisher, 'Treatment of the Crimean Wounded', pp.33–44

5

Diseases

The principal sources of statistical information on disease and wounds and injuries in the public domain are found in the *Medical and Surgical History*, the contents of which have been summarized in Section 1.6. Of the many tables in the two volumes it is General Return A that provides the most comprehensive numerical overview of what took place during the Eastern campaign. That Return summarizes the reasons for the primary admission of NCOs and men into the 'hospitals of the Army of the East' during each month,[1] together with the deaths that 'occurred in regimental and general hospitals, in hospital ships, or suddenly, or from violence, with the exception of those which occurred in action with the enemy'. The 121 reasons for admission and deaths are listed in 19 categories with some 7,344 items of information – including nil returns. The two sets of data, which are printed side by side for each month, are not directly comparable, however, as they were prepared from separate sources. This means that mortality rates cannot be determined by expressing the deaths in any month as a proportion (percent) of the admissions because individuals may have died some weeks after admission to hospital (see Section 5.7), and at a location other than the Crimea.[2]

Nevertheless, the calculation of the ratio (percent) of 'total deaths' to 'total admissions' does provide an approximation of the overall mortality rate and these are included in the right hand column of Table 5.1. The highest ratio was 59.5 percent for cholera. It was 19.5 percent and 8.5 percent for two scourges of the first winter (frostbite and scurvy) and about 10 percent over the whole campaign for fever, gastrointestinal diseases, and wounds or injuries. Incidentally, several conditions which occurred infrequently (<0.5 percent of admissions) also had high ratios. For example: apoplexy (80.5 percent), tetanus (60), pulmonary tuberculosis (41.5), enteritis, gastritis, and

---

1   The totals in General Return A did not include 5,113 primary admissions for disease when the month was not known; and there is 'no reference to commissioned officers or men of the Land Transport Corps, Mounted Staff Corps, and the Medical Staff Corps.'
2   The time between admission and death are given in the *Medical and Surgical History*, 2, General Return C.

peritonitis (34.5), pneumonia (27), erysipelas (27), gangrene (25), paralysis (24), heart disease (22), dropsy (21.5), and small pox (21). However, as these only accounted for 1.2 percent of admissions and 3.3 percent deaths from disease between them they will not be considered further, with the exception of erysipelas and gangrene which, being potentially nosocomial or hospital acquired infections, will be discussed in the Section 5.5.1.

The twenty most prevalent diseases are summarised in Table 5.2, and, of these, four, diarrhoea, continued fever, dysentery, and cholera accounted for 85,029 (60 percent) of the admissions for disease and 13,212 (81 percent) of the deaths. Conversely, the ratio of deaths to admissions was 2.7 percent or less for catarrh, abscesses, rheumatism, ulcers, eye disease, venereal diseases (syphilis and gonorrhoea), intermittent fever, colic, sore throat, dyspepsia, and jaundice. These eleven diagnostic categories represented 39,895 (28 percent) of admissions with the ratio of deaths to admissions overall being 1.25 percent. Further details of some of these illnesses will be presented in Section 5.5.

Tables 5.1 and 5.2 include entries for wounds, injuries, and punishment as a comparison; and these will be covered in more detail in Chapter 6.

The monthly incidence of admissions and mortality were summarized in General Return B and these are presented in Table 5.3 and graphically in Figures 5.1 and 5.2. Primary admissions for disease peaked during the summers of 1854, the winter of 1854–55, and the summer of 1855 before declining to low levels after the fall of Sevastopol until the end of the campaign. On the other hand, primary admissions for wounds or injuries reflected the periods of greatest military activity, viz. September to November 1854 and from the spring of 1855 until the fall of Sevastopol.

Most of deaths from disease occurred between July 1854 and August 1855 with the worst months being from December 1854 to March 1855 while deaths from wounds or injuries were far fewer and corresponded with admissions.

5.1 Diarrhoea and dysentery

Over the centuries armies on active service had been plagued by epidemics of gastrointestinal diseases, particularly diarrhoea and dysentery.[3] The Eastern campaign was no different. However, the situation was complicated by cholera which, because of its devastating impact, will be covered separately in Section 5.2, although reference to it will be made to herein for comparative purposes.

Gastrointestinal diseases accounted for 55,765 (34 percent) of 162,673 primary hospital admissions listed in General Return A, and 5,950 (33 percent) of 18,058 deaths (Table 5.1) – the proportion being 36.5 percent if the 1,761 deaths from wounds

---

3 See G.C. Cook, 'Influence of Diarrhoea Disease on Military and Naval Campaigns', *Journal of the Royal Society of Medicine*, 94 (2001), pp.95–7.

Table 5.1 Principal reasons for primary admissions into the hospitals of the Army of the East and also the deaths which occurred in the regimental and general hospitals and hospital ships with the exception of those killed in action, April 1854–June 1856

Diagnostic category*	Number of conditions	Admissions to hospitals	Proportion (%) of all admissions	Number of deaths	Proportion (%) of all deaths	Ratio (%) of deaths to admissions (c5/c3)*100
I Fever	4	31,204	19	3,446	19	11
II Eruptive fever	4	29	–	6	–	20.5
III Respiratory disease	9	12,382	7.5	644	3.5	5
IV Cardiovascular disease	6	266	–	41	–	15.5
V Diseases of liver and spleen	4	1,138	0.5	40	–	3.5
VI Gastrointestinal disease	13	55,765	34	5,950	33	10.5
VII Nervous disease	7	736	0.5	160	1	21.5
VIII Cholera	1	7,574	4.5	4,512	25	59.5
IX Rheumatic disease	5	5,131	3	233	1.5	4.5
X Boils and ulcers	4	12,542	7.5	37	–	–
XI Venereal disease	7	3,717	2.5	4	–	–
XII Urogenital disease	9	270	–	6	–	2
XIII Wounds and injuries	8	18,283	11	1761	10	9.5
XIV Punishment (*Punitis*)	1	1,733	1	0	–	–
XV Frostbite	2	2,398	1.5	463	2.5	19.5
XVI Scurvy	1	2,096	1.5	178	1	8.5
X VII Eye disease	1	3,307	2	0	–	–
XVIII Skin disease	1	749	–	1	–	–
XIX Other diseases	34	3,353	2	576	3	17
Totals	121	162,673	100	18,058	100	11

* Listed in the order in the Return.

(Summarized from *Medical and Surgical History*, 2, General Return A)

Diseases 197

Table 5.2 Twenty most common reasons for the admission of NCOs and men into hospital for disease, April 1854–June 1856

Condition	Total admissions (% of disease total)	Total deaths (% of total deaths)	Ratio of deaths: admissions (%)
Diarrhoea	44,164 (31)	3,651 (22.5)	8.5
Continued fever	25,013 (17.5)	2,790 (17)	11
Catarrh	10,083 (7)	240 (1.5)	25
Dysentery	8,278 (6)	2,259 (14)	27.5
Abscesses	7,922 (5.5)	23 (0.1)	0.3
Cholera	7,574 (5.5)	4,512 (27.5)	59.5
Rheumatism	4,906 (3.4)	132 (0.8)	2.7
Ulcers	4,090 (2.9)	11 (0.1)	0.3
Eye diseases	3,307 (2.3)	0	–
Venereal diseases	2,959 (2.1)	3 (<0.1)	0.1
Remittent fever	2,957 (2.1)	311 (1.9)	10.5
Intermittent fever	2,406 (1.7)	60 (0.4)	2.5
Frostbite (Gelatio)	2,398 (1.7)	463 (2.4)	19.5
Scurvy (Scorbutus)	2,096 (1.5)	178 (1.1)	8.5
Colic	1,514 (1.1)	5 (<0.1)	0.3
Bronchitis	1,111 (0.8)	103 (0.6)	9.5
Sore throat (Cynanche)	924 (0.6)	9 (0.1)	1.0
Dyspesia	906 (0.6)	2 (<0.1)	0.2
Jaundice (Icterus)	878 (0.6)	22 (0.1)	2.5
Typhus	828 (0.6)	285 (1.7)	34.4
All other 93 conditions	8,307 (6)	1,238 (7.5)	14.9
Wounds & injuries*	18,279	1,761	9.5
Punishment (Punitis)*	1,773	0	–
Totals for disease	142,621	16,292	11.5

* Included for comparative purposes.
(Adapted from the *Medical and Surgical History*, 2, General Return A)

Table 5.3 Ratio percent to strength during each month of admissions and deaths in General Return B

Date		Admissions (%)			Deaths (%)		
		Disease	Wounds & injuries	Total admissions	Disease	Wounds & injuries	Total deaths
1854	April	3.5	0.4	3.9	0.1	0.0	0.1
	May	9.3	0.9	10.2	0.1	0.0	0.1
	June	8.5	0.8	9.3	0.1	0.0	0.1
	July	17.0	0.5	17.5	1.3	0.0	1.3
	August	27.8	0.4	28.2	2.8	0.0	2.8
	September	16.6	5.7	22.3	2.8	0.3	3.1
	October	21.2	2.4	23.6	2.1	0.4	2.5
	November	21.3	6.5	27.8	3.2	1.0	4.2
	December	31.5	0.9	32.4	5.7	0.3	6.0
1855	January	34.2	0.6	34.8	9.5	0.2	9.8
	February	22.6	0.4	23.0	8.0	0.1	8.2
	March	18.5	0.8	19.3	4.6	0.1	4.7
	April	12.4	1.9	14.3	1.7	0.2	1.9
	May	14.5	1.7	16.2	1.6	0.1	1.7
	June	22.4	5.9	28.3	2.1	0.5	2.7
	July	21.1	2.5	23.6	1.0	0.3	1.3
	August	19.5	3.5	23.0	1.1	0.4	1.5
	September	11.7	5.0	16.7	0.4	0.6	1.0
	October	10.5	1.0	11.5	0.3	0.1	0.4
	November	8.8	1.0	9.8	0.4	0.1	0.5
	December	10.2	0.9	11.1	0.2	0.0	0.3
1856	January	8.6	0.7	9.3	0.2	0.0	0.2
	February	7.0	0.7	7.7	0.1	0.0	0.1
	March	7.3	0.8	8.1	0.1	0.0	0.1
	April	6.2	0.8	7.0	0.1	0.0	0.1
	May	5.4	0.6	6.0	0.1	0.0	0.1
	June	3.2	0.4	3.6	0.0	0.0	0.0

(Adapted from the *Medical and Surgical History*, 2, General Return B. The proportions (%) were calculated using the monthly strengths furnished by the regimental surgeons in the regimental summaries in the *Medical and Surgical History*, 1)

Diseases 199

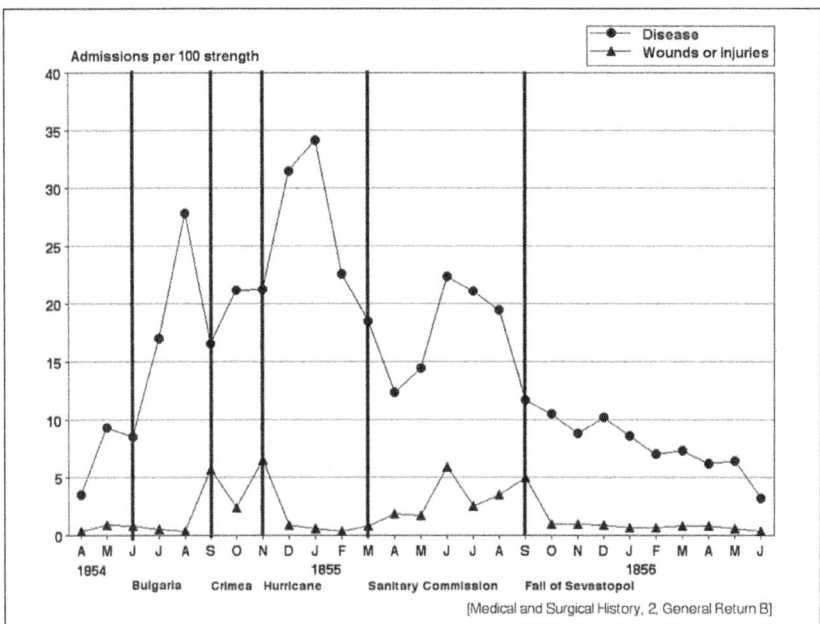

Figure 5.1 Primary admissions of NCOs and men to hospitals in Turkey, Bulgaria, and the Crimea, April 1854–June 1856.

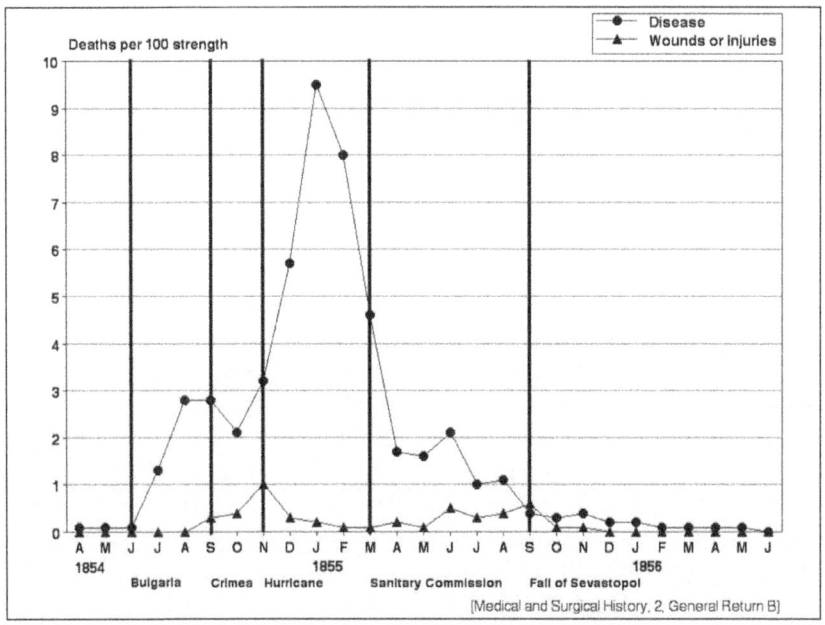

Figure 5.2 Deaths of NCOs and men in regimental and general hospitals and on board ship, April 1854–June 1856.

and injuries are excluded. Details of eleven conditions listed as 'Diseases of stomach and bowels' are listed in Table 5.4. The admissions were dominated by diarrhoea (79 percent) followed by dysentery (15 percent), and they accounted for 62 percent and 38 percent respectively of all deaths, with dysentery having a case-fatality rate about three times greater than that for diarrhoea (Table 5.4, col. 6).

Table 5.4 Gastrointestinal diseases, excepting cholera, diagnosed in NCOs and men, April 1854–June 1856

Gastrointestinal disease (in the order listed)	Primary admissions to regimental hospitals	Proportion (%) of all admissions	Deaths in regimental and general hospitals and on ships	Proportion (%) of all deaths	Ratio (%) of deaths to admissions (c4/c2*100)
Peritonitis	16	–	9	–	56
Enteritis	36	–	11	–	30.5
Dysentery*	8,278	15	2,259	38	27.5
Diarrhoea	44,164	79	3,651	62	8.5
Colic	1,514	3	5	–	–
Gastritis	29	–	8	–	27.5
Constipation	348	0.5	0	–	–
Haematemesis	15	–	2	–	13.5
Haemorrhoids	358	0.5	0	–	–
Hernia	101	–	2	–	2
Dyspepsia	906	1.5	3	–	–
Total	55,765		5,950		10.5

* Includes acute, chronic dysentery and scorbutic dysentery.

(Adapted from the *Medical and Surgical History*, 2, General Return A)

Diarrhoea and dysentery can be associated with several infectious and non-infectious diseases. Shepherd questioned the value of attempting to distinguish between them given the absence of adequate diagnostic criteria at the time.[4] The patterns of admissions and deaths on a monthly basis were broadly similar and the data have been combined in Figure 5.3. There were two periods of increased prevalence; the first from June 1854 to March 1855 and the second from May 1855 until the end of the year. The incidence was considerably reduced after the fall of Sevastopol and neither proved troublesome during 1856. Mortality was only exceptionally high between November 1854 and March 1855 and nearly 80 percent of the deaths occurred during this period (Figure 5.4). The figure also illustrates the difference in the patterns of mortality for cholera and the fevers.

4 Shepherd, *Crimean Doctors*, 1, p.317.

Diseases 201

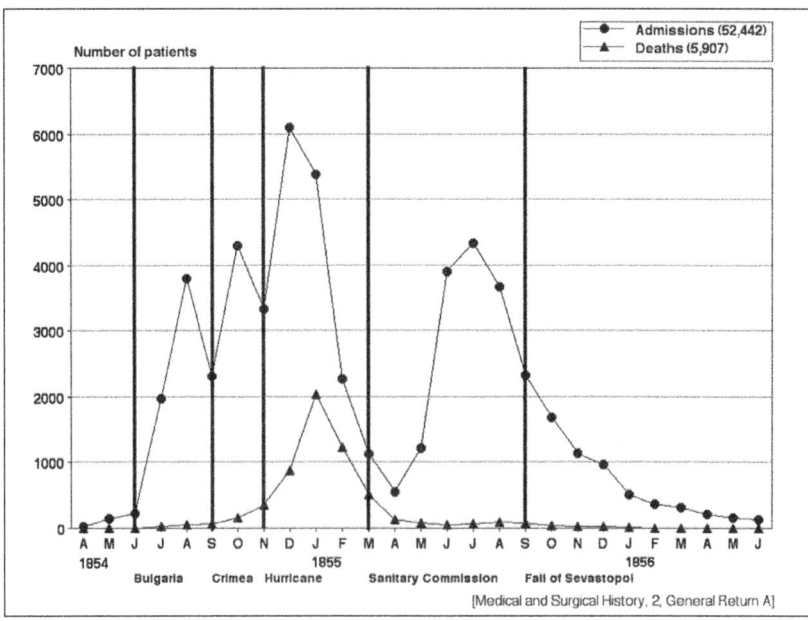

Figure 5.3 Admissions for, and deaths from diarrhoea and dysentery, fevers, and cholera among NCOs and men, April 1854–June 1856.

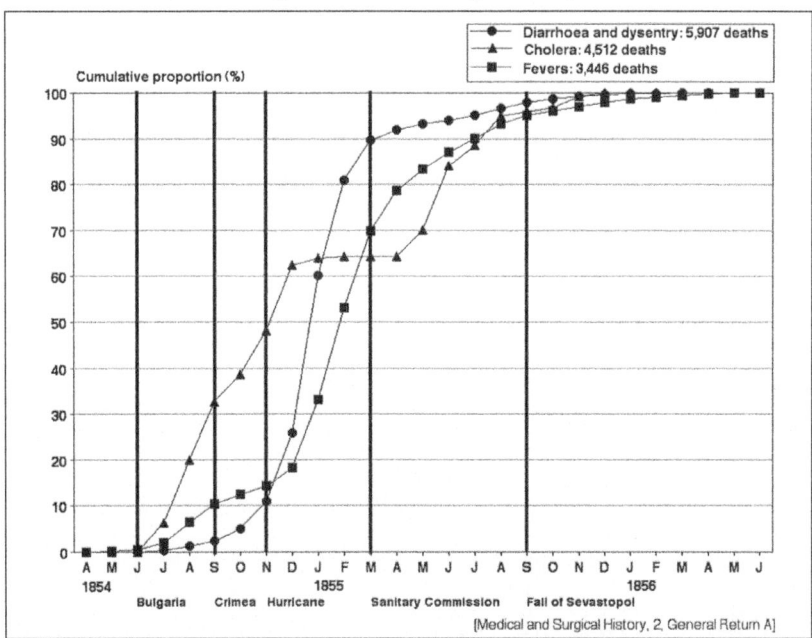

Figure 5.4 Cumulative proportion (%) of deaths from diarrhoea and dysentery, fevers, and cholera among NCOs and men, April 1854–June 1856.

5.2 Cholera

Cholera was present in Europe during 1854 and it had been recognized for over 20 years that the movement of people was of importance in spreading the disease.[5] It is not surprising, therefore, that it followed the allied armies eastwards; and 'visited' Piraeus, Gallipoli, and the Bosphorus. The infection was probably introduced into Bulgaria by the French[6] with the first fatal case in the British troops occurring on 17 June 1854.[7] The British public was informed by *The Times* on 17 July.[8] The development of these epidemics during the next 18 months are discussed in this section.[9]

5.2.1 *Clinical features*

The clinical presentation of cholera were described by Dr W. Linton[10] and it is likely that most fatalities with pronounced pathognomonic symptoms would have been recorded accurately but the milder form (now known to occur during epidemics) may have been returned simply as diarrhoea. It is unlikely that many of the deaths due to diarrhoea represented a misdiagnosis of cholera as the 1854 epidemic was effectively over when fatalities from diarrhoea were at their worst. Similarly, the return of relatively few deaths from diarrhoea during the 1855 cholera epidemic suggests that cholera was not confused with other gastrointestinal diseases.

In his official report on the health status of the Army for June 1855 Hall noted that Raglan died of choleraic diarrhoea,[11] a condition that was recorded in the reports of regimental surgeons in 34 of the 66 cavalry and infantry regiments.[12] Hall also used the term in his summary of the '*Avon*' affair', viz. 'The greater proportion of the sick sent on board were cases of cholera, or choleraic diarrhoea, but twenty-two of them were wounded.'[13] In December 1854 the term was used to describe Major General Pennefather's illness that left him in a critical condition for two days before he eventually recovered.[14]

---

5 *The Lancet* (1831), pp.241–84.
6 A naval surgeon suggested that cholera was brought by a French vessel arriving on 14 July; *Medical Times and Gazette*, 30 September 1854.
7 Hall to Smith, 2 July 1854; RAMC: 397/F/CO/1/1/277 and Smith, *Précis of Letters*.
8 *The Times* 17, 18 & 21 July include further despatches dated 21 & 22 June and 8 July 1854, while a letter dated Malta, 21 July, reported cholera in Gallipoli and Dardanelles; *The Times*, 28 June 1854.
9 The *Medical and Surgical History*, 2, pp.45–89 provides a contemporary account. For a recent review see M. Hinton, 'Cholera in the British Army and Navy during the Crimean War', in M. Holland, G, Gill, and S. Burrell (eds.), *Cholera in Conflict*, (Leeds: Medical Museum Publishing, 2009), pp.160–203.
10 *Medical and Surgical History*, 2, p.60.
11 TNA: WO 17/1731.
12 *Medical and Surgical History*, 1, pp.5–542.
13 Mitra, *Life and Letters*, p.350.
14 Letter from the Crimea dated 16 December 1854; *The Times*, 10 January 1855.

When these reports are considered together it is clear that a proportion of the medical officers regarded choleraic diarrhoea as a separate clinical entity. It was not included as a specific diagnosis in the summary tables in the *Medical and Surgical History* though the symptoms were described:

> The dejections were watery, though generally coloured, and more or less foeculent, and often voided several times in twenty-hours. In most instances borborygmi [audible sounds of intestinal movements] and griping pains in the bowels were felt, and these sensations frequently preceded the calls to evacuate them. There was little or no constitutional disturbance, but there was more or less sinking or depression, and the spirits were often dull or anxious [and there was no] great disposition of diarrhoea of this kind to pass into dysentery [though there was a] tendency [for] choleraic diarrhoea to run into cholera.[15]

The illness was fatal on occasions but its course was not as rapid as cholera, and severe dehydration, the passing of rice-water stools, vomiting, and the suppression of urine formation were not characteristic of the syndrome.

Half the patients with cholera died within two days of the admission to hospital with about a tenth surviving beyond a week. The fatality rates in the regiments, and on naval ships, were within the range previously recorded in epidemics though the incidence might have been relatively higher as the medical officers would have reported a greater proportion of the patients with 'symptoms [...] pathognomonic for the disease', than their civilian counterparts.[16]

The symptoms were similar to those in previous epidemics and the fatality rates were not affected by the troops being located 'on a dry elevated mountain ridge, in a swampy malarious locality, or a filthy overcrowded town',[17] or being managed in an efficient, common-sense manner, as in the Naval Brigade.[18] Anecdotal opinion suggested that severe diarrhoea made its appearance before cholera which implies that a fall in standards of camp hygiene facilitated the spread of the disease.

5.2.2 Contemporary views on the cause, treatments and prevention

Ignorance of the cause of cholera meant that many of the suggestions for risk factors, treatment and prophylaxis would now appear bizarre. Those factors included accommodation in bell tents, the climate, the vicissitudes of temperature, heavy dews, defective diet, unripe fruit, and sour wines, and, only occasionally, the consumption of impure and dirty or muddy water. It would seem that not many medical officers were 'impressed [...] with the idea that the disease was transmissible' although some were

---

15 *Medical and Surgical History*, 2, p.92.
16 *Medical and Surgical History*, 2, p.80.
17 *Medical and Surgical History*, 2, p.55.
18 HCPP 1857 Session 1 (71) IX.797: *Medical Statistical Returns of the Baltic and Black Sea Fleets, during the Years 1854 and 1855*, p.40.

'disposed to regard it as possessing some power of self-extension' and that it had an 'eminently contagious nature under certain conditions.'[19]

Calomel, opium, mineral acids, turpentine, quinine, chloroform, arsenic, hydrocyanic acid, lead acetate, and stimulants were all prescribed, while 'the saline treatment has not apparently put to the test of experiment.'[20] A tragedy given that several contemporary reports had recorded the beneficial effect of that specific therapy.[21] This omission probably reflected the prevailing attitude of the medical establishment as a whole, rather than hard pressed medical officers eschewing what would now be accepted as an early example of an approach to treatment that was evidence-based.

Wearing cholera belts was considered beneficial for preventing the onset of symptoms. For example, Panmure, through the Military Undersecretary, requested Smith on 13 March 1855 to impress on PMOs the necessity of the men wearing woollen shirts and cholera belts. Smith concurred and wrote to Hall on the 19 March requiring him to direct medical officers to ensure that in changeable and bad weather the men wear cholera belts, as 'excellent protection and a comfortable support.' Hall replied on 5 April stating that the men wear woollen undergarments but cholera belts 'are not much in repute as they preferred the broad woollen sash worn outside their clothes; Smith then ordered a supply of sashes.[22] A further example of an ineffective approach to prophylaxis was provided by a memorandum issued on 1 June 1855: 'Salt taken [...] with food, to the extent one salt-spoonful night and morning, two salt-spoonfuls at dinner, is said by Dr Beaman to prevent cholera. This quantity may be doubled [...] and the addition of a small quantity of Cayenne pepper is useful. The use of this simple precaution is recommended, as well as that of constantly wearing a cholera belt next the skin.'[23]

After the war Panmure issued instructions for medical officers to follow when cholera was suspected or diagnosed.[24] It is clear that thinking on this matter remained unresolved since the provision of a clean water supply was not among the recommendations. This is surprising perhaps given that the General Board of Health's Medical Officer concluded in the same year that Londoners drinking dirty water were more likely to contract cholera than those receiving a cleaner supply.[25]

19   *Medical and Surgical History*, 2, p.8.
20   *Medical and Surgical History*, 2, pp.63–4.
21   For example, *Medical Times and Gazette*, 21 August 1853. Incidentally, the restoration and maintenance of fluid and electrolyte balance remains a treatment of first choice to this day.
22   Smith, *Précis*.
23   TNA: WO 28/191.
24   Anon, *Instructions to Army Medical Officers for their Guidance on the Appearance of Spasmodic Cholera in the United Kingdom*, (London: Eyre and Spottiswoode, 1856).
25   HCPP 1856 [2103] LII.257: *Report of the Last Two Cholera-Epidemics of London as Affected by the Consumption of Impure Water*. Incidentally, it was suggested when tackling the cholera epidemic in Haiti that priority should have been given to sanitation and providing a clean water supply, rather than introducing a vaccination programme; Wampler, 'Pick Sanitation over Vaccination', p.175.

Investigations into cholera in the United Kingdom: A Council with the brief to investigate the ongoing cholera epidemic was convened by the General Board of Health in London during August 1854 under the chairmanship of J.A. Paris, President of the Royal College of Physicians. The report, published the next year, would not have proved of much practical value to the medical officers in the Crimea as none of the treatments prescribed 'could be confidently recommended [...] a few treatments – calomel, castor oil, and sulphuric acid – were associated with higher than expected mortality, and others – opium and chalk – [...] with lower than expected rates of death.'[26]

The report has been reviewed critically by Dean who pointed out that 'Snow's empirically plausible explanation' for the spread of the disease was ignored since they concluded that 'the theory that infection occurred by swallowing water and other items contaminated with faeces of choleraic patients as having been disproved "beyond the possibility of reasonable doubt."' Dean also provided evidence to suggest that the Council suppressed the more favourable recovery rates recorded at the London Homeopathic Hospital.[27]

Another committee under the chairmanship of Dr J. Simon reported the next year on 13 May 1856 and concluded that 'faecalised drinking water and faecalised air equally may breed and convey the poison; and that this whether in one vehicle of another, may be expected to prevail most forcibly against the feeble and ill-nourished part of the population,' though the committee did note that 'the fatal disease [cholera] had been more prevalent among the drinkers of foul water than among the drinkers of clean water.'[28]

This, and other reports, such as a letter from the President of the Board of Health to Viscount Palmerston which included a report from Dr J. Sutherland, who was later to be appointed one of the Sanitary Commissioners,[29] did recognize that cholera was associated with unsanitary living conditions and impure water, and that there was need to provide improved infrastructure and a clean water supply. However, none of these so-called specialists espoused Snow's hypothesis that water was of crucial importance in the epidemiology of the disease. Accordingly, they failed to formulate more positive recommendations on the control of the disease.

26 HCPP 1854–5 [1901] XLV.41: *Report on the Results of Different Methods of Treatment Pursued in Epidemic Cholera throughout England and Scotland in 1854.*
27 M.E. Dean, 'Selective Suppression by the Medical Establishment of Unwelcome Research Findings: the Cholera Treatment Evaluation by the General Board of Health', *Journal of the Royal Society of Medicine*, 109:5 (2016), pp.200–5.
28 HCPP 1856 [2103] LII.257.
29 HCPP 1854–55 [1893] XLV.69: *Letter of the President of the General Board of Health to Viscount Palmerston Accompanying a Report from Dr Sutherland on Cholera in the Metropolis in 1854.*

5.2.3 Observations in camp

There were several references to the unsanitary nature of camp sites. Presumably the disregard of basic rules of hygiene 'helped [cholera] sweep through the allied army and navy.'[30] A point effectively made by Dr W. Cattell, 5th Dragoon Guards:

> Horses being watered at the fountains (which should have been reserved for other use) made a puddle around. [...] thirsty men in a blazing sun and already suffering from diarrhoea [...] would eagerly lap up water from the puddle [...] The latrine was a deep trench, but Mosaic sanitation or use of dry earth was neglected and the pit was a hot bed of flies innumerable which spent their days between ordure of all kinds and our food. In the river men washed, washed clothes and bathed, and the butchers found it a convenient place for offal. Yet it still formed the chief supply for cooking, and what was of far more consequence it was eagerly drunk by men whose thirst became excessive. In vain was warning given against such practices.[31]

Another eyewitness, Private Harry Blishen, Rifle Brigade, appreciated these events rather differently:

> We have harder work against the cholera, dysentery and lake fever, than we should have had against five times our number of the enemy in Russia. The number of deaths [have] been fearful [...] dear mother, if you can give me a better example of the 'frailty of life' than many of my comrades have offered me of late; that of being in robust health one hour, and the next hour groaning in the agonies of death; one poor fellow invoking the Almighty to forgive him his sins, and another raging with fever.[32]

A naval surgeon suggested that the 'dreadful calamity was attributed to drinking water from wells that had been poisoned by throwing in putrid carcasses.'[33] He also provided some support to the theory that water is the medium by which 'cholera poison is conveyed' when he observed 'soldiers, wearied by marching from a focus of cholera infection [...] washing their persons and clothing in the streams from which all the French ships of war, and the majority of the English fleet, obtained their water; and following this 'the disease burst out with great violence among the crews of several

---

30   Royle, *Crimea*, p.176. The author suggested without providing evidence that there was an outbreak of amoebic dysentery at this time. This is unlikely since *Entamoeba histolytica* is usually associated with a tropical climate.
31   RAMC: 391 and quoted by Cantlie, *History*, 2, p.26.
32   H.B., *Letters from the Crimea during the Years 1854 and 1855* (London: Emily Faithfull, 1856), pp.26–8. (Henry Blishen, Rifle Brigade, was killed on 8 September 1855.)
33   Letter to Dr J.T. Veitch dated Baljik, 23 August 1854; *Medical Times and Gazette*, 30 September 1854.

ships.'[34] The possibility of the spread of cholera being influenced by the 'impurity of the water' was also mentioned by Cattell although he was probably a miasmatist as he noted that there was an 'offensive odour drifted over the place from some weeds which grew in the vicinity.'[35]

There are several references in the *Medical and Surgical History* suggesting filtering polluted river water and water for hospital use but there is no suggestion in this document, or the 52 recommendations issued by Smith in 1853, that water should be boiled or filtered as a control measure.[36] The value of improving hygienic standards was recognized, however, but principally because this reduced the 'emanation of miasmas', rather than as a means of breaking the cycle of infection.

5.2.4 Cholera in the Army, 1854–1856

Cholera accounted for 7,574 (4.5 percent) of 162,673 primary hospital admissions, and 4,512 (25 percent) of 18,053 deaths, with the proportion being 28 percent if the 1,761 deaths from wounds and injuries are excluded (Table 5.2)

The primary admissions for the specific gastrointestinal diseases listed in the General Return A were dominated by diarrhoea (70 percent) followed by dysentery (12.5) and cholera (12). Cholera was the principal cause of all deaths (43), with diarrhoea and dysentery accounting for 35 and 20.5 percent respectively (Table 5.2). The pattern of mortality in cholera is clearly different from that of diarrhoea and dysentery (Figure 5.4).

The 1854 epidemic lasted longer than might have been expected following the invasion, presumably because of the arrival of new and susceptible regiments and the unsanitary conditions that developed in the trenches and camp during the autumn. There was a definite break of a few weeks between the epidemics of 1854 and 1855, which proved less serious, and there was no recrudescence of the disease in 1856 (Figure 5.5), although the few cases diagnosed during the first quarter may represent a carry-over from 1855.

Infantry regiments besieging Sevastopol: The incidence of cholera among regiments destined to do duty on the trenches reached a peak in August 1854, and, after a decrease it increased again after the siege was joined with a further peak in December, before petering out in the New Year. Regiments going directly to the Crimea during November and December suffered more severely than those that had spent time in Bulgaria or landed in September with those arriving in November being the worst affected. The 1854 epidemic was nearly over by the time three regiments arrived in January and only a few cases were recorded in those.

34 *Medical Times and Gazette*, 30 September 1854
35 RAMC: 391.
36 *Medical Times and Gazette*, 1 October & 10 December 1854, pp.369 & 596–7.

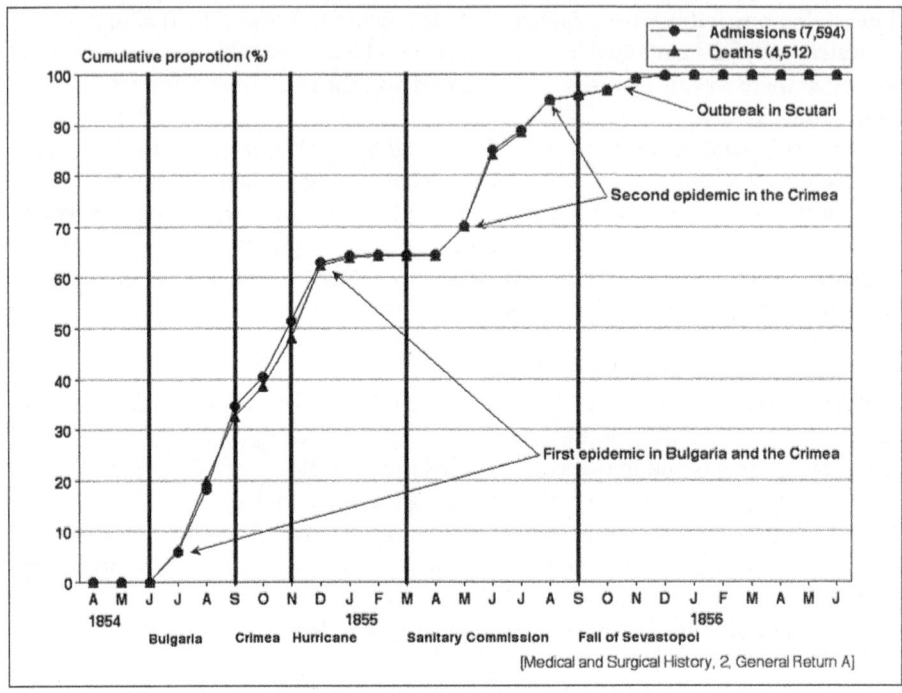

Figure 5.5 Admissions for, and deaths from cholera among NCOs and men, April 1854–June 1856.

The epidemic in 1855 was shorter and proved more serious in the regiments arriving after the end of the winter. A few cases were recorded during the months after the fall of Sevastopol but cholera ceased to be problem in the Crimea thereafter.

Highland Brigade and Cavalry Division: These troops were spared duty in trenches during the winter if 1854/55 and this may explain why there was no recrudescence of cholera following the invasion despite suffering similarly to the other regiments when in Bulgaria.

Cholera 'visited' both corps during 1855 with the problem being rather greater in the four cavalry regiments that arrived during that year. Thirteen of the fourteen cavalry regiments relocated to Turkey in the autumn of 1855 and cases of cholera occurred in several of those located near Scutari during November (Figure 5.6).[37]

---

37   For details see M. Hinton, 'A Short-lived Cholera Epidemic in Scutari during November 1855', *Soldiers of the Queen*, No. 171 (2018), pp.22–8.

Diseases 209

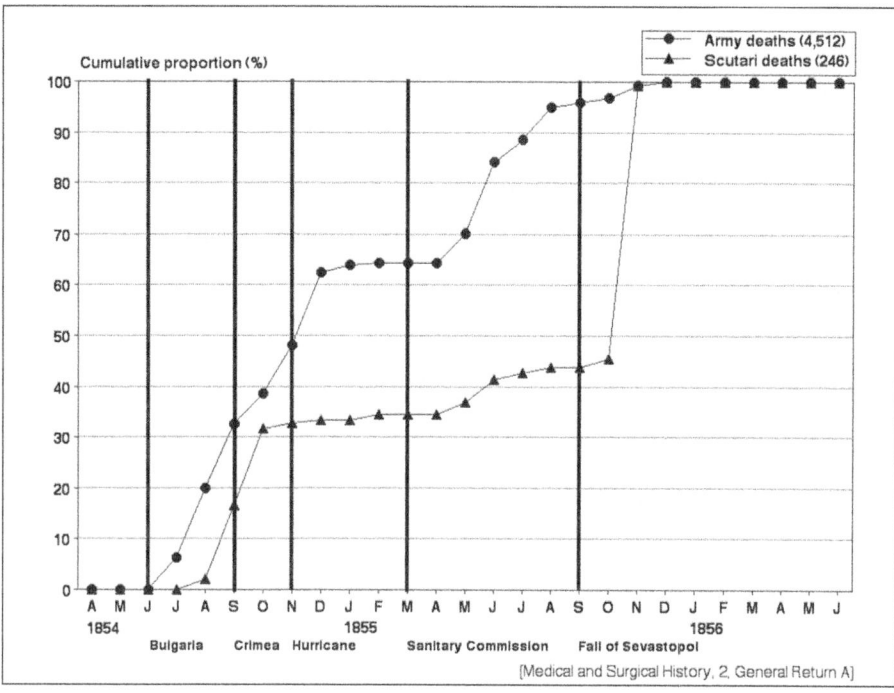

Figure 5.6 Deaths among NCOs and men from cholera in the Army as a whole and the hospitals at Scutari, April 1854–June 1856.

Royal Artillery and Royal Sappers and Miners: The *Medical and Surgical History* provided few details about disease in the RA and RS&M although the records for these Corps combined (the Ordnance) for the first and second cholera epidemics indicated that the mortality tended to be higher in the Ordnance than the cavalry and infantry in both years.[38]

Military and medical officers: The incidence of cholera in officers was not recorded but the loss of individuals, both senior and junior, would have made the management of the Army problematical, particularly during 1854. An early casualty was Lieutenant Colonel Maule, a brother of Lord Panmure, while other senior officers included Brigadier Tylden, Lieutenant Colonel Hoey, 30th Regiment, Purveyor Ward, Major General Estcourt, General Marmora of the Sardinian Army, Rear Admiral Boxer, and Lieutenant Colonel Vico, the French Commissioner at the British Headquarters.[39]

38 *Medical and Surgical History*, 2, pp.86–8.
39 *Gentleman's Magazine*, 1854 & 1855: Maule, October, p.390; Tylden, November, p.534; Ward, March, p.328; Marmora & Boxer, July. pp.93 & 95; Estcourt, August, p.199; and

Several contemporary reports, and later commentaries, have suggested that Lord Raglan died of cholera, although the evidence of for this is not compelling.

The obituaries in *Gentleman's Magazine* recorded that cholera caused the death of four lieutenant colonels, six majors, ten captains, fourteen lieutenants, and three ensigns, while sixteen staff or regimental surgeons, two civilian surgeons, and one dispenser died of the disease.

Cholera in the hospitals on the Bosphorus: Cholera was never a serious problem in the troops located in Turkey as there were 246 (0.5 percent) deaths among 43,288 admissions. About a third of the deaths occurred during the summer of 1854 and over half during November 1855 (Figure 5.6). This topic is considered further in Section 7.2.

Cholera during 1856: One incentive for repatriating troops as quickly as possible after hostilities ceased was the apprehension of an epidemic of cholera during 1856.[40] In the event only thirteen cases were recorded in the Army during the first six months of the year.[41] Eleven occurred during the first quarter and these may represent the final cases of the 1855 epidemic.

5.2.5 Concluding remarks
The epidemics of cholera in 1854 and 1855 were described at length in the *Medical and Surgical History*.[42] That and other contemporary accounts generally agreed that the British Army and Royal Navy were cholera-free when they arrived in Turkey, and later in Bulgaria, and that the 'pestilence' was brought to the region by French troops.[43] It was suggested at the time that the infection may have lain dormant following an epidemic in the Danubian Principalities some years previously. That is unlikely in view of what is now known on the subject, while an unreferenced suggestion made by Miles that it was brought to the East by British troops that passed through London is not supported by contemporary accounts.[44]

The epidemic was relatively simple to describe while the Army was in Bulgaria, but following the invasion it was more difficult to determine any pattern as the troops 'enjoyed too constant intercourse with every part of the camp to favour accurate analysis.' This is a fair conclusion given that the men who manned the trenches were exposed to 'an atmosphere, often unavoidably vitiated by the excretions of the masses engaged on such duty,' and were also employed collecting supplies from Balaklava, a

  Vico, September, p.318; and *The Times*, 21 October 1855 (Hoey).
40 *Medical and Surgical History*, 2, p.45.
41 *Medical and Surgical History*, 2, General Return A.
42 *Medical and Surgical History*, 2, pp.45–89.
43 *Medical and Surgical History*, 2, pp.46–7.
44 Miles, *Accidental Birth*, p.113.

place 'eminently favourable to the development and extension of cholera,'[45] and had contact with the camps of the French and Turkish armies, and the sutlers' bazaars.

There was a break of a few weeks between the epidemics of 1854 and 1855 when the weather was at its coldest. *Vibrio cholerae* is now known to persist in the environment in a viable but non-culturable state and this provides a scientific explanation for what was suggested in the *Medical and Surgical History*:

> No case [of cholera] was returned in March [1855]; it unfortunately, however, soon became apparent that the principle of this awful scourge was merely in a dormant state, for in April, instances of the disease were again presented [...] the pestilence had only slumbered in the work of death, to burst forth again with fresh acquired vigour and still greater power of destruction.[46]

It was concluded that once 'the choleraic poison had nearly exhausted itself on those who had been [...] exposed to its influence [...] it required [...] fresh subjects upon which to develop its effects,'[47] while the 'most powerful predisposing cause' was considered to be the 'recent arrival of the soldiers.'[48] There is considerable anecdotal evidence to support this assertion though multivariate analyses yielded limited statistical evidence suggesting a link between outbreaks and the receipt of drafts of new troops (the 'virgin soil' model).[49] This may be more a reflection of the inadequacy of the data available for analysis than an accurate assessment of events.

During the height of the epidemic in Bulgaria a naval surgeon noted that 'this alarming visitation, which may appear [...] quite unprecedented [has] conformed to laws already ascertained.'[50] This conclusion prompts the question: Was the cholera epidemic worse in the British forces than might be expected in civilian populations? Did the exigencies of campaigning influence the course of the epidemics? The short answer is a qualified 'No'; for the following reasons: The role of shipping in the transmission of cholera was well recognised as it frequently appeared in ports and then spread inland along trade routes. That this obtained in Bulgaria was confirmed in

---

45   *Medical and Surgical History*, 2, pp.75–6.
46   *Medical and Surgical History*, 2, p.72.
47   *Medical and Surgical History*, 2, p.66. This can be explained by the development of immunity in those suffering mild symptoms or remaining asymptomatic.
48   *Medical and Surgical History*, 2, p.74.
49   M. Smallman-Raynor and A.D. Cliff, 'The Geographical Spread of Cholera in the Crimean War: Epidemic Transmission in the Camp Systems in the British Army of the East, 1854–55', *Journal of Historical Geography*, 30 (2004), pp.32–69.
50   *Medical Times and Gazette*, 30 September 1854. The correspondent's view reflected that of Sutherland expressed a few years earlier, viz. 'cholera is by no means so capricious in its attacks as has generally been supposed [...] on the contrary it is propagated according to certain fixed laws, although the limits of these have not yet been precisely defined;' J. Sutherland, *Appendix (A) to the Report of the General Board of Health on the Epidemic of Cholera of 1848 and 1849* (London: HMSO, 1850).

the *Medical and Surgical History* in which it was noted 'that the pestilence strongly affects the estuaries of sea coasts, the towns built upon them, the courses of rivers [...] for its extension' but as the distance from the sea and rivers increased 'the tendency of the disease to spread and commit ravages reduced', although this did not always hold good since the 'extraordinary fact was noticed' that the Highland Brigade quartered 'nearest the lake on [ground previously] occupied by the Light Division, suffered much less [...] than the Brigade of Guards.'[51] Cholera subsequently accompanied the Army to the Crimea with deaths occurring on board ship and during the march to Sevastopol. The course of the secondary epidemic, which was in part associated with the arrival of new regiments, followed the typical pattern and was over in early 1855.

Small outbreaks may last a few days or weeks, but larger epidemics usually persist for two or three months before gradually petering out. This situation occurred in the epidemics involving the cavalry and ordnance in Bulgaria, and the whole army in the Crimea in 1855. Cholera would not be expected to persist year on year in non-endemic regions like the Crimea. Thus, the recording of only a few cases during the last months of the occupation is not unexpected, while the few cases involving Royal Navy personnel were associated with time spent ashore in Malta and Lisbon.

Despite the hype occasioned at the time, the commentary in the *Medical and Surgical History* began with the following simple statement: 'Hitherto [...] cholera was entirely an exceptional occurrence, the pestilence confining itself to small bodies of troops in camp, or on the line of march, appearing only for short periods, and generally in detached positions, but seldom constituting itself an agent of a widespread destruction.'[52] Although this retrospective assessment may not be far from the truth, it would be naïve to suggest that cholera is not a devastating disease. An illness that can kill a healthy soldier within hours would have a profound effect on morale and strike fear into the hearts of even the bravest of men. However, to suggest that cholera 'decimated' the Army, i.e. killed one in 10, is an exaggeration,[53] especially as several other diseases, particularly diarrhoea and dysentery, coupled with the effects of exposure, overwork, and malnutrition, exacted a even more terrible toll than cholera on the hapless soldiery, particularly during the autumn and winter of 1854–55.[54]

The *Medical and Surgical History* was published in 1857 and it is perplexing that Smith and his colleagues were seemingly unaware of Snow's publications.[55] From a

---

51 *Medical and Surgical History*, 2, p.55.
52 Kaufman, *Surgeons at* War, p.165.
53 'Decimation' was used Smallman-Raynor and Cliff, 'The Geographical Spread of Cholera' while C. Lloyd, and J.L.S. Coulter, *Medicine and the Navy 1200–1900. Volume 4. 1815–1900* (Edinburgh: E & S Livingstone, 1963), p.141 concluded 'cholera, and not malaria, which nearly destroyed the Army and Navy before hostilities began.'
54 H.B., *Letters*, pp.26–8.
55 For example, J. Snow, *On the Mode of Communication of Cholera* (London: Churchill, 1855). Dr Buzzard, who served with the Turkish Contingent was aware of Snow's work when in the Crimea: 'Whenever possible I refrained from drinking water that had not been boiled

modern perspective the 'concluding observations'[56] are of limited value for explaining the epidemic as this possibility of spread was not used to inform the discussion. Similarly, there is no evidence that the Sanitary Commissioners had espoused Snow's hypothesis. They published their report in the same year and concluded that 'a more striking example of the deadly effects of impure air cannot be imagined' while Burnetts's official account of cholera in the Royal Navy 'constantly speaks about air, and never about water.'[57]

It is clear, therefore, that the majority of the medical profession, both at home and serving with the Army were in ignorance how the 'pestilence' was transmitted and this meant that the cholera bacillus was given a free rein to wreak havoc among the armies of all the nations involved in the campaign. A misfortune indeed, since, (with hindsight) it is easy to appreciate that the number of fatalities could have been reduced by the simple expedient of boiling drinking water and following the basic rules of good hygienic practice in the camps and on board ship.

5.3 Fevers

Fevers accounted for 31,204 (19 percent) of 162,673 primary admissions to hospital and for 3,446 (19 percent) of 18,058 deaths (Table 5.1).[58] An analysis of data in General Return B demonstrates that they were more prevalent in the summer of 1854 and, in a biphasic form during the spring and summer of 1855 (Figure 5.7), with the pattern of mortality differing from those of diarrhoea and dysentery, and cholera (Figure 5.4). The incidence of fevers fell progressively after the fall of Sevastopol until the evacuation of the Crimea. The majority (61 percent) of all fatalities were recorded during the four-month period January to April 1855 as compared to two percent during the last six months of the campaign.

The fevers were recorded in the *Medical and Surgical History* as either common continued, remittent, and intermittent fever, or typhus, though, as Shepherd pointed out, these diagnoses must be regarded with circumspection as fever is merely a symptom and thus labelling them on 'purely clinical observations' makes for a classification that is 'utterly confusing.'[59] Irrespective of the precise aetiology fevers were particularly enervating, and this accounts for the following conclusions: 'in the circumstances of camp life recovery from fever was an extremely slow process, […] that relapses were

>   […] and if not taking tea or coffee' drank 'a light ale;' T. Buzzard, *With the Turkish Army in the Crimea and Asia Minor* (London: John Murray, 1915), p.81.
> 56 *Medical and Surgical History*, 2, pp.70–2 & 84–5.
> 57 *Medical and Surgical History*, 2, p.56 and Lloyd, and Coulter, *Medicine and the Navy*, p.142. Sir William Burnett was the Director General of the Naval Medical Department.
> 58 *Medical and Surgical History*, 2, General Return A. For a detailed contemporary discussion see pp.129–67.
> 59 Shepherd, *Crimean Doctors*, 1, p.318.

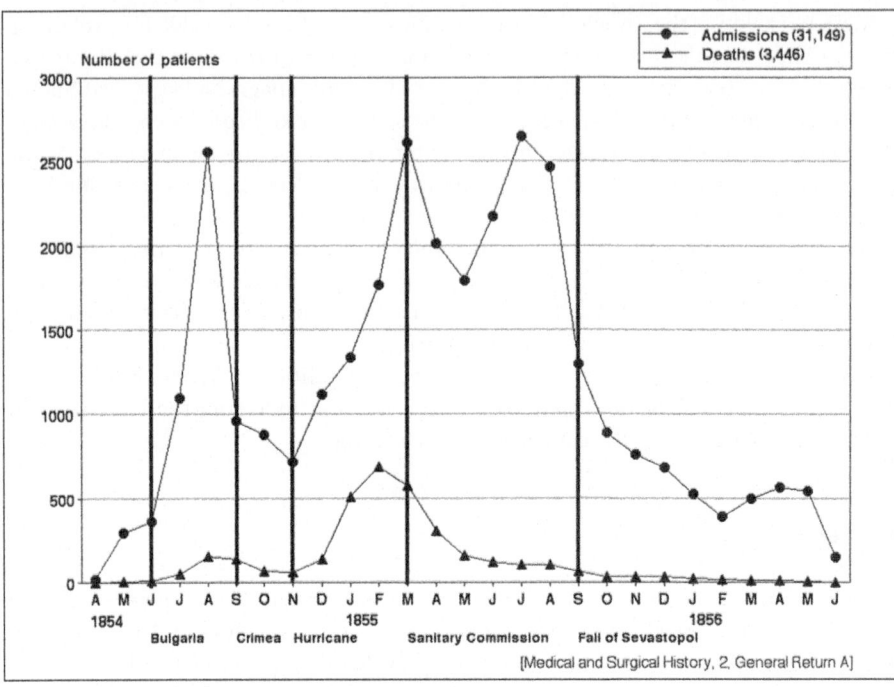

Figure 5.7 Admissions, for, and deaths from fevers among NCOs and men, April 1854–June 1856.

[...] numerous, and the efficient treatment of the disease would have required removal [...] to a purer air, and to more natural conditions of life, to a much greater extent than was at all practicable.'[60]

It is possible the continued fevers (25,013 admissions; 2,790 deaths) could have been enteric fever or typhoid, while remittent fevers (2,957; 311), may be those that responded to dosing with quinine, for example malaria, and intermittent fever (2,406; 60) was an undulant fever, such as that associated with *Brucella melitensis*, an infection which was not uncommon in the Mediterranean littoral. The characteristic clinical presentation of typhus (828; 285) meant that it is probably the most reliable diagnosis.

Typhus was a recognized hazard in over crowded and unsanitary prisons during the 18th and 19th centuries, hence the soubriquet 'jail fever'. However, it did not become rife in the British Army as might have been expected given the extremely unsatisfactory living conditions experienced by the troops during the first winter with the result and was the least common of the four categories of fever recorded although the case-fatality rate was high at 34.5 percent. By comparison the rates for continued, remittent, and intermittent fevers were 11, 10.5, and 10.5 percent respectively (Table 5.2).

60 *Medical and Surgical History*, 2, p.157.

Hospitals in Turkey: Typhus was never an issue in the hospitals on the Bosphorus with only six (0.015 percent) cases among 42,288 admissions, though after the war Nightingale incorrectly suggested otherwise: 'Scutari buildings were, in their unimproved state, like the jails of old, pest houses of typhus fever.'[61] Similarly, Kaufman claimed that over 100 patients died from a 'particularly virulent form of typhus' at Smyrna when the official history recorded were only nine cases with three deaths.[62] On the other, hand it proved a serious problem in the French hospitals during the second winter with over 7,000 cases being admitted in February and March 1856.[63]

5.4 Scurvy and Frostbite

Scurvy develops after a prolonged period on an inadequate diet particularly during long sea voyages,[64] while frostbite, or gelatio as it was termed, only afflicted the troops in the Crimea, Both conditions were most prevalent during the first winter with the peaks for primary admissions for scurvy and frostbite being recorded in February and January respectively with the greatest mortality for both occurring during February (see Figures 5.8 and 5.9). Both conditions recurred during the second winter, but to a much lesser extent, and with very much lower mortality.

Scurvy: As early as July 1854 Hall informed HQ that the troops were receiving 'indifferent rations owing to a want of vegetables' with the implication that they should be provided,[65] while shortly afterwards the PMO at Scutari went as far as recommending the issue of lime juice for the same reason.[66]

The first cases of scurvy in the Crimea were diagnosed in the 1st Battalion Rifle Brigade during October 1854[67] and Dumbreck recommended to HQ that fresh vegetables should be obtained from neighbouring ports.[68] Scurvy then made its appearance in many of the regiments though there were considerable differences between them. A reflection on the effectiveness of the regimental staff in provisioning the men during

---

61 *Medical and Surgical History*, 2, General Hospital Returns I and L. McDonald (ed.), *Florence Nightingale. The Crimean War*, 14, p.146.
62 Kaufman, *Surgeons at War*, p.165 and *Medical and Surgical History*, 2, General Hospital Returns VIII.
63 For details on typhus in the French hospitals on the Bosphorus see Bryce, *England and France before Sebastopol*, pp.96–121.
64 See *Medical and Surgical History*, 2, pp.171–86.
65 Hall to Military Secretary, 15 July 1854; RAMC: 397/F/CO/1/1/337; Smith, *Précis*, 1, Appendix I; and Royal Commission Report, Appendix LXXIX, pp.99–100.
66 PMO, Scutari to Commandant, 11 August 1854; Royal Commission Report, Appendix LXXIX, p.200.
67 The corps travelled from the Cape of Good Hope arriving on 14 September after two months at sea.
68 Dumbreck to AG, 24 October 1854; Royal Commission Report, Appendix LXXIX, p.161.

216 Victory Over Disease

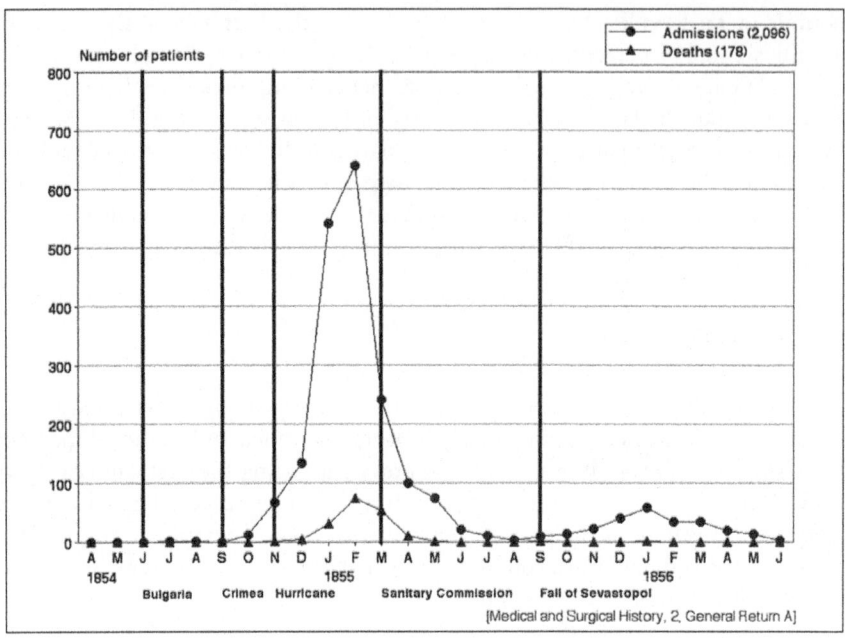

Figure 5.8 Admissions, for, and deaths from scurvy among NCOs and men, April 1854–June 1856.

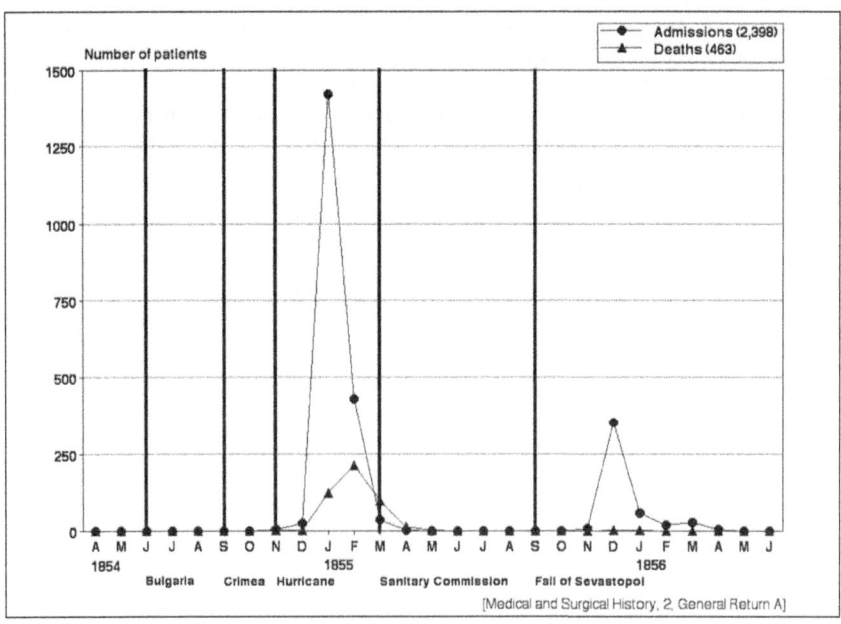

Figure 5.9 Admissions, for, and deaths from frostbite among NCOs and men, April 1854–June 1856.

the late summer or the failure of some medical officers to recognize so called 'land scurvy', such as occurred during the Great Irish Famine of the 1840s.[69]

Scurvy proved a minor problem in the regiments arriving in December 1854 and January 1855, presumably as they had an adequate diet during their journey to the East and continued to do so after their arrival by which time the level of nutrition for the Army as a whole was improving. The incidence in the Highland Brigade was lower than those on the plateau, presumably as the duties were less arduous and it was easier to obtain supplies as the regiments were closer to Balaklava.

Lime juice was landed for clinical use at the end of October,[70] while in his monthly report for December Hall noted that it was being 'freely issued medicinally' and that 'fresh meat and vegetables should be acquired at any price' as a preventative measure.[71]

Following a report from Hall, Smith wrote to the Military Secretary, Horse Guards on 17 November stressing the 'urgent necessity of immediately transmitting a supply of lime or lemon juice for the use of the forces in the Crimea.'[72] Inevitably it took several weeks to obtain sufficient supplies from countries where citrus fruits were grown and hence the issue of lime juice to all the troops for prophylaxis did not commence until February 1855.[73] The beneficial effect of this policy was obvious and its continued use during the remainder of the campaign, coupled with the provision of a more adequate diet, resulted in only a few cases being diagnosed during the winter of 1855/56.

Scorbutic dysentery: This diagnostic term was considered 'obscure' by Shepherd but it is not unreasonable to presume that it was a complication of scurvy since the 396 cases with 116 deaths were recorded between December 1854 and May 1855 in General Return A; the period when scurvy was most prevalent and when 1,734 (83 percent) of all admissions and 174 (98 percent) of the deaths were recorded.[74]

Frostbite: The majority of cases of frostbite were recorded during January; and to a lesser extent February 1855. The incidence was highest in the infantry regiments doing duty in the trenches and lower in the Highland Brigade and Cavalry Division, which had been withdrawn from the plateau before the end of 1854 to a more sheltered valley near Kadikoi.

69   J. Geber, 'The Kilkenny Workhouse Mass Burials' *Current Archaeology*, May 2013, pp.12–7.
70   Medical Department Memorandum, 30 October 1854; RAMC: 397/F/RT/2.
71   TNA: WO 17/1730; RAMC: 397/F/RT/1/1 (in Hall's hand); and Supplies Commission Report, p.159.
72   TNA: WO/32/2A and Royal Commission Report, Appendix LXXIX, pp.18 & 20
73   General Order, 16 February 1855; TNA: WO 28/130. An earlier order dated 31 January stipulated that for every 100 men five pints of lime juice should be mixed with eight pints of rum, 18 pints of water together with four lbs of sugar. This would equate to over 300 gallons, or over one and a quarter tons, of juice each day for an army of 50,000 men.
74   Shepherd, *Crimean Doctors*, 1, p.83.

Frostbite was 'frequently the result of protracted application of cold and wet' rather than 'the direct or specific effect of an extremely low temperature.' The feet and toes were frequently affected, and thus it was more akin to trench foot which proved so troublesome during the First World War.[75]

Improvement in the weather and general living conditions were associated with a dramatic fall in the number of admissions during February 1855. Frostbite was also diagnosed during the second winter but during this time it was more typical and commonly affected the exposed parts of the body such as the ears and digits, the tissues of which having become frozen.[76]

It was suggested in several reports in the *Medical and Surgical History* that the debility caused by fevers and intestinal disease predisposed to the development of gangrene of the toes, presumably due to the blood flow to the extremities being compromised. What proportion these cases formed of the whole cannot be ascertained from the records that survive.

Incidentally, scurvy and frostbite also proved serious problems for the French Army, especially after the November storm as the 'men had only their miserable *tentes d'abri* for shelter, and their clothing was [...] insufficient for the season.'[77]

5.5 Other diseases

5.5.1 Nosocomial (hospital acquired) infections

The Supplies Commissioners drew the following conclusion from their analysis of the medical records:

> The mortality [...] was further increased by the diseases which broke out at Scutari, and carried off many men who had entered the hospital with a prospect of speedy recovery, or who had actually recovered from the diseases for which they were admitted. Had the sanitary condition [...] been from the first what it afterwards became, there can be little doubt that the mortality would have been perceptibly reduced.[78]

This suggestion is not unreasonable given that when things were at their worst the men were: 'put on board in such a frightful state of vermin and filth, and so [...] when they land [...] they carry the filth and vermin into hospitals with them.'[79] However, no proof was provided for the inference that there was a problem with nosocomial infections, and it is not now possible to test the hypothesis as few records of individual

---

75 *Medical and Surgical History*, 2, p.189.
76 For further commentary see Shepherd, *Crimean Doctors*, 1, p.323.
77 G. Milroy, 'On the Sickness and Mortality in the French Army'.
78 Supplies Commission Report, p.37.
79 Special correspondent, 23 January; *The Times*, 8 February 1855.

patients survive. However, indirect evidence that nosocomial infections were not as important as implied can be obtained by assessing data on hospital gangrene and erysipelas, both of which may be associated by poor standards of hospital hygiene.

Hospital gangrene: Gangrene is a potentially fatal complication of surgery, particularly amputations before the introduction of antiseptic operating techniques.[80] It is contagious and frequently associated with overcrowding. There were advantages in early amputation after injury as this 'shortened hospital stays, reduced the risk of infection, and reduced the trauma of transportation.'[81] This explains why Smith's predecessor, McGrigor, advocated the distribution of the wounded to regimental rather than general hospitals, and this was given as one reason give for keeping the wounded in the Crimea,[82] where hospital gangrene was not recorded as a problem.[83]

The PMO at Scutari appreciated the risks of overcrowding and he 'dispersed the wounded as far as circumstances allowed.' In all, only 67 cases were diagnosed specifically as gangrene in the hospitals on the Bosphorus, of which 17 (25 percent) were fatal.[84] Almost all of the cases were recorded during the three months from November 1854 (Figure 5.10). The absence of a serious epidemic, which had been predicted by some commentators,[85] was confirmed by Dr Macleod, a civilian surgeon, who noted that: 'Hospital gangrene was not common in the East. During the first winter it prevailed a good deal in a mild form at Scutari, but it never became either general or severe. It did not appear to pass from bed to bed, but rose sporadically over the hospitals. [...] Whenever it appeared, the patients were [...] sent into wards set apart.'[86]

Macleod pointed out that: 'The French suffered most dreadfully from hospital gangrene in its worst form' and he ascribed this in part to their policy of transferring surgical cases to general hospitals. This opinion was confirmed by Milroy, a Sanitary Commissioner, who analysed some French medical data:

---

80 Incidentally, the mortality rate following amputation at Scutari was relatively low by the standards of the day at 74 (27 percent) of 274 cases' *Medical and Surgical History*, 2, General Hospital Returns I.
81 C.K. Murray, M.K. Hinkle, and H.C. Yun, 'History of Infections Associated with Combat-Related Injuries', *Journal of Trauma*, 64 (2008), pp.S221–31.
82 *Medical and Surgical History*, 2, p.254. Incidentally, Nightingale suggested that there may be an advantage for doing without general hospitals as they may become 'pest houses' if improperly managed; McDonald, *Florence Nightingale. The Crimean War*, p.685 and McDonald, *Florence Nightingale at First Hand*, p.88
83 *Medical and Surgical History*, 2, p.275.
84 Cantlie, *A History*, 2, p.87 and *Medical and Surgical History*, 2, General Hospital Returns I.
85 For example, C. Kidd and E. Cullen to Editor; *The Times*, 18 October 1854 & 24 January 1855; and implied incorrectly by Kaufman, *Surgeons at War*, p.143, that: 'Because of overcrowding, outbreaks of hospital gangrene occurred were highly contagious, and rapidly spread to other patients.'
86 G.H.B. Macleod, *Notes on the Surgery of the War in the Crimea with Remarks on the Treatment of Gunshot Wounds* (London: John Churchill, 1858), pp.152–3.

In February [1855] the state of things was even more dreadful. Beside scorbutic diseases, utterly intractable, typhus and hospital gangrene were frequent in the hospitals, and the medical officers could do nothing to prevent their spreading. [After the fall of Sevastopol] the huts and tents were crowded, and, ere long, hospital gangrene became very prevalent. Scurvy [...] continued to add [...] to the sick list, and cholera had not ceased to attack the fresh arrivals.[87]

Erysipelas: This condition, now known to be caused by *Streptococcus pyogenes*, was recognized as a potentially fatal complication of wound infections. It was uncommon, according to the *Medical and Surgical History*, and was not associated with any deaths following a gunshot wound in the Crimea[88] though Macleod noted that at Scutari: 'there were a good many cases of erysipelas, at the time the men were most depressed by their hardships; but it was seldom virulent.'[89] Small numbers of cases of were diagnosed sporadically throughout the campaign with 46 cases being recorded in the hospitals on the Bosphorus with ten fatalities (Figure 5.10).

Despite the small number of cases of gangrene and erysipelas it is clear that their epidemiological characteristics differed. The majority of admissions for, and deaths from, gangrene were recorded between November 1854 and March 1855 while erysipelas occurred sporadically throughout the campaign, with the majority of deaths recorded during the first half of 1855 (Figures 5.10 and 5.11). Incidentally, the ratio of deaths to admissions for both conditions was very similar in Scutari as it was for the Army as a whole, suggesting that no special factors were operating in those hospitals.

5.5.2 Other infectious diseases

Venereal diseases: These were most prevalent in new recruits, although this may reflect in part the relative ease of detection by superficial examination. Cases were diagnosed throughout the campaign and 3,717 men were admitted to the 'hospitals of the Army'.[90] Of those, a third was diagnosed before the invasion of the Crimea, with the highest rates in May and June 1854 (18 per thousand of strength). The rates were also somewhat higher than in previous months during May to October 1855 (4.2–5.8 per thousand), presumably as a result of the augmentation of the Army with new regiments, and drafts for others.[91]

---

87 Milroy, 'On the Sickness and Mortality in the French Army'.
88 *Medical and Surgical History*, 2, p.274.
89 Macleod, *Notes*, p.157.
90 *Medical and Surgical History*, 2, General Return A.
91 It is not improbable that 'ladies of the night' frequented the bazaars, and they would have been at risk from their clients and vice versa. However, there are no references to prostitution in the Crimea in the indexes of books by Shepherd, *Crimean Doctors*: Gill, *Nightingales*: Rappaport, *No Place for Ladies* (London: Arum Press, 2005); and Bostridge, *Florence Nightingale*.

Diseases 221

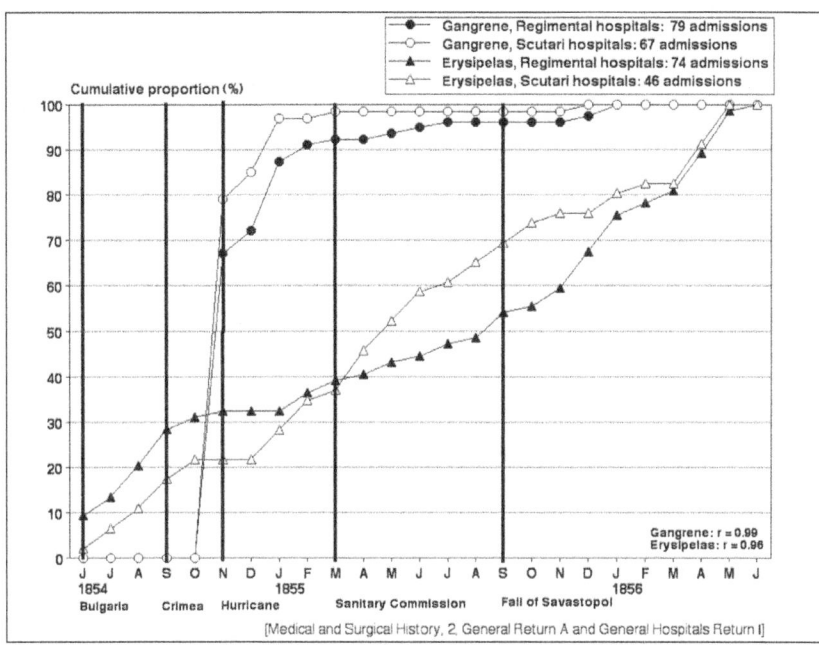

Figure 5.10 Admissions of NCOs and men to hospital with gangrene or erysipelas, June 1854–June 1856.

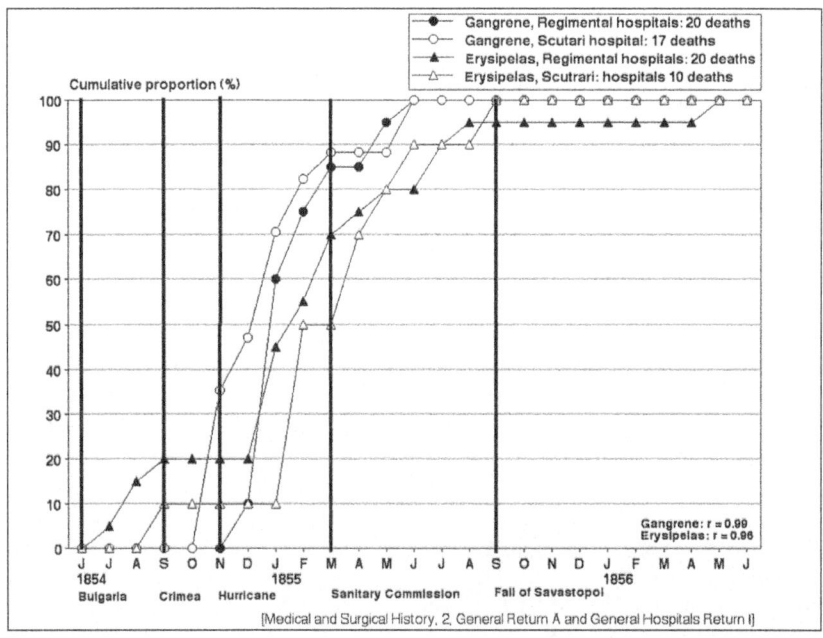

Figure 5.11 Deaths of NCOs and men from gangrene or erysipelas, June 1854–June 1856.

Of the admissions in this category 1,546 (42 percent) and 622 (17 percent) were for syphilis and gonorrhoea respectively while other diagnoses included ulcerated penis (266; seven percent), *bubo* [swollen lymph nodes] (525; 14), *verrucae et condylomata* [genital warts] (76; 2), and *hernia humoralis* [testicular swelling associated with gonorrhoea] (682; 18). Only two deaths were recorded and these involved men with syphilis.

Tuberculosis: This infection was endemic in the British Isles during the 19th century but the disease did not prove a serious clinical problem in the field as only 279 cases were admitted to the 'hospitals of the Army', and no more than 20 in any month. On the other hand, phthisis was not an uncommon reason for discharge from the Army (see Chapter 8).

Eye disease: This was recorded in the summary tables as *morbus oculorum*, a generic term that gives no indication of the cause though Shepherd suggest most were probably 'various types of conjunctivitis of a severe or chronic nature.'[92]

Infectious ophthalmia proved troublesome in the infantry during the autumn of 1855 and the decision to utilize the Monastery Hospital for the more severe cases was reflected in a dramatic increase in admissions. In contrast, the Castle Hospital admitted few eye cases during this period until patients from the Monastery were transferred to there following its closure on 17 June 1856.

Incidentally, of 9,899 men discharged from the Army at Chatham in the 27 months up to 31 March 1857 633 (seven percent) were for eye disease.[93]

Tetanus: Ten cases were recorded in the General Return A of which eight died; though the commentary on wounds indicated that the number was at least 26.[94] Nevertheless, the incidence was low suggesting that the spores of the causative organism, *Clostridium tetani*, were uncommon in the uncultivated steppe and farmland in the Crimea.[95]

Respiratory diseases: There were 12,382 admissions designated as respiratory disease and these were dominated by catarrh (9,506 cases) and bronchitis (1,111), while pneumonia and pleuritis (pleurisy) accounted for only 854 (seven percent) though the mortality rate was relatively high at 184 (22 percent).

It is not known how much use was made of stethoscopes in the diagnosis of respiratory disease as there are only two references to them in the *Medical and Surgical History*. Nevertheless, it should have been possible for at least one to have been available in each regimental and general hospital because 248 were sent to the East during the campaign.[96]

92 Shepherd, *Crimean Doctors*, 2, pp.577–8.
93 *Medical and Surgical History*, 2, p.239.
94 *Medical and Surgical History*, 2, pp.279–85.
95 Shepherd, *Crimean Doctors*, 2, p.475.
96 *Medical and Surgical History*, 2, pp.560–1.

5.5.3 Conditions typically associated with low mortality

Several conditions in General Return A had more than 100 primary admissions but the ratio of deaths to admissions was less than one percent. A total of 26,408 cases (18.5 percent of 142,621 admissions for disease) satisfied these criteria, and of these 53 died (0.3 percent of 16,292 deaths). The results are summarized in two parts in Table 5.5 in order to present those for the first winter separately. The mortality was slightly higher during this period in several instances, but it is unlikely that this would have prompted any comment as the deaths were not numerous and would have occurred sporadically in different locations.

This analysis suggests that the deterioration in the living and working conditions did not render these afflictions more life-threatening, in contrast to diarrhoea, dysentery and continued fever, the results for which are included for comparison in Table 5.5. A comparable analysis for the hospitals on the Bosphorus revealed that there were 3,664 cases (nine percent of 37,227 admissions for disease), and of these 19 died (0.4 percent of 5,009 deaths). This result indicates that the situation in Turkey was not dissimilar to that in the Army as a whole (see Chapter 7 for further discussion).

5.6 Non-medical hospital admissions and miscellaneous topics

The most notable reasons for admission to the 'hospitals of the Army' in this category are the consequence of intemperance and punishment by being flogged, although both were uncommon.

Intemperance: The records of courts martial[97] confirm that alcoholic beverages must have been readily obtainable as drunkenness was 'a great vice of English soldiers which no punishment will put an end to.'[98] Romaine's opinion was echoed by Russell who noted that '25 lashes, or even 50, are all insufficient to wean the British soldier from his favourite vice.'[99]

Panmure expressed his concern about intemperance to Codrington after the fall of Sevastopol. A survey of the proceedings of courts martial was then instituted and it was concluded that drunkenness was not as serious as might be supposed and: 'the Army will bear a comparison with many towns, many villages; many populations of Great Britain.'[100] This opinion was echoed by Private William Baillie, 68th Light Infantry, who pointed out that though drunkenness did occur it was not the universal problem suggested in *The Times*. He concluded that it was an: 'insult to the soldiers

---

97　TNA: WO 28/126.
98　Romaine to Mulgrave, 28 June 1854; Robins, *Romaine's Crimean War*, p.13.
99　*The Times*, 29 October 1855.
100　Codrington to Panmure, 27 December 1855; TNA: WO 1/380 and *London Gazette*, 9 January 1856.

Table 5.5 Conditions typically associated with low mortality listed in the *Medical and Surgical History*, 2, General Return A, April 1854–June 1856

Condition*	Apr.–Oct. 1854 and Apr. 1855–June 1856			Nov. 1854–Mar. 1855		
	Primary admissions	Deaths in all locations	Ratio Admissions/ Deaths (%)	Primary admissions	Deaths in all locations	Ratio Admissions/ Deaths (%)
Ulcers/abscesses	6,679	9	0.15	1,243	14	1.1
Eye diseases	3,060	0	–	247	0	–
VD (6)	2,722	0	–	313	3	0.95
Hernia†	1,486	1	<0.1	102	2	2.0
Punishment	1,461	0	–	312	0	–
Luxations	1,395	2	0.15	138	0	–
Colic	1,387	3	0.2	127	2	1.6
Sore throat	863	3	0.35	81	6	7.5
Dyspepsia	829	1	0.1	77	2	2.6
Skin diseases	688	0	–	61	1	1.5
Paronychia	355	0	–	46	0	–
Burns	353	0	–	46	0	–
Haemorrhoids	322	0	–	36	0	–
Constipation	311	0	–	37	0	–
Scabies	239	0	–	18	0	–
Headache/vertigo	119	0	–	9	0	–
Anal fistula	104	1	0.95	25	2	8.0
Otitis	101	0	–	6	1	16.5
Total	22,474	20	<0.1	3,934	33	1.1
Diarrhoea	42,662	566	1.3	14,502	3,085	21.5
Continued fever	19,457	1,106	5.5	6,156	1,684	27.5
Dysentery	4,568	343	7.5	3,710	1,913	51.5

* The selection depended on there being more than 100 primary admissions and the ratio of deaths to admissions being less than one percent.
† Entered with both gastrointestinal and venereal diseases.

here, as I am positive there is less drunkenness here than amongst soldiers and civilians at home.'[101]

Nevertheless, despite the perceived problem of excessive alcohol consumption delirium tremens was an uncommon reason for admission to hospital; 281 (0.2

101 *Bradford Observer*, 31 January 1855

percent) cases among 162,673 admissions, with 44 deaths. Forty-two (15 percent) of the admissions occurred during the first eleven months of the campaign up to February 1855; thereafter the incidence increased, presumably as a reflection of an increased supply of alcoholic beverages. Over half (56 percent) of the admissions took place after the fall of Sevastopol, when the men had more free time and a greater chance of spending their pay in the various bazaars located within the lines of the allied armies.

Punishment: By today's standards flogging is considered a barbaric punishment but in that period it was an established feature of army life. Presumably the soldiers were prepared to take the risk when committing an offence known to be punishable by this means.

Admissions into the 'hospitals of the Army' for punishment comprised 1,773 (one percent) of the total. No men died, which confirms that any complications of the wounds were not life-threatening. The maximum number of floggings in any one month was 178, in October 1855, while over the whole campaign the median monthly total was 60, or, expressed another way, the median (range) incidence per 1,000 strength was 0.18 (0.03–0.36).

Sun Stroke: Only twelve cases were recorded in the General Return A. This Shepherd considered an underestimate as it was the reason why many men collapsed from exhaustion during the advance towards the Alma on 19 September; a day that was very hot. In addition, the men were wearing 'thick and uncomfortable uniform' and the amount of water available to them was extremely limited.[102]

Flies: The surgeon of the Coldstream Guards recorded that: 'One great source of annoyance was the myriads of common flies which abound [...] Fly nets for the sick, and a weak solution of creosote for the wounded appeared to be the best means of alleviating this intolerable nuisance.'[103] Another commentator noted that flies became a 'regular pest' in the summer and 'no matter how a wound was excluded from air [...] larvae [were frequently found] on the surface of wounds,' while 'the most rigid enforcement of cleanliness and burial of offal or refuse [...] failed to do no more than check the evil.' Various preventative treatments met with variable success, such as the application of solutions of creosote, while gauze curtains, though used extensively, were 'not liked generally by the patients' 'in consequence of the increased temperature caused by their use.'[104]

Assistant Surgeon W. Cattell, 5th Dragoons Guards, pointed out the importance of maintaining the latrine trenches by either 'Mosaic sanitation or [the] use of dry earth'

---

102 Shepherd, *Crimean Doctors*, 1, p.120.
103 *Medical and Surgical History*, 1, p.119.
104 *Medical and Surgical History*, 2, p.274.

as otherwise the 'pit [became] a hot bed of flies innumerable which spent their days between ordure of all kinds and our food.'[105] In addition, the large numbers of horses in the Crimea resulted in substantial quantities of dung; an excellent breeding ground for flies and other vermin.

Three letters written during the summer of 1855 also provide further comments on the scourge, viz.:

- Assistant Surgeon E.M. Wrench: 'I don't suppose Lord Raglan has telegraphed that flies are very plentiful and increase visibly every daily. My tent is covered with them and they are a great pest in the hospital as they won't allow the men sleep.'[106]
- Captain F.B. Ward, RA: 'The weather here is really delightful, the great nuisance is [a] plague of flies which settle in myriads upon eatables of all kinds.[...] In our hospitals it is terrible to see the flies settling upon the faces of the sick, and we are obliged to keep orderlies constantly employed in brushing them away. Our horses also suffer dreadfully from them. They are the common house fly. In our tents we are obliged to use veils or mosquito nets for our beds.'[107]
- Newspaper letter: 'One of the greatest curses of the camp at the present moment is the multitude of flies. It is really an Egyptian plague. In every hut and tent they swarm in myriads.'[108]

5.7 Intervals between admission and death

General Return C in the *Medical and Surgical History* summarized the 'duration of diseases, wounds and injuries that proved fatal' among the men in the cavalry and infantry regiments.

The time to death for cholera, stomach and bowel diseases, respiratory diseases, fevers, other diseases, and wounds or injuries are summarized on a weekly basis in Table 5.6. The time to death of patients with cholera was recorded for 3,481 deaths with half occurring within two days of admission and three-quarters within four.[109] In contrast, half of the deaths in the other four disease categories were recorded during the second or third week with 10–15 percent of patients lingering for six weeks or

---

105 Quoted by Cantlie, *History*, 2, p.26.
106 Letter home, 5 June 1855; University of Nottingham: Wr C/59
107 Letter dated 11 June 1855; K. Smith (ed.) *Letters from Francis Beckford Ward*. (Unpublished typescript, 1994).
108 Letter dated 3 August; *The Examiner*, 18 August 1855.
109 It is presumed the returns refer to hospitalized patients, although this is not stated, and hence these figures may or may not include those who died on the line of march, in the trenches, or elsewhere.

more. A tenth of those with wounds or injuries died with two days of admission; over half by the end of the first week and nearly three-quarters by the end of the second.

Table 5.6 Number of patients in cavalry, Guards and infantry regiments dying each week during the weeks following admission to hospital

Time to death (days)	Number (Cumulative %)					
	Cholera	Bowel diseases*	Fevers	Respiratory diseases	Other diseases	Wounds and injuries
≤6	3,104 (89)	490 (16)	437 (20)	100 (28)	206 (29)	652 (54)
7–13	372 (100)	690 (38)	648 (49)	66 (47)	93 (43)	217 (72)
14–20	0	626 (58)	412 (68)	46 (60)	100 (57)	115 (82)
21–27	0	377 (71)	253 (79)	37 (70)	76 (68)	54 (86)
28–34	0	291 (80)	150 (86)	31 (79)	58 (76)	61 (92)
35–41	0	203 (86)	91 (90)	19 (84)	62 (85)	26 (94)
≥42	0	419 (100)	213 (100)	55 (100)	104 (100)	75 (100)
Total†	3,476	3,906	2,204	354	699	1,200

* Nearly all would have been due to diarrhoea or dysentery; see *Medical and Surgical History*, 2, General Return A.
† Each category included a number of individuals for whom this information was unavailable; these have not been included in these totals.

(Adapted from the *Medical and Surgical History*, 2, General Return C)

5.8 Accidental deaths

Inevitably there were a number of fatalities associated with accidents. But, as these occurred sporadically, they did not necessarily merit detailed comment in the *Medical and Surgical History* – although on occasions there was considerable loss of life. For example, the destruction by fire of the transport ship *Europa* shortly after she sailed for the East with a detachment of the 6th Dragoons,[110] and the French frigate, *Sémillante*, that sailed from Toulon for the Black Sea and struck a reef in the Straits of Bonifacio, with the loss of all 700 on board.[111]

Fire engulfed several huts housing Commissariat labourers on 17 March 1856 resulting in the death of 14 or 15 men.[112] The heating of poorly ventilated tents with charcoal was not without risk and there were several reports of 'suffocation' by what

---

110 The tragedy was reported in *The Times* on 17, 19, & 20 June 1854. For further details see M. Boxall, 'Devotion to Duty at the Expense of Life: The Fire on the Troopship *Europa*', *The War Correspondent*, 34:2 (2017), pp.32–3.
111 *Malta Times*, 13 March 1855; TNA: CO 163/28.
112 TNA: WO 28/143.

is now known to be carbon monoxide poisoning during January 1855.[113] Two soldiers were found frozen to death during December 1855; one had 'drunk himself into insensibility' and the other was a sentry who 'fell asleep on his post.'[114] There were also reports of death by drowning associated with the wrecking of ships, as occurred during the hurricane of 14 November 1854, the capsizing of smaller boats or their destruction by larger vessels, flash-flooding, and bathing in fresh and sea water.[115]

5.9 Concluding remarks

Gastrointestinal disorders other than cholera, dominated the sick lists for most months from mid-summer 1854 until the fall of Sevastopol with two major peaks in the winter of 1854–55 and the summer of 1855, though it was only during the first winter that they were associated with high mortality.

Fevers were recorded principally during the summer in Bulgaria and at an increased incidence during the spring and summer of 1855, while there were epidemics of cholera, in 1854 and 1855, with the first being the more serious.

Scurvy was a feature of the first winter, while frostbite was diagnosed during both winters, although to a much lesser extent during the second. In contrast, rheumatic diseases (aches pains in the muscles and joints) occurred throughout the campaign though the incidence was higher during the winter of 1854–55. As expected, respiratory diseases were more prevalent during the two winters while ocular disease appeared more frequent in the summer, particularly during 1856.

Venereal diseases were more common in the troops sent to the East early in the campaign, while there was a slight increase in the spring and summer of 1855 when several regiments joined the Army. The low incidence of hospital gangrene and erysipelas throughout the Army suggests that these potential nosocomial infections did not pose a serious threat in the Scutari hospitals or elsewhere. Similarly, mortality from gunshot wounds at Scutari was not sufficiently great to suggest that there was any epidemic of fatal wound infections.

Trends in the incidence of these diseases followed a generally predictable pattern. It was the number of cases and the fatality rate that made them exceptional. A point that was made effectively in the *Medical and Surgical History*: 'Nearly all the diseases [...] were of a kind more or less incidental to troops employed on active service in the field, and familiar to the conditions of camp life. [The occurrence] of fevers and fluxes [...] was merely remarkable for the amazing prevalence and mortality which, for a considerable period, they obtained.'[116]

---

113 M. Hinton, 'Death by Charcoal', *The War Correspondent*, 18:4 (2001), pp.33–7.
114 TNA: WO 28/143.
115 M. Hinton, 'Death by Drowning during the War with Russia', *The War Correspondent*, 34:3 (2014), pp.5–13.
116 *Medical and Surgical History*, 2, p.45.

The pattern of disease changed month by month with the fatal illnesses experienced during the first winter being superseded by less life-threatening maladies during the second. The principal diseases diagnosed during the campaign were the 'traditional killers encountered in civil populations', with the exception of plague and measles which were not a problem.[117] The suggestion that it was: 'The surgeon's knife, along with frostbite, killed thousands. But the deadliest killers were diseases including pneumonia and tuberculosis,' [118] is patently incorrect; and this reflects the misinformation on the subject put about by several other commentators who have obviously chosen not to consult primary sources of information.[119]

Bell concluded in a BBC broadcast that: 'Infections are the true beneficiaries of war' as 'history has repeatedly shown that contagion makes an easy bedfellow with human conflict' and hence 'war and insurgency provide the ideal conditions for bacteria and viruses to take a foothold.' Some of Bell's examples of the devastating effects of natural infections in these circumstances are listed in Table 5.7.[120] On the other hand, Martineau pointed out that though: 'Disease from exposure, fatigue, and want is more fatal than shot and shell, and bayonet' it is when 'disease arrives in the form of epidemics, the troops in fact sustain at once the horrors of war, and the two evils should not be mixed up together, and laid at the door of war.'[121] Similarly, Cooter questioned whether a 'fatal partnership' between pathogens and war should be assumed, and suggested that 'many, perhaps most, epidemics are not rooted in war.' Certainly, from the British perspective diseases such as small pox, tuberculosis, and typhus did not become rife during the campaign despite the privations endured by the troops. On the other hand, cholera which had been present in several countries in Europe before war was declared, merely spread to Bulgaria and the Crimea by the movement of the troops. In addition, the fact that it petered out during the winter of 1854/55 when the many problems confronting the Army were at their most serious supports Cooter's proposition that a 'pathogenic price' does not necessarily have to be 'paid for the devastation caused by military action.'[122]

---

117 M.R. Smallman-Raynor and A.D. Cliff, *War Epidemics* (Oxford: University Press, 2004), pp.176 & 230.
118 Edgerton, *Death and Glory*, p.123.
119 For a commentary on misinformation see M. Hinton 'Reporting the Crimean War', *19: Interdisciplinary Studies in the Long Nineteenth Century*, 20 (2015), DOI: http://doi.org/10.16995/ntn.711
120 J. Bell, 7 December 2013; <www.bbc.co.uk/news/health-24962331> consulted on 7 November 2017.
121 Martineau, *England and Her Soldiers*, p.270.
122 R. Cooter, 'Of War and Epidemics: Unnatural Couplings, Problematic Conceptions', *Journal of the Society of the Social History of Medicine*, 16:2 (2003), pp.283–302.

Table 5.7 Chronicles of contagion, AD 165–1918

Date	Campaign	Abstract
165	Parthian war	Roman soldiers returning from the war sparked the Antonine Plague (probably smallpox) that ravaged the Roman Empire.
1618–48	Thirty Years war	Typhus fever led to the cancellation of some battles.
1804–15	Napoleonic wars	Typhus fever killed more French soldiers than the war effort itself.
1853–56	Crimean war	British forces were decimated by cholera outbreaks.*
1870–71	Franco-Prussian war	Smallpox originating in France was introduced into Prussia by French prisoners and spread through the civilian population, but not to the Prussian soldiers who had been protected.
1914–18	First World War	An influenza pandemic killed millions. In Russia, peace was followed by widespread famine with cholera, dysentery, malaria, typhoid and typhus being spread by refugees.

* This is an exaggeration as cholera was responsible for about of a quarter of deaths from disease.

(Adapted from www.bbc.co.uk/news/health-24962331)

The serious losses from disease during the first winter received widespread publicity though matters were distorted when the 'home newspapers regaled their readers with accounts of the Scutari hospitals' which tended to be exaggerated, while the medical press considered that the fault lay not with the AMD but with the military authorities who had neglected medical affairs for many years and had not improved the supply and commissariat system since the Napoleonic War.

The improvement of living standards in the camps during the spring of 1855 was associated with a reduction in mortality and this was reflected in a simultaneous improvement in the Scutari hospitals during the weeks before the arrival of the Sanitary Commission. The close correlation between the mortality rates recorded during the first winter for several diseases in the Army in the Crimea and in the hospitals on the Bosphorus is remarkable. That the facilities in the hospitals in Turkey may have been less than adequate is not at issue, but without doubt they were less important in influencing the outcome for the evacuees than the seriousness of their condition on arrival from the Crimea. A conclusion which was supported by Nightingale when she informed Panmure on 19 August 1855: 'The physically deteriorating effect of Scutari has been much discussed, but it may be doubted. The men sent down in the winter died because they were not sent down till half dead – the men sent down now live because they are sent in time.'[123]

---

123 Douglas & Ramsey (1898), 1, pp.356–7. The same point was also appreciated by another nurse, Miss Terrot; Cantlie, *A History*, 2, p.125.

6

Casualties consequent upon action with the enemy

There has been considerable interest in the battles of the Alma, Balaklava, and Inkerman, principally from a military point of view,[1] while the *Medical and Surgical History* included a section on battle field injuries and their management.[2] Losses from enemy action were lower than those associated with disease, but significant nevertheless because of the temporary or permanent loss of manpower, and the resources required to care for the wounded, particularly following the principal engagements.

The conveyance of the seriously wounded from the front line to the rear was inevitably going to be traumatic for the patient and challenging and potentially hazardous for the stretcher bearers and ambulance personnel, at least until the action was over (Figures 6.1 and 6.2). In the case of a major engagement there was the additional possibility that advanced dressing stations might be overwhelmed by the number of patients or from attack by the enemy.

The situation was at its most unsatisfactory after the battle of the Alma as there had been no time to set up even rudimentary casualty clearing stations, and it had not been possible to requisition sufficient wheeled vehicles locally to substitute for the ambulance waggons left behind at Varna.[3] The provision for the immediate care of the wounded improved as the campaign progressed, as summarized in Table 6.1,

1   For example: W. Baring Pemberton, *Battles of the Crimean War* (London: Pan Books, 1968); M. Barthorp, *Heroes of the Crimean War. The Battles of Balaklava and Inkerman* (London: Blandford, 1991); M. Adkin, *The Charge. The Real Reason Why the Light Brigade was Lost* (London: Leo Cooper, 1996); T. Brighton, *Hell Riders. The Truth about the Charge of the Light Brigade*, (London: Viking, 2004); D. Watson, *Battlefield Detectives* (London: Grenada Publishing, 2003), pp.150–78; D. Buttery, *Messenger of Death. Captain Nolan and the Charge of the Light Brigade* (Barnsley: Pen & Sword Military, 2008); I. Fletcher and N. Ishchenko, *The Battle of the Alma 1854* (Barnsley: Pen & Sword Military, 2008); P. Mercer, *Inkerman 1854. The Soldiers' Battle* (Westport, Ct: Praeger, 2008); and J. Grehan, *Voices from the Past. The Charge of the Light Brigade* (Barnsley: Frontline Books, 2017).
2   *Medical and Surgical History*, 2, pp.253–396.
3   The carnage would have reminded the older participants of the aftermath of the battles in the Peninsular War and Waterloo.

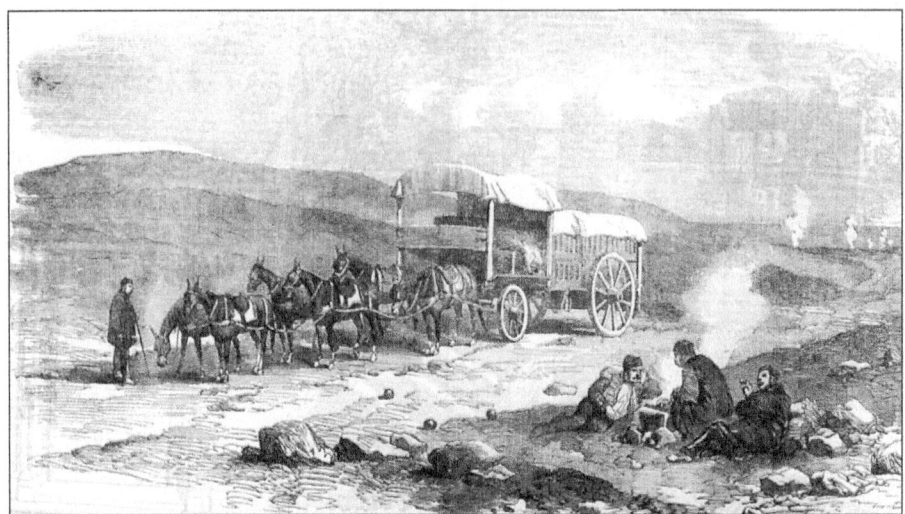

Figure 6.1 Near Sebastopol – Ambulance waiting for the wounded. (*Illustrated London News*, 2 June 1855, p.540.

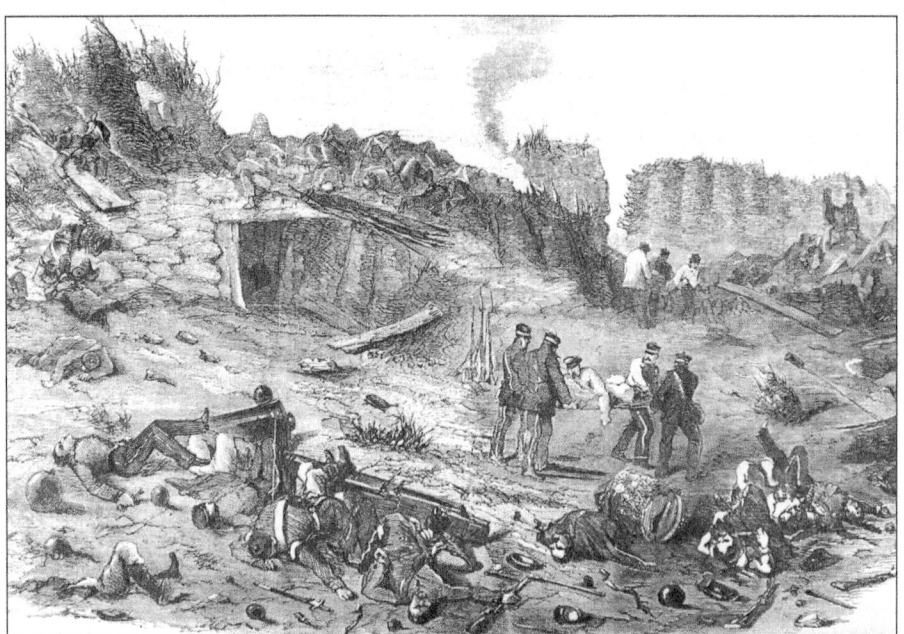

Figure 6.2 The Redan at sunset, September 8 – removing the wounded. (Sketched by E.A. Goodhall. *Illustrated London News*, 6 November 185, p.416)

although, as outlined in Section 2.2.6, the development of a satisfactory ambulance service remained elusive throughout the whole campaign.

Table 6.1 Management of men suffering battlefield injuries

	Battles		Siege operations		
	Alma 20 Sep. 1854	Balaklava 26 Oct. 1854	Inkerman 5 Nov. 1854	Redan 18 June 1855	Redan 9 Sep. 1855
Location for treatment					
Battlefield/front line	•	•	•	•	•
Casualty clearing stations	–	–	–	•	•
Regimental hospitals	–	•	•	•	•
General hospitals	–	?	•	•	•
Transport for casualties					
Stretchers	•	•	•	•	•
Ambulance waggons	–	?	•	•	•
Railway	–	–	–	•	•
Evacuation by sea	•	•	•	(•)	(•)

•, Utilized;
(•), available if required.

This chapter presents analyses from the three most comprehensive sources of data, consulted,[4] viz. the *Medical and Surgical History*; an unpublished copy of the Adjutant General's ledger of the daily number of officers and other ranks who were killed, wounded in action or reported missing;[5] and a summary of a selection of official despatches and papers relevant to the topic published by Captain F. Sayer.[6] Descriptions of the wounds and how they were treated have been dealt with in extenso in the *Medical and Surgical History* and Shepherd's monograph.[7]

4   Other publications on this topic that were not utilized include: HCPP 1854–55 (204) XXXII, 387: *Return of the Total Number of Officers and Men in the Army who have been Killed in the Crimea; and Like Return of the Number Wounded* […] *up to 15th Match 1855*; W.B. Hodge, 'On the mortality arising from military operations', *Journal of the Statistical Society of London*, 19 (1856), pp.219–71; HCPP 1857 Session I, (42) IX.1: *Return Concerning the Late Army of the East*; and R. T. Thomson, 'Mortality among Officers of the British Army in the Crimea', *Journal of the Statistical Society of London*, 20 (1857), pp.54–60.
5   RAMC: 397/F/RM/17/7. The original has not been found in TNA: WO 28.
6   Sayer, *Despatches*.
7   *Medical and Surgical History*, 2, pp.253–396 and Shepherd, *Crimean Doctors*, 2, pp.468–84.

234 Victory Over Disease

The admission of NCOs and men to hospital, and deaths from, with wounds or injuries during each month is illustrated in Figure 6.1. The rate was greatest during the time when action with the enemy was most intense, viz. following the invasion when the battles of the Alma, Balaklava, and Inkerman were fought, and during the spring and summer of 1855 with numbers being greatest when the engagements of 7 and 18 June, and 8 September took place.

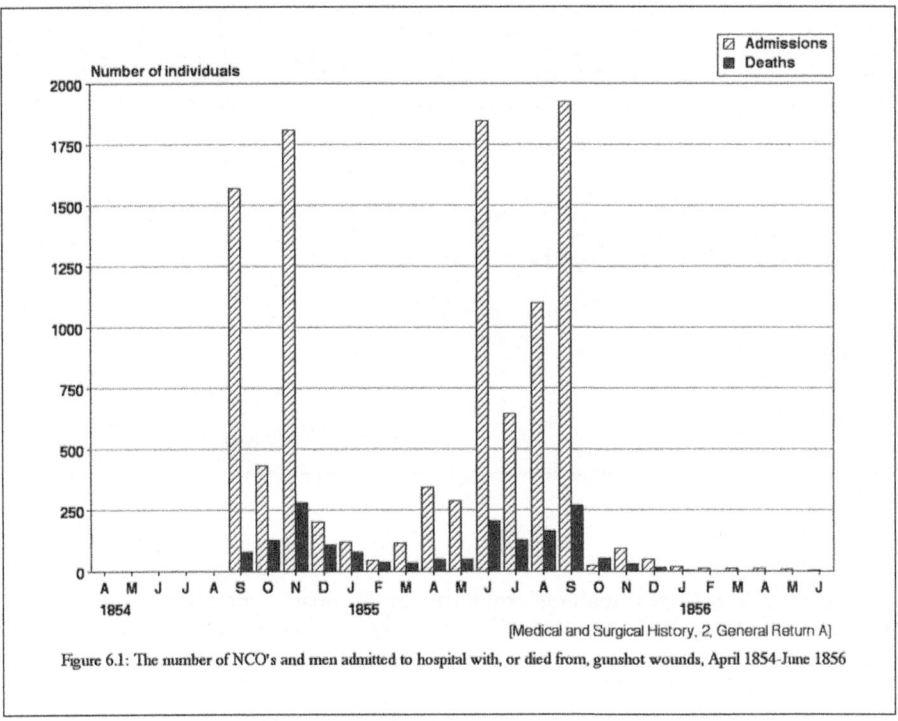

Figure 6.1: The number of NCO's and men admitted to hospital with, or died from, gunshot wounds, April 1854–June 1856
[Medical and Surgical History, 2, General Return A]

Figure 6.3 The number of NCOs and men admitted to hospital with, or died from, gunshot wounds, April 1854–June 1856.

In all 10,691 (58 percent) of the 18,283 admissions for wounds or injuries were for gunshot wounds (*Vulnus sclopitorum*),[8] of which 1,706 (16 percent) died. By comparison there were 55 (0.7 percent) deaths among 7,592 patients with other injuries including incised wounds (*Vulnus incisum*), burns, contusions, luxations, and fractures.

Nearly all (97.5 percent) of the gunshot wounds were sustained between September 1854 and September 1855 (Table 6.2). On the other hand, the other categories of

---

8   The precise nature of the injuries is not give in the summary tables, and presumably included those caused by musket balls, grape, round shot, shell, and blast.

injury were recorded throughout the whole campaign which included fourteen months of camp and garrison duties. A finding that confirms that soldiers were at risk of incurring injuries, particularly contusions, irrespective of whether it was a time of war or peace.

Table 6.2 The wounds and injuries sustained by NCOs and men during the Eastern campaign, April 1854–June 1856

	Gunshot wound	Incised wound	Burns	Contusion	Fracture	Luxation
Periods 1 & 3*	246	714	242	1,931	202	954
Period 2†	10,445	556	157	2,075	178	579
Totals	10,691	1,270	399	4,006	380	1,533
Proportion (%) in Period 2	97.5	44	39	52	47	38
Proportion (%) of the 18,279 admissions‡	58	7	2	22	2	8.5

* April–August 1854 and October 1855–June 1856.
† September 1854–September 1855.
‡ Four cases of concussion have been omitted from the table.

(Summarized from the *Medical and Surgical History*, 2, General Return A)

6.1 General hospitals in the Crimea and Turkey

The majority of those injured during action were admitted to regimental hospitals (Table 6.3) but the initial lack of facilities in the Crimea resulted in nearly 3,000 being evacuated to Turkey between September and November 1854. Although this was inevitable, some surgeons deplored the hurried transfer of the severely wounded and favoured undertaking primary surgery before evacuation. However, this policy, which reduced the risk of overcrowding in the regimental hospitals, was later excused on the grounds that Raglan was determined to evacuate all men thought unlikely to return to duty in a short time, or be unable to march.[9] In the event, the hospitals on the Bosphorus received three-quarters of all the admissions for gunshot wounds during that time (Table 6.3). The winter of 1854–55 saw relatively little direct action and only 89 patients were sent to Turkey between February and May 1855, while the majority of those evacuated between April and September were probably convalescent as only eight (two percent) of 586 patients died.[10]

9   *Medical and Surgical History*, 2, p.254 and Shepherd, *Crimean Doctors*, 1, p.237.
10 *Medical and Surgical History*, 2, General Hospital Returns I.

Table 6.3 Numbers of NCOs and men admitted to hospitals in the Crimea and Turkey with gunshot wounds (*Vulnus sclopitorum*), September 1854–September 1855 and October–December 1855

Month (1854/55)	Crimea					Turkey*		
	Regimental hospitals	Balaklava General	Castle†	Camp General	Monastery	Bosphorus hospitals	Abydos	Renkioi
September	1,560	–	–	–	–	1,013	–	–
October	280	9	–	–	–	444	–	–
November	1,748	11	–	–	–	1,431	–	–
December	192	0	–	–	–	116	43	–
January	118	4	–	–	–	196	0	–
February	48	4	–	–	–	33	1	–
March	113	2	0	–	–	34	1	–
April	307	1	107	4	–	16	3	–
May	313	1	52	4	–	6	0	–
June	1,778	8	480	279	–	91	0	–
July	601	2	194	21	0	31	0	–
August	1,003	1	388	12	0	259	0	–
September	1,776	1	392	293	0	183	0	–
Totals	9,937	44	1,613	613	0	3,853	48	–
October–December†	154	3	168	117	1	122	0	61

* In addition, five cases were admitted to the hospital at Smyrna between February and July 1855.
† Principally convalescent patients.

(Summarized from the *Medical and Surgical History*, 1, Regimental histories, and 2: General Hospital Returns I & III–VII)

The Camp General Hospital, being close to the front received recently injured men,[11] while the Castle Hospital, set apart from the main centres of population, was used to the care for convalescent wounded soldiers. This difference in function was reflected by the fact that the ratios of deaths to admissions for gunshot wounds for these two hospitals were 25 and 4.5 percent respectively. The Balaklava General Hospital was utilized principally for treating the sick as there were only 44 (one percent) cases among 4,278 patients admitted in the period October 1854 to December 1855.

The hospital at Abydos received 44 of a total of 48 wounded patients during December 1854, the month it opened, when matters were still pressing in the Crimea.

---

11 Of 1,005 patients admitted between April and November 1855 730 (73 percent) were for gunshot wounds; *Medical and Surgical History*, 2, General Hospital Returns V.

Four cases only were admitted at Smyrna while the 61 cases sent to Renkioi during the last three months of 1855 were almost certainly convalescents (Table 6.3).

6.2 Fatalities due to wounds or injuries

Of 1,761 fatalities for wounds or injuries recorded in the General Return A 1,706 (97 percent) were due to gunshot wounds and only 18 (one percent) to incised wounds (Table 6.4).

Table 6.4 The number of deaths among NCOs and men who sustained wounds and injuries, April 1854–June 1856

	Gunshot wound	Incised wound	Burns	Contusion	Fracture	Luxation
Admissions*	10,691	1,270	399	4,006	380	1,533
Deaths	1,706	18	0	21	14	2
Ratio of deaths to Admissions (%)	16	1.5	–	0.5	3.5	0.1

* Four non-fatal cases of concussion have been omitted.

(Summarized from the *Medical and Surgical History*, 2, General Return A)

The interval between admission and the death from wounds and mechanical injuries for 1,200 NCOs and men in the cavalry and infantry was tabulated in General Return C and summarized in Table 6.5. The data in Table 6.4 confirms that most of these would have been associated with gunshot wounds. Nearly 40 percent of the patients died within three days. It is probable that many of these early deaths would have been associated with a: 'want of power to withstand the shock to the general system of a severe injury.'[12] Shepherd pointed out, the improvement in the general health of the Army during 1855 would have resulted in better wound healing, while the policy to keep the injured in the Crimea was also beneficial.[13]

12 *Medical and Surgical History*, 2, p.260.
13 Shepherd, *Crimean Doctors*, 2, p.472.

Table 6.5 Time to death from fatal wounds and mechanical injuries

Days to death	Corps			Total	
	Cavalry	Foot Guards	Infantry	Number	%
<1	4	1	160	165	14
1–3	6	23	306	335	28
4–6	0	10	142	152	13
7–13	1	19	197	217	18
14–20	1	21	93	115	10
21–27	2	7	45	54	4
28–34	1	11	49	61	5
35–41	1	4	21	26	2
≥42	4	12	59	75	6
Total	20	108	1,072	1,200	100
Time unknown	33	161	400	594	
Grand totals	53	269	1,472	1,794	

(Summarized from the *Medical and Surgical History*, 2, General Return C)

6.3 Adjutant General's ledger

The Adjutant General's ledger covered the affair on the Bulganek on 19 September 1854 until the final assault on Sevastopol on 8 September 1855, together with three additional days in September, and the explosion in the magazine of the Right Attack on 25 November 1855.

The ledger only noted the losses on a particular day. The number who died later was not known at the time, but was probably in the region of 16 percent.[14] The total number of individuals in action on each day was not recorded and so the casualty rates as a proportion of the number of individuals at risk cannot be estimated.

This document is valuable, however, as it lists the number of casualties among officers, sergeants, drummers, and rank and file separately for the siege operations, the battles of the Alma, Balaklava, Little Inkerman, and Inkerman, and the assaults on the Quarries (7/8 June) and Sevastopol (18 June and 8 September 1855).

Battles, assaults, and siege operations: The casualties totalled 15,189, viz. 767 (five percent) officers, 840 (six) sergeants, 102 drummers (<one), and 13,480 (89) rank and file. Of these 2,728 (18 percent), 12,033 (79), and 428 (three) were killed, wounded, or missing respectively. The officers suffered relatively more battlefield fatalities than the

---

14 *Medical and Surgical History*, 2, General Return A.

other ranks, viz. 177 (23 percent) of 767 casualties as opposed to 2,551 (18) of 14,422 (Table 6.6).

Table 6.6 Casualties according to rank, 18 September 1854–8 September 1855

Rank	Killed		Wounded		Missing		All casualties
	No.	%	No.	%	No.	%	No.
Officers	177	23	574	75	16	2	767
Sergeants	163	19.5	653	77.5	24	3	840
Drummers	20	19.5	82	80.5	0	–	102
Rank and File	2,368	17.5	10,724	79.5	388	3	13,480
Total	2,728	18	12,033	79	428	3	15,189

(Summarized from RAMC: 397/F/RM/7/17)

Two thirds of all casualties were sustained during the seven days of direct action (battles and assaults) and the remainder during the eleven months of the siege. Three quarters of the casualties among the officers and sergeants occurred during the battles and assaults, suggesting that they may have taken greater risks thereby setting an example to the men. The drummers were employed in assisting the wounded and four fifths of their casualties were recorded during the battles and assaults. In contrast, proportionally more of the casualties suffered by the rank and file occurred in the trenches (Table 6.7).

Table 6.7 Number of casualties resulting from action with the enemy, 18 September 1854–8 September 1855

Action	Officers		Sergeants		Drummers		Rank & File		All casualties	
	No.	%	No.	%	No.	%	No.	%	No.	%
Battles*	288	38	305	36	53	52	4,419	33	5,065	33
Siege ops	185	24	213	26	20	20	5,033	37	5,451	36
Assaults†	294	38	322	38	29	28	4,028	30	4,673	31
Total	767	100	840	100	102	100	13,480	100	15,189	100

* Alma, Balaklava, Little Inkerman, and Inkerman.
† 7/8 and 18 June, and 8 September 1855.

(Summarized from RAMC: 397/F/RM/7/17)

The chances of a casualty being killed tended to be higher during the three battles (22 percent of casualties) than in either the siege operations or assaults on the Sevastopol garrison when the proportion of casualties killed was 15 and 17 percent respectively (Table 6.8).

Table 6.8 The proportion of officers and men killed during battles, siege operations, and assaults on Sevastopol, 18 September 1854–8 September 1855

Month (1854/55)	Battlefield casualties (% killed in action)											
	Battles			Siege ops			Assaults			Total		
	Total	Killed	%	Total	Killed	%	Total	Killed	%	Total	Killed	%
September	1,983	352	18	–	–	–	–	–	–	1,983	352	18
October	509	124	24	380	61	16	–	–	–	889	185	21
November	2,573	632	25	151	27	18	–	–	–	2,724	659	24
December	–	–	–	250	59	24	–	–	–	250	59	24
January	–	–	–	121	23	19	–	–	–	121	23	19
February	–	–	–	42	8	19	–	–	–	42	8	19
March	–	–	–	187	33	18	–	–	–	187	33	18
April	–	–	–	541	106	20	–	–	–	541	106	20
May	–	–	–	366	66	18	–	–	–	366	66	18
June	–	–	–	691	98	14	2,226	391	18	2,917	489	17
July	–	–	–	843	105	12	–	–	–	843	105	12
August	–	–	–	1,493	184	12	–	–	–	1,493	184	12
September	–	–	–	386	73	19	2,447	386	16	2,833	459	16
Total	5,065	1,108	22	5,451	843	15	4,673	777	17	15,189	2,728	18

(Summarized from RAMC: 397/F/RM/7/17)

The stage of the campaign: The Army encamped before Sevastopol at the beginning of October 1854 and the Adjutant General's ledger covered the period from 5 October until 8 September 1855, a period of 333 days of trench warfare if the days of battles of the Balaklava and Inkerman and the three main assaults on the Sevastopol garrison on the 8 and 18 June and 9 September 1855 are excluded.

The number of casualties remained low until March 1855 (median six or less per day for each month) although there were four days when the number was 50 or more. Thereafter, losses increased so that those sustained during six weeks before the fall of Sevastopol accounted for a third of all siege casualties (1,879 of 5,451; Table 6.9).

There were no casualties on 35 (11 percent) of the 333 siege days while there 1–10, casualties, including fatalities, on 150 (45 percent) with 51 or more casualties recorded on 28 (eight percent); (Table 6.10: left hand side). No person was killed on 119 (36 percent) days while there were 1–4 fatalities on 161 (48 percent) and 17 or more on five (1.5 percent) (Table 6.10: right hand side).

Table 6.9 Minimum, maximum, and median number of casualties sustained each day during siege operations, exclusive of the three principal assaults on Sevastopol, October 1854–September 1855

Month (1854–55)	Number of casualties/day			Total casualties	No. of days with ≥50 casualties
	Minimum	Maximum	Median		
October	0	116	6	380	2
November	0	30	2	151	0
December	0	78	4	250	1
January	0	22	3	121	0
February	0	7	1	42	0
March	0	78	4	187	1
April	3	72	14.5	541	1
May	3	43	10	366	0
June	4	58	23	691	2
July	9	63	27	843	2
August	13	141	44	1,493	13
September	37	63	55	386	6
Total	0	141	8	5,451	28 (8.4%)/333

(Summarized from RAMC: 397/F/RM/7/17)

Table 6.10 Distribution of casualties among officers and men according the number that were recorded on each day of the siege

Casualties including fatalities			Officers and men killed		
Number per day	Number of days	Proportion (%) of total	Number per day	Number of days	Proportion (%) of total
0	35	11	0	119	36
1–5	98	29	1–2	95	28
6–10	52	16	3–4	66	20
11–15	38	11	5–6	19	6
16–20	18	5	7–8	11	3
21–25	18	5	9–10	9	2.5
26–30	12	4	11–12	5	1.5
31–40	22	7	13–14	3	1
41–50	12	4	15–16	1	0.3
51–85	26	8	17–18	1	0.3
116	1	0.3	19–20	3	1
141	1	0.3	21	1	0.3
Total	333	100	Total	333	100

(Summarized from RAMC: 397/F/RM/7/17)

242 Victory Over Disease

The maximum number of casualties recorded was 141 (19 killed) on the first day of the 5th Bombardment on 17 August 1855. The next highest was 116 (21 killed) on the 17 October 1854 when the 1st bombardment commenced, while attacks by the British on 20 November 1854 and 14 April 1855 and Russian sorties on 20 December 1854 and 22 March 1855 resulted in higher than usual casualties.

6.4 Captain Sayer's analyses

Captain F. Sayer served in the Crimea and published a book based on official documents available at Horse Guards. A summary of some of his data is presented in Table 6.11. Of 3,905 officers in the Army a total of 154 (4%) 84 (2.2%), and 420 (11%) were either killed, died of wounds, or were wounded. The comparable figures for 93,959 NCOs and men were 2,598 (2.8%), 1,933 (2.1%), and 9,428 (10%) respectively.

Table 6.11 Number of officers, sergeants and men who served in the cavalry, infantry, Royal Artillery, and RS&M during the Crimean campaign, together with the numbers who were killed and wounded

Rank	Corps	Total served	Killed in action	Died of wounds	Wounded*	Total casualties
		(Proportion (%) in each column)				
Officers	Cavalry	427 (11)	9 (6)	4 (5)	22 (4.5)	35 (5.5)
	Infantry	2,995 (76.5)	125 (81)	73 (87)	362 (86)	560 (85)
	RA	388 (10)	11 (7)	1 (1)	29 (7)	41 (6)
	RS&M	95 (2.5)	9 (6)	6 (7)	7 (1.5)	22 (3.5)
	Total	3,905	154	84	420	658
Sergeants and men	Cavalry	8,293 (9)	114 (4.5)	26 (1.5)	211 (2.5)	351 (2.5)
	Infantry	73,399 (78)	2,331 (90)	1,832 (95)	8,574 (91)	12,737 (91)
	RA	10,723 (11.5)	121 (4.5)	52 (2.5)	580 (6)	753 (5.5)
	RS&M	1,644 (1.5)	32 (1)	23 (1)	63 (0.5)	118 (1)
	Total	93,959	2,598	1,933	9,428	13,959

* This value was obtained by subtracting the number wounded (pp.428–9) from the number dying of wounds (pp.420–3).

(Summarized from Sayer, *Desptches*, pp.420–3, 428–9, and the endpaper. A similar table was published in the *Medical and Surgical History*, 2, p.388, though it differs in some details)

The infantry regiments bore the brunt of the casualties in all categories when compared with the cavalry (which played little part in the battles of the Alma and Inkerman and were spared duty in the trenches), Royal Artillery, and Royal Engineers/Royal Sappers and Miners. However, despite the small size of the corps, the numbers of RE officers who were killed or died of wounds was relatively high at

68 percent of the 22 casualties, as compared with 37, 35 and 29 percent for the cavalry, infantry and RA respectively. This difference probably reflects the need for them to work in exposed positions during the construction and maintenance of the siege works (Table 6.12).

Table 6.12 Number of officers, sergeants and men who served in the cavalry, infantry, Royal Artillery, and RS&M during the Crimean campaign, together with the numbers who were killed and wounded

Rank	Corps	Total served	Killed in action	Died of wounds	Wounded*	Total casualties
		(Proportion (%) in each row)				
Officers	Cavalry	427	9 (2)	4 (1)	22 (5)	35 (8)
	Infantry	2,995	125 (4)	73 (2.5)	362 (12)	560 (18.5)
	RA	388	11 (3)	1 (0.25)	29 (7.5)	41 (10.5)
	RS&M	95	9 (9.5)	6 (6.5)	7 (7.5)	22 (23)
	Total	3,905	154	84	420	658
Sergeants and men	Cavalry	8,293	114 (1.5)	26 (0.5)	211 (2.5)	351 (4.5)
	Infantry	73,399	2,331 (3)	1,832 (2.5)	8,574 (11.5)	12,737 (17)
	RA	10,723	121 (1)	52 (0.5)	580 (5.5)	753 (7)
	RS&M	1,644	32 (2)	23 (1.5)	63 (4)	118 (7.5)
	Total	93,959	2,598	1,933	9,428	13,959

* This value was obtained by subtracting the number wounded (pp.428–9) from the number dying of wounds (pp.420–3).

(Summarized from Sayer, *Desptches*, pp.420–3, 428–9, and the endpaper. A similar table was published in the *Medical and Surgical History*, 2, p.388, though it differs in some details)

6.5 Outcome for wounded personnel

A survey of nearly 7,000 NCOs and men treated for gunshot wounds is summarized in Table 6.13. Nearly two thirds were injured in the arms or legs. About a tenth of these patients died and this followed amputation in nearly a half (217). The case-fatality rate was highest for injuries to the trunk, and in particular the abdomen. On the other hand, the chances of survival were greatest for injuries to the head and neck, although this may be because those with serious wounds were more likely to die before hospitalization could be effected.[15]

---

15 No survey of the nature of fatal battlefield injuries has been found but these will include those individuals who suffered a direct hit from round shot, fragments of shell, and grape and canister shot fired at close range.

Table 6.13 The outcome for NCOs and men with gunshot wounds

Location of wound	Deaths (c2/c5*100)	Discharged to duty (c3/c5*100)	Discharged or transferred (c5/c5*100)	Totals (% in column)
Head	170 (20)	594 (70)	87 (10)	851 (12)
Face	14 (3)	445 (83)	74 (14)	533 (8)
Neck	4 (3)	108 (84)	16 (13)	128 (2)
Chest	118 (28)	226 (54)	76 (18)	420 (6)
Abdomen	131 (56)	71 (30)	33 (14)	235 (3)
Perineum/genitals	17 (31)	23 (42)	15 (27)	55 (1)
Spine	45 (14)	225 (69)	56 (17)	326 (5)
Extremities	471 (11)	2,553 (57)	1,420 (32)	4,444 (64)
Totals	970 (11)	4,245 (60)	1,777 (18)	6,992

(Adapted from *Medical and Surgical History*, 2, p.258)

Amputation: The only practical treatment available at the time for severe comminuted fractures was amputation and many of the operations would have been performed on the battlefield or close by, and would have been completed within a few minutes. This means that the assertion by Edgerton that the 'surgeons had no time for the sick, who lay unattended for days and even weeks. All their time was spent amputating limbs, with singular lack of success,'[16] is a flight of fancy given that the official number of amputations performed in the Army as a whole was 824 during a period of about a year. Probably many of those would have been carried out on the days of the principal actions to which reference has been made.[17] A further comment in the same vein is provided by Taylor who suggested that the harbour at Balaklava, which was a considerable distance from the front, contained: 'Piles of arms and legs amputated after the battles [which] had been thrown into the almost tide less lagoon-like harbour, and could be seen in the clear water from the jetty.'[18] This statement is rendered even more bizarre because there are several valid reports of the disgusting state of the water, and the pollution would have rendered it anything but clear.

Discharge from hospital: A survey of 4,015 wounded men who survived their injury indicated that nearly three quarters (72 percent) were hospitalized for less than a month while a small proportion (four percent) took more than three months to recover (Table 6.14).[19] No time was recorded for a further 2,344 patients; perhaps because the information was not recorded by the hospital or they had been sent elsewhere to convalesce in order to vacate hospital beds.

16   Edgerton, *Death or Glory*, p.138.
17   *Medical and Surgical History*, 2, pp.368–9.
18   E. Taylor, *Wartime Nurse: One hundred Years from the Crimea to Korea 1854–1954* (London: Robert Hale, 2001), p.28.
19   *Medical and Surgical History*, 2, p.388

Table 6.14 Length of time taken for 4,015 NCOs and men to return to duty after treatment for wounds

	Period of treatment							
	≤1 week	<1 month	<2 months	<3 months	<4 months	<5 months	<6 months	>6 months
Number treated	1,476	1,408	709	263	101	40	11	7
Proportion (%)	37	35	17.5	6.5	2.5	1	0.25	0.2

(Adapted from the *Medical and Surgical History*, 2, p.388)

Maimed soldiers: During January 1856 a surgeon in 23rd Regiment suggested that men rendered unfit 'for duties of soldiers in the ranks' by minor wounds or injuries should not be discharged but redeployed on other duties, and thus spare men capable of 'all duties'. The proposition was seemingly accepted by the GOC of the Light Division,[20] although it has not been ascertained whether it became a general policy throughout the Army.[21]

Discharge from the Army: Seventy percent of 3,011 men discharged in England had gunshot wounds with the infantry accounting for 1,942 (92 percent) of 2,118 men in this category. Incised wounds accounted for only 1% of those discharged with 19 (61 percent) of 31 being in cavalry regiments. Other injuries, including luxations, contusions, fractures, burns, and surgical complications, accounted for nearly half of the men discharged from the Royal Artillery, but they were less significant reasons in the other corps (Table 6.15).

Table 6.15 NCOs and men disabled and discharged the service for wounds and other injuries

Reason for disablement or discharge	Cavalry		Infantry		Royal Artillery		RS&M		Total	%
	Total	%	Total	%	Total	%	Total	%		
Gunshot wound	56	51	1,942	72.5	101	49	19	79	2,118	70.5
Incised wound	19	17	11	0.5	0	–	1	4	31	1
Other injuries*	35	32	718	27	105	51	4	17	862	28.5
Total	110	100	2,671	100	206	100	24	100	3,011	100

* These included luxations, contusions, fractures, burns, and surgical complications.

(Summarized from the *Medical and Surgical History*, 2, pp.241–245)

20 TNA: WO 28/90 & 163.
21 See M. Hinton, 'A Recommendation that Maimed Men be Employed in the L.T.C.', *The War Correspondent*, 31:4 (2014), pp.31–2.

6.6 Concluding remarks

The lack of adequate hospital facilities during the first few months after the invasion resulted in the evacuation of large number of wounded men to the base hospitals in Turkey, particularly after the battles of the Alma, Balaklava and Inkerman. The progressive improvement in the provision for the sick and wounded, including the opening of a hospital close to the front line and a convalescent hospital, meant that emergency and follow-up treatment could the be carried out in the Crimea. As a result from beginning of 1855 the majority of evacuees would either have been convalescents or were not suffering life threatening injuries.

About two thirds of all the casualties, which were principally gunshot wounds, occurred during the six principal engagements while in her commentary on the campaign Martineau opined that 'life in the trenches was life face to face with death. Shot and shell hurtled without ceasing.'[22] However, the data in Table 6.10 suggests that this is an overstatement given that on forty percent of the siege days the number of casualties was five or less. These numbers would have been easily managed by the medical officers on routine duty in the trenches. On days when firing was more active, as during the bombardments, or when a sortie by the Russians had to be repulsed additional personnel from the camp could be called upon at short notice. This meant that there was no priority for a formalized scheme of what is now termed triage. On the other hand, simple casualty clearing stations were utilized during the assaults of 18 June and 9 September 1855 and this would have permitted patient selection. The advantage of treating of the wounded close to the front, as was amply demonstrated during the First World War, was obviously recognized by Hall and his colleagues.[23]

---

22   Martineau, *England and Her Soldiers*, p.172
23   Harrison, *The Medical War*, p.297.

7

Hospitals on the Bosphorus

7.1 Mortality from disease in the Crimea and at Scutari

There is an extensive literature on Miss Nightingale, both her own writings and numerous biographies, and this has resulted in a tendency for the problems in the Barrack Hospital at Scutari to be considered by several commentators to be exceptional and unusual. However, it was merely one of the several general hospitals utilized during the campaign (Table 1.4), and since the majority of the patients came from the Crimea there is justification in considering it as an integral part of the Army, rather than a special case.

It is the purpose of this chapter to consider this possibility. The testing of this hypothesis will involve a comparison of the pattern of mortality recorded in the regimental hospitals in the Crimea with what occurred in the hospitals on the Bosphorus. The cumulative mortality caused by diarrhoea and dysentery, continued fever, scurvy and frostbite during the eleven months after the invasion in the Crimean and Scutari are illustrated in Figures 7.1–7.4. These reveal that the curves for both locations were similar, and very highly correlated, with correlation coefficients (r) of 0.999, 0.993, 0.999, and 0.989 respectively.

These comparisons, together with similar ones for typhus, pneumonia and pleurisy, and bronchitis, which are not shown, together with the findings for the nosocomial infections illustrated in Figures 5.10 and 5.11, provide extremely strong circumstantial evidence that the situation in Turkey merely reflected that which obtained in the Army before Sevastopol. It was, therefore, the amelioration of the health problems in the Crimea which led to the reduction in mortality in the hospitals on the Bosphorus during the spring of 1855. As a consequence, the arrival of the Sanitary Commissioners in Turkey in early March 1855, the time of which is indicated in Figures 7.1–7.4, had little or no impact on the principal causes of mortality in either the camps before Sevastopol or the general hospitals in Turkey and elsewhere.

248 Victory Over Disease

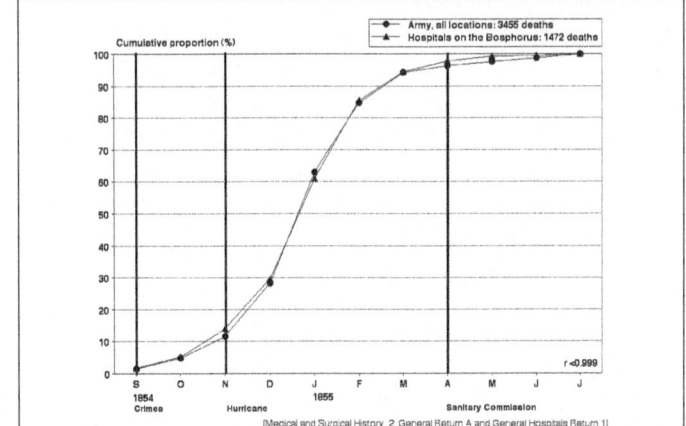

Figure 7.1 Deaths from diarrhoea and dysentery in regimental hospitals and the hospitals on the Bosphorus, September 1854–July 1855.

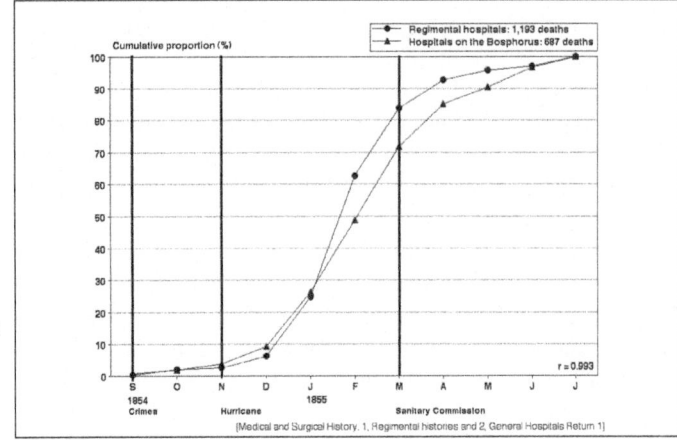

Figure 7.2 Deaths from continued fever in regimental hospitals and the hospitals on the Bosphorus, September 1854–July 1855.

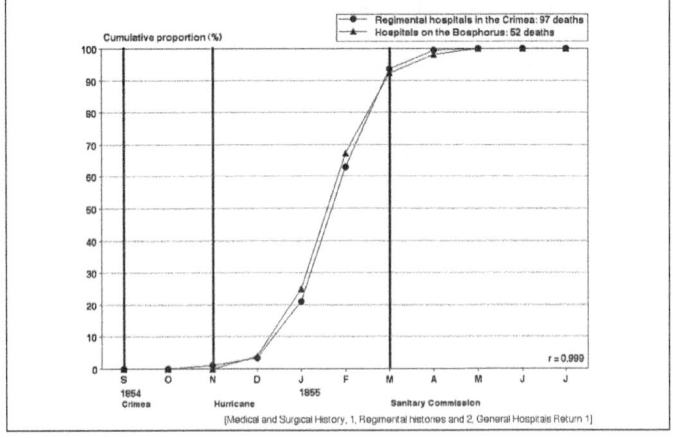

Figure 7.3 Deaths from scurvy in regimental hospitals and the hospitals on the Bosphorus, September 1854–July 1855.

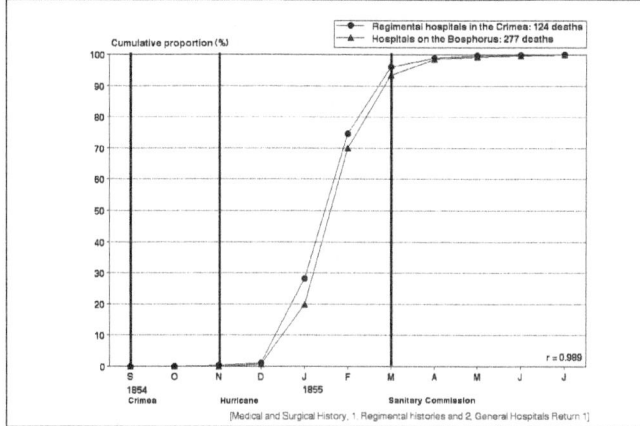

Figure 7.4 Deaths from frostbite in regimental hospitals and the hospitals on the Bosphorus, September 1854–July 1855.

7.2 Cholera

Cholera was not as serious a problem in Turkey as it was in the Army when in Bulgaria and the Crimea. The patterns on mortality in the Army as a whole and in the hospitals on the Bosphorus are illustrated in Figure 5.6 and were very different. The epidemic in Turkey during the summer of 1854 lasted for only a couple of months after which there were then only a few admissions until November 1855 when there was an outbreak in the locality which was not mirrored by one in the Crimea.[1]

Cholera was clearly most prevalent at Scutari at a time when the Army was not actively engaged with the Russians and this means that published statements that suggest that: 'wounded soldiers lay packed in corridors along side hundreds of cholera cases' indicate woeful lack of appreciation of the facts.[2]

7.3 Gunshot wounds (*Vulnus sclopitorum*)

The lack of hospital facilities during the first few weeks after the invasion resulted in the need to evacuate large number of battlefield casualties to Turkey. Nearly three quarters of those sent away during the campaign had arrived there by the end of November. The rate slowed during the winter as static siege warfare resulted in fewer casualties, and these could be treated in the Crimea. The intensity of fighting increased during the spring and summer of 1855. This resulted in an increase in the numbers of men admitted to the regimental hospitals. On the other hand, there was no corresponding increase in the number of patients evacuated as these could be catered for

---

1 Hinton, 'Cholera Epidemic'.
2 Taylor, *Wartime Nurse*, p.27.

locally in regimental hospitals and the Camp General Hospital. This opened in April 1855 and up to the end of September over 600 battlefield casualties were admitted, with 152 (25 percent) deaths.

Over ninety percent of the 315 deaths on the Bosphorus had been registered by the end of March 1855. Thereafter, the evacuees were mainly convalescent. In contrast, seventy percent of the deaths in the regimental hospitals took place during the spring and summer of 1855 prior to the fall of Sevastopol, after which time fighting effectively ceased.

7.4 Conditions typically associated with low mortality

Several conditions in General Return A accounted for more than a hundred primary admissions but for which the ratio of deaths in all locations to primary admissions was less than one percent. A total of 26,408 cases (16.2% of 162,673 admissions) satisfied these criteria, and of these 53 died (0.3% of 18,053 deaths) (Table 6.3). The mortality was somewhat higher during the first winter (November 1854–March 1855) in several instances (Table 7.1, col. 7 cf. col. 4), but it is unlikely that this would have prompted any comment as the deaths occurred sporadically over several months. This analysis also suggests that the deterioration in the living and working conditions did not in themselves render these afflictions more life-threatening. This is in contrast to diarrhoea, dysentery and continued fever; the comparable results for which are included for comparison.

It is unlikely that men suffering from the diseases listed in Table 7.1 would have been evacuated to Turkey for treatment and so the patients in this category would have been stationed in the army depots in the locality. The comparable analysis for these hospitals is summarized in Table 7.2. In all there were 3,664 cases (8.5% of 43,288 admissions), and of these 19 died (0.35% of 5,432 deaths). This result suggests that the situation in Turkey was not dissimilar from that in the Army as a whole, and that there was no persuasive evidence that the environmental conditions in these hospitals resulted in a higher than expected mortality rate.

7.5 Concluding remarks

Analyses presented in this chapter question a commonly held assumption that is was the contribution of Nightingale and the Sanitary Commission that caused the reduction in mortality in the hospitals at Scutari (see Table 7.3 for some examples of this misconception).

Table 7.1 Conditions typically associated with low mortality listed in the *Medical and Surgical History*, 2, General Return A, April 1854–June 1856

Condition*	Apr.–Oct. 1854 and Apr. 1855–June 1856			Nov. 1854–Mar. 1855		
	Primary admissions	Deaths in all locations	Ratio of Deaths/ Admissions (%)	Primary admissions	Deaths in all locations	Ratio of Deaths/ Admissions (%)
Ulcers/abscesses	6,679	9	0.15	1,243	14	1.1
Eye diseases	3,060	0	–	247	0	–
VD (6)	2,722	0	–	313	3	0.95
Hernia†	1,486	1	<0.1	102	2	2.0
Punishment	1,461	0	–	312	0	–
Luxations	1,395	2	0.15	138	0	–
Colic	1,387	3	0.2	127	2	1.6
Sore throat	863	3	0.35	81	6	7.5
Dyspepsia	829	1	0.1	77	2	2.6
Skin diseases	688	0	–	61	1	1.5
Paronychia	355	0	–	46	0	–
Burns	353	0	–	46	0	–
Haemorrhoids	322	0	–	36	0	–
Constipation	311	0	–	37	0	–
Scabies	239	0	–	18	0	–
Headache/vertigo	119	0	–	9	0	–
Anal fistula	104	1	0.95	25	2	8.0
Otitis	101	0	–	6	1	16.5
Total	22,474	20	<0.1	3,934	33	1.1
Diarrhoea	42,662	566	1.3	14,502	3,085	21.5
Continued fever	19,457	1,106	5.5	6,156	1,684	27.5
Dysentery	4,568	343	7.5	3,710	1,913	51.5

* The selection depended on there being >100 primary admissions and the ratio of deaths in all locations to primary admissions being <1%.
† Entered with both gastrointestinal and venereal diseases.

Table 7.2 Conditions typically associated with low mortality listed in the *Medical and Surgical History*, 2, General Hospital Returns I, April 1854–June 1856

Condition*	June–Oct. 1854 and Apr. 1855–June 1856			Nov. 1854–Mar. 1855		
	Admissions	Deaths	Ratio of Deaths/Admissions (%)	Admissions	Deaths	Ratio of Deaths/Admissions (%)
Ulcers/abscesses	270	1	0.4	69	2	2.9
Eye diseases	474	0	–	68	1	1.5
VD (6)	1,145	1	<0.1	126	2	1.6
Hernia†	164	0	–	41	1	2.4
Punishment	57	0	1	11	0	–
Luxations	90	0	–	29	0	–
Colic‡	108	0	–	8	2	25
Sore throat	89	1	1.1	27	1	3.7
Dyspepsia	174	1	0.6	46	3	6.5
Skin diseases	136	0	–	29	2	7
Paronychia	33	0	–	9	0	–
Burns	30	1	3.3	5	0	–
Haemorrhoids	46	0	–	7	0	–
Constipation	25	0	–	12	0	–
Scabies	170	0	–	0	0	–
Headache/vertigo	68	0	–	1	0	–
Anal fistula	48	0	–	17	0	–
Otitis	30	0	–	2	0	–
Total	3,157	5	0.15	507	14	2.8
Diarrhoea‡	5,037	207	4.1	3,787	1,313	34.5
Continued fever	4,394	185	4.2	2,822	562	20
Dysentery‡	1,850	163	9	1,805	952	52.5

* The conditions selected are those listed in Table 7.1.
† Entered with both gastrointestinal and venereal diseases.
‡ Amended totals; see Table 1.3.

Table 7.3 Examples of misinformation on the state of the hospitals on the Bosphorus

In 1856 (*sic*), six months after arriving in Scutari, Albania (*sic*), she [Nightingale] cut the military hospital mortality rates from 42.7% to 2.2%. (I. B. Cohen, *Scientific American*, 250, pp.128–36 (1984) quoted by Iezzoni, *A Cautionary Ta*le, pp.1079–85.)

The second Sanitary Commission, headed by Dr John Sutherland, also produced quick results by insisting on immediate improvements to the conditions endured by troops in Balaklava. The death rate fell rapidly once the narrow harbour had been cleared of corpses and filth, and a strict regime had been introduced for the troops' hygiene. (Royle, *Crimea*, p.502.)

The mortality rate in wards dropped from the awful 42 per 100 to 22 per 1,000 – thanks to the insistence of absolute cleanliness. (Taylor, *Wartime Nurse*, p.38.)

Florence and her team scrubbed the wards clean and changed the dirty bed-sheets. Far more wounded soldiers stayed alive while in their care. (J. Shuter, *Florence Nightingale and Crimean War* (Oxford: Heinemann Library, 2004), p.15)

In two weeks, the death rate had dropped by 80%. Pettenkoffer would have been proud of her [Nightingale]. (I.W. Sherman, *The Power of Plagues* (Washington, D.C.: ASM Press, 2006), p.184.)

The Barrack Hospital at Scutari 'had to be re-engineered by a team of visiting experts before the death rate could be brought down. (McDonald, *Florence Nightingale at First Hand*, p.72.)

Overcoming the hostility from the military, she set about organising the hugh barrack hospital and, with discipline and good sanitary practices, drastically reduced the mortality rate. (B. Best, *The Luckless Tribe. The Golden Age of British War Reporters* (Peterborough: FastPrint Publishing, 2012), p.14)

The honour of actually reducing death rates at the war hospitals must go primarily to the sanitary commission and also the supply commission. (L. McDonald, *History Today*, September 2012, p.16.)

A Scottish Engineer (*sic*), Dr John Sutherland, and his team arrived in March to flush out the sewers, repair the building and supply clean water. Only then did the death rate begin to fall. (K. Nixon and C. Worthington, *Florence Nightingale Museum* (London: Florence Nightingale Museum, Undated), p.21.)

Compelling evidence has been presented in Figures 7.1–7.4 that show that the mortality at Scutari mirrored that at the front and hence it was the improvement in the health of the troops in the Crimea that was the principal factor that lead to the reduction in mortality in the base hospitals. And, on this point, Nightingale agreed; as this extract from Gill's book attests:

> As Nightingale told Sidney Herbert unequivocally, Scutari was only a symptom of the army's malady, not a cause, and once things began to improve at Balaclava, things improved at Scutari. Once the men on the plains below Sevastopol began to get better food and the weather became warmer, their strength increased, they became more resistant to disease, the number arriving at Scutari went down, the wards became less crowded, and the medical personnel were under less pressure[3]

It would be unfair to suggest that Nightingale was not extremely influential and that very many people the world over have benefited in some way from her later achievements. Similarly, it would be churlish to suggest that the Commissioners, who were

---

3   Gill, *Nightingales*, p.393–4.

able and industrious individuals, did not play a part in the scheme of things. However, in the context of the Crimean War their contribution was probably much less than some would wish to think. For example, Deputy Medical Inspector D. Deas informed the Director General of the Naval Medical Department on 19 February 1855 that, though he admired Nightingale, he saw 'dozens of things placed at her credit which [...] she had nothing to do with; but such is the fashion of the day [she] now gets credit for having both suggested and executed.'[4] Similarly, Bostridge concluded: 'A [...] notion, prevalent among an older generation of historians, [and] found in popular historical writing today, is that the dramatic decrease in mortality at Scutari in the first months of 1855 is directly attributable to Florence Nightingale herself. This was transparently not so.'[5] In like manner, Ponting surmised: 'She did not institute many of the reforms ascribed to her [...] in medical terms she accomplished little [...] apart from providing basic comforts.'[6] However, as Major Bennett, RAMC, opined, these views should not 'detract for her' rather they do 'remind us that other people were contributing to reform.'[7]

To summarize, the principal cause of the high mortality recorded at Scutari during the first winter was a consequence of the need to evacuate from the Crimea large numbers of serious ill and wounded patients which had a very poor or hopeless prognosis. When health of the Army improved the patients evacuated had a better prognosis and the rates of mortality then fell dramatically.

4   Select Committee, 2nd Report, p.723
5   Bostridge, *Florence Nightingale*. pp.248–9.
6   Ponting, *The Crimean War*. pp.194–5.
7   Bennett, 'The Medical Service in the Crimea', pp.3–10.

8

Repatriation and discharge from the Army

The *Medical and Surgical History* included the following statement on repatriation:

> It might naturally be supposed that, as the number of deaths which occurred in the Crimea, and the various secondary hospitals in the Bosphorus and elsewhere, was so considerable, the proportion of men sent to England would be similarly large. We find, however, that the total number of men invalided to England only amounted to 9,544. [...] this is to be explained [in part] by the fact, that the pressure of service was for a time so great, that all the men likely to prove fit for duty in the ranks were detained at the seat of war [while many of those who died may have survived under different circumstances and could have been invalided.]'[1]

Some of the men who returned with their regiments may also have been candidates for repatriation if the occupation of the Crimea had continued beyond June 1856; and a proportion of them would have been sent to Chatham for assessment or further treatment. In addition, from September 1856: 'invaliding was increased by the reduction of the army [and this included those] who from slight wounds and other causes, it was deemed undesirable to retain [...] although they could not could not be said to be totally unfit.'[2]

Section XII in the *Medical and Surgical History* deals with the discharge of 'men from the service in consequence of disease incurred during the war.' The information presented was drawn from several different sources, and discrepancies can be found between them, particularly with respect to the numbers involved. The general conclusions that can be drawn are unaffected and are summarized in this abstract from the opening page:

---

1 *Medical and Surgical History*, 2, p.227.
2 *Medical and Surgical History*, 2, p.237.

The number of men discharged [...] on account of disease [until] the end on March 1857, amounted to 3,120; of which nearly three-quarters were discharge at Chatham, and the remainder in Ireland. [In] England, the proportion of men discharged was, with reference to strength, nearly equal in the cavalry and infantry – 391 [...] in the former, and 2,446 in the Guards and Infantry, while 283 only were incapacitated [...] in the Ordnance. [...] Thus it appears that, although fever proved [...] so fatal disease in the army [no soldier was discharged for] that disease, while only 194 were discharged [for] disability incurred by the fluxes, and four from unfitness referred to as scurvy. [However] it was noticed that many of the instances of rheumatism, paralysis, mental derangement, debility, impaired health, and even phthisis, were primarily the result of fever, the fluxes, and scurvy.[3]

The main purpose of this chapter is to illustrate the differences in the reasons why NCOs and men were admitted to hospital in the Crimea and then for their selection for evacuation to the base hospitals in Scutari, repatriation to England, and their final discharge from the Army. The sections on repatriation and discharge were based on data in the *Medical and Surgical History* that were presented in a format as used for General Return A and General Hospital Returns I.

Unlike the general hospitals in the Crimea and Turkey no detailed monthly tables were published for the hospitals in England although some anecdotal observations were published, as was the average number of beds available each day in each week between 21 February and 25 July 1855 (Figure 8.1).[4] The increase in the July was presumable in anticipation of an increased requirement following the return of the Army during June and July 1855.

8.1 Repatriation for disease

The seven most common diseases in each of the four categories of patient have been included together in Table 8.1. The most common reasons for primary admissions to the hospital for disease in the Crimea and referral to Scutari were broadly similar, although there were differences in the order of their importance, particularly abscesses and ulcers, while the small number of cases of cholera at Scutari would have been admitted from men stationed locally. No patient was evacuated for cholera. In those repatriated there was a reduction in the relative importance of abscesses/ulcers, while chronic rheumatism followed by common continued fever and diarrhoea headed the list with conditions such as eye disease, frostbite, and phthisis being among the top seven diseases.

3   *Medical and Surgical History*, 2, p.236.
4   *Medical and Surgical History*, 2, pp.231–5 & 241–5.

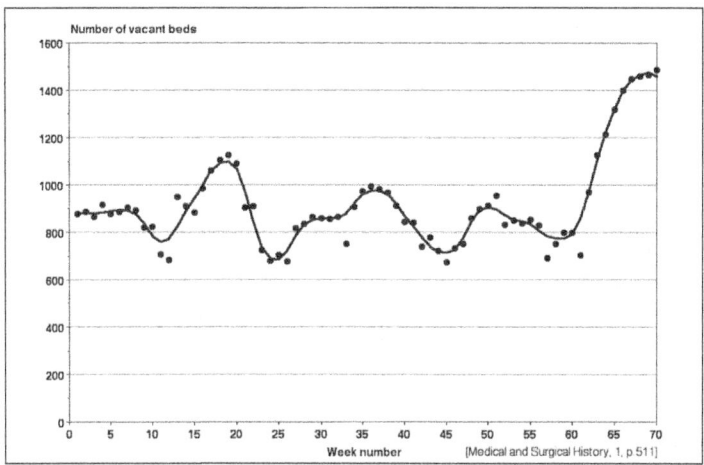

Figure 8.1 The average daily number of vacant beds in the hospitals at Chatham, Chichester, Plymouth, and Portsmouth for each week from 21 February until 25 July 1856.

Table 8.1 The seven most common disease conditions recorded for the primary admission of NCOs and men into the hospitals of the Army and for their selection for evacuation to Turkey and England, and discharge from the Army

Disease	Number of cases in each category (% of the total and the ranking in top seven)			
	Primary admissions to hospital*	Admissions to Scutari hospitals†	Repatriation to England‡	Discharged from the service§
Diarrhoea	44,164 (31: 1st)	8,571 (22: 1st)	1,533 (14: 3rd)	14
Continued fever	23,013 (16: 2nd)	7,216 (19: 2nd)	1,466 (14: 2nd)	0
Abscesses/ulcers	12,012 (8: 3rd)	743 (2: 7th)	175	63
Catarrh	10,083 (7: 4th)	1,742 (5: 5th)	513 (5: 5th)	32
Dysentery	8,278 (6: 5th)	3,381 (9: 4th)	945 (9: 4th)	20
Cholera	7,574 (5: 6th)	388	0	0
Rheumatism	4,906 (3: 7th)	3,463 (9: 3rd)	2,094 (20: 1st)	275 (9: 2nd=)
Frostbite	2,289	811 (2: 6th)	266 (2.5: 7th=)	171 (5.5: 6th)
Eye diseases	3,307	542	483 (4.5: 6th)	226 (7: 5th)
Phthisis	185	197	266 (2.5: 7th=)	234 (7.5: 4th)
Debility	214	507	278 (2.5: 7th=))	760 (24: 1st)
Diseases of lungs	Not recorded	Not recorded	Not recorded	274 (9: 2nd=)
Varicose veins	58	23	34	183 (6: 7th)
Totals	144,390	38,345	10,672	3,120

* *Medical and Surgical History*, 2, General Return A
† *Medical and Surgical History*, 2, General Hospital Returns I.
‡ *Medical and Surgical History*, 2, pp.231–5.
§ *Medical and Surgical History*, 2, pp.241–5.

After return to England diarrhoea, dysentery, common continued fever, and catarrh ceased to feature while conditions such as debility, chronic rheumatism, eye disease, phthisis, frostbite, and varicose veins proved to be relatively important reasons for discharge from the Army, as was 'lung disease'; though this term was only used in this category and hence cannot be compared with the other returns.

8.2 Repatriation for wounds and injuries

Primary admissions to hospital in this category were dominated by gunshot wounds (58.5 percent) and contusions (22 percent) and there was bias towards men with gunshot wounds being selected for evacuation to Scutari, and it was these patients who formed the majority of those who were repatriated and subsequently discharged.

This is in contrast to amputees, who formed a relatively small proportion of referrals to Scutari but were an important reason for discharge as they were obviously unfit for active service and opportunities for alternative employment in the Army were few. On the other hand, contusions and incised wounds would have tended to heal and these patients formed a smaller proportion of patients as time progressed, presumably because the men would have been able to return to duty following their recovery (Table 8.2).

Table 8.2 The number of NCOs and men with wounds and injuries who were admitted to hospital, repatriated to England, and discharged from the Army

Nature of injury	Number of cases (%)			
	Primary admissions to hospital*	Admissions to Scutari hospitals†	Invalided to England‡	Discharged from the service§,¶
Gunshot wounds	10,691(58.5)	3,690 (74.5)	2,405 (72)	2,118 (70.5)
Incised wounds	1,270 (7)	200 (4)	35 (1)	31 (1)
Contusions	4,006 (22)	494 (10)	89 (2.5)	54(2)
Amputations/ resections	No data**	277 (5.5)	658 (19.5)	682 (22.5)
Other injuries††	2,316 (12.5)	282 (6)	162 (5)	126 (4)
Totals	18,283	4943	3,349	3,011

* *Medical and Surgical History*, 2, General Return A.
† *Medical and Surgical History*, 2, General Hospital Returns I.
‡ *Medical and Surgical History*, 2, pp.231–5.
§ *Medical and Surgical History*, 2, pp.241–5.
¶ No details about the award of pensions is given in the *Medical and Surgical History*.
** These are treatments and would not have been recorded as a reason for admission to hospital.
†† These totals include, inter alia, luxations, fractures, and burns.

8.3 Mortality among repatriated patients

No information on mortality was included in the returns used in the preparation columns 4 and 5 in Table 8.1. The data on 452 fatalities summarized in Table 8.3, was drawn from other tables and shows that overall two thirds of the deaths were associated with gastrointestinal and respiratory diseases, and fever (39, 30.5, and 11 percent respectively).

Of 3,318 men repatriated with wounds 13 (0.5 percent) died on the voyage to England. This low figure suggests that the patients had been retained in the East until they were not in a critical condition; and this provides 'evidence of the general sufficiency of the arrangements' that were made for them.[5]

Table 8.3 The number of NCOs and men who died of disease during the voyage to England or after arrival

Disease category	Men dying on passage home*		Dying after arrival to end of 1856†	
	Number	Proportion (%) of total	Number	Proportion (%) of total
Gastrointestinal disease	72	39.5	103	38
Respiratory disease	36	20	102	38
Fever	29	16	22	8
Rheumatic disease	12	6.5	1	<0.5
Cardiovascular disease	5	2.5	9	3.5
All other diseases	28	15.5	33	12
Total	182		270	

* *Medical and Surgical History*, 2, pp.229–30.
† *Medical and Surgical History*, 2, p.236.

8.4 Reasons for discharge

In all 15,707 invalids were received at Chatham during the 27 months up to March 1857 and of these 9,899 (63 percent) were discharged, 5,054 (32) returned to duty, 283 (2) died, 23 (0.15) deserted, and 14 (<0.1) transferred.[6] Of those discharged 2,695 (27 percent) left the service 'on reduction' as merely 'undesirable to retain,' while 2,296 (23 percent), 1,880 (19), and 1,306 (13) were for battlefield injuries, thoracic diseases, and chronic rheumatism and infirmity.

5   *Medical and Surgical History*, 2, pp.259 & 388.
6   *Medical and Surgical History*, 2, pp.237–8.

8.5 Potential future employment

With regard to the longer term it was suggested that many men declared unfit for military service would be 'capable of duties where steady habits of discipline, trustworthiness, and obedience are required [and would be] well suited to act as private watchmen, gate-keepers, porters, warehouse-keepers, and as porters in attendance upon passengers at railways.'[7]

No detailed statistics on the ultimate fate of discharged soldiers have been found. Reference to the obituary columns in the *Gentleman's Magazine* and other journals record the premature death of a relatively large number of officers whose health had been compromised by war service. In all probability a similar fate befell a proportion of NCOs and men; particularly because many of them would have been exposed to more hardship then the officers.

8.6 Concluding remarks

Protracted wars have been associated with epidemics of infectious disease which may subsequently be spread by prisoners and returning soldiers. Examples in the 19th century include typhus fever in Napoleon's Russian campaign, and small pox after the Franco-German War 1870–1, while in the American Civil War measles and typhoid were widespread.[8] However, there were no serious outbreaks of disease in the British troops after they returned home and this was a reflection of good health they enjoyed when they left the Crimea. Some men were discharged from the Army on account of disease but by and large these were causes that would not have represented a serious threat to the civilian population. In contrast, Emperor Napoleon ordered the establishment of several extensive quarantine camps for returning troops on account of the presence of typhus in the French Army.[9]

---

7 *Preston Guardian*, 3 March 1855.
8 F. Prinzing, *Epidemics Resulting from Wars* (Oxford: The Clarendon Press, 1916), pp.1–10.
9 Report to the Emperor, 8 September; *Daily News*, 28 October 1856.

9

Commissions and committees of enquiry

The serious health problems in the Army during the winter of 1854–55 prompted the government to send three Commissions of enquiry to the East to investigate matters on the spot, while a Select Committee of the House of Commons chaired by John Roebuck, MP, was convened after the resignation of the Earl of Aberdeen's administration to ascertain what had been going wrong, and who was to blame.[1] A Royal Commission, with Sidney Herbert as the president, was then convened in 1857 to enquire into the health of the Army. Its influential report was published the following year, although it was more concerned with making recommendations for the future development of the Army Medical Department (AMD), and thus did not provide a retrospective assessment of what took place in the Black Sea theatre.[2] In addition, as referred in Section 2.2.8, a select committee of the House of Commons under the chairmanship of Mr Augustus Stafford, MP, was convened on 28 April 1855 to consider the future development of the AMD, and it reported during July of that year.

9.1 Hospital Commission

The first of the Commissions comprised Dr A. Cumming, P.B. Maxwell, a barrister, and Dr T. Spence, who drowned on *Prince* on 14 November 1854, and was replaced by Dr P.S. Laing. Their brief was to make recommendations rather than institute reforms and the matters addressed in their report included, inter alia, staffing levels, particularly hospital orderlies, the duties of the purveyor, laundry facilities, and the preparation and distribution of food, while with respect to Scutari they suggested the acquisition of a ship for a store; a steamer to ply between Scutari and Constantinople; and open boats to assist the landing of evacuees.

---

1 For further details see Shepherd, *Crimean Doctors*, 2, pp.373–411.
2 Royal Commission Report, Appendix LXXIX.

Much criticism has been levelled against the hospitals at Scutari and part of the problem was the lack of an overall command structure, as enunciated by Stratford: 'Sillery [Commandant], Boxer [Port Admiral], and Menzies [PMO] are excellent well-intentioned men, but they are not of the most clear-headed or energetic race, and the great obvious want is that of a head.'[3] Nevertheless, despite these shortcomings Spence was able to report on the day that Nightingale arrived in Constantinople, viz. 4 November 1854: 'Just returned from Scutari perfectly delighted to find things so well managed. A great number of sick and wounded from Balaklava just landing, those unable to walk carried to hospital on stretchers and put to bed immediately they arrive. All beds on trestles have a neat and comfortable appearance, 400 excellent iron bedsteads have lately been obtained for the Turks.'[4]

Maxwell, another of the commissioners, was critical of several aspects of management when he visited on 10 November though his 'first impression [was] favourable [...] I found ample ventilation, comfortable bedding, and healthy looking convalescents. The fine weather, the ample building, and abundant supply of water may have contributed to give the place an air of cheerfulness.'[5] Similarly, the PMO reported to Hall that Nightingale's initial reaction was encouraging: 'The hospitals are [...] in tolerable order as regards cleanliness and comfort, and this opinion has been expressed [...] by various officers of our own and Naval service, and [...] Nightingale, [...] stated that on her arrival here that after all she had heard she was surprised at the regularity and comfort which appeared in our wards.'[6] Similarly, she reported to Hebert on 25 November that: 'The wounded were bathed every night according to Dr McGrigor's orders in slippers baths.'[7]

Clearly things deteriorated when large numbers of seriously ill and wounded patients arrived during the next few weeks, but that was more a reflection of the facilities being overwhelmed than anything else. By the time the Sanitary Commissioners arrived in March 1855 conditions had improved once again (see below).

Maxwell also confirmed that the wards and latrines were not as bad as has been stated by some critics, and that the PMO was not to blame: 'I have been backwards and forwards in that [Barrack] hospital for three months; though I found sometimes the effluvium from the privies offensive [...] I never found anything positively offensive in

---

3   Stratford to Raglan, 16 November 1854; S. Lane-Poole, *Life of the Right Honourable Stratford Canning Viscount Stratford de Redcliffe* (London: Longman, Green, & Co., 1888), 2, pp.381–2.
4   Spence to Smith, 4 November 1854; Wiltshire and Swindon History Centre: 2057/F8/III/B/315.
5   Maxwell to Herbert, 10 November 1854; Wiltshire and Swindon History Centre: 2057/F8/III/B/356.
6   Cantlie, *History*, 2, pp.123–4. Incidentally, Bostridge, *Florence Nightingale*, p.224 suggested that Nightingale, showed self-discipline by 'making a tactical move designed to disarm [the PMO, Menzies].' It is difficult to know how this could have been the case given the remark was made soon after her arrival and the hospital had yet to be overwhelmed.
7   Quoted by Bennett, 'The Medical Service in the Crimea', pp.3–10.

any of the wards or corridors.'[8] It transpired that the unsatisfactory state of the latrines at Scutari was due principally to their construction, and the misuse to which they are put, as explained by Hall and the resident military engineer:[9]

> Hall: The water closets [...] speedily got choked up from the men recklessly thrusting old shoes and other articles down them. When [...] put right, I advised small iron gratings to be placed over them, so as to prevent [this], but it was not attended to; hence the disgusting scene, described by Mr Osborne, in the Barrack Hospital. Nothing of that kind existed when I was there in October, but to become so would only require a few days.[10]

> Resident engineer: The soil, etc., was, conveyed from the closets [...] by means of earthenware piping 7 inches in diameter, protruding from the inner side of the walls of the building. The whole system of drainage was most defective, and constant repairs were therefore needed [...] About the middle of September 1854 a general repair of [...] the closet pipes in the Barrack Hospital was made [and] up to the 5th December [they] underwent a general repair no less then three separate times. [...] caused chiefly by the obstruction of the pipes from [...] throwing old clothing, bones, and other refuse matter down them, thus completely stopping the passage or bursting the pipes, and thereby causing most offensive smells. In one instance [...] the obstruction was [...] caused by the body of a newly born infant.[11]

The 'evil' may not have been solved completely, however, as Spencer Wells, a civilian surgeon noted in June 1855 that: 'The system of drainage and privies is still very imperfect and objectionable.'[12]

Incidentally, the resident military engineer also reported on 5 December 1854 that: 'The pipes conveying the water supply were entirely renewed from its source, a distance of upwards of four miles, and sedimentary wells were formed at intervals along its course.'

9.2 Select Committee of the House of Commons

The Roebuck Committee investigated the 'Condition of the Army before Sebastopol' and produced five reports with four containing the answers to 21,431 questions posed

---

8   Cantlie, *History*, 2, p.100.
9   Capt. E.A. Gordon, RE.
10 Letter to Editor, 9 July; *The Times*, 27 July 1855.
11 Elphinstone, *Journal*, Appendix LIII, p.291.
12 *Medical Times and Gazette*, 30 June 1855, pp.648–50.

to witnesses and other evidence.[13] The responses provided by senior commanders who had returned home suggested that overwork, and not a shortage of food, was the principal factor that caused the breakdown in the health of the troops (Table 9.1), and this view was endorsed in general terms by Maxwell.[14]

Table 9.1 Responses of senior officers to questions posed by the Roebuck Committee during March 1855 on the health of the troops under their command

Officer	Question number	Abstract of the response
Sir De Lacy Evans, 2nd Division	717	[The troops'] suffering [was] mainly attributable to exposure and overwork [...] not so much a want of clothing.
	914	The main cause [of the misery] was overwork and exposure at night [...] we [in the 2nd Division were] never really [...] deprived of any regular issue of provisions [...]
Major General H.J.W. Bentinck, Guards Brigade	1,209	[The troops suffered] from hard work, not want of food
	1,323	[Illness was due] principally [to] over-work in the trenches and on picket; exposure to damp and wet, over exertion, in short.
	1,361	[Mortality was] principally to exposure more than the want of clothing.
H.R.H. Duke of Cambridge, 1st Division	3,860	I conceive that the men were worked to a degree that no man could stand it without being seriously affected in their health by it.
	4,090	I think [the medical men] were very efficient in deed. I have no fault to find what ever in that respect.
Lt. Col. J.P. Sparks, 38th Regiment, 3rd Division	5,305	The duty became very severe latterly; [...] the extreme severity of the weather and [...] more duty to than usual, was what caused the disease.
	5,306–7	Not badly [off for provisions] for troops in the field. We had a good deal of fresh provisions in the 3rd Division.

(Select Committee, 2nd Report)

The fifth report, which provided a short summary of some of the problems that faced the Army, opened with the following obvious realistic conclusions, although they were only made after making allowance for difficulties resulting from a long period of peace, and the storm of 14 November 1854:

> An army encamped in hostile country, at a distance of 3,000 miles from England, and engaged in a severe winter in besieging a fortress which for want of numbers,

---

13   Select Committee, 2th, 3th, 4th, & 5th Reports.
14   Anon [Maxwell], *Whom Shall We Hang?*, pp.149–160.

it could not invest, was necessarily placed in a situation where unremitting fatigue and hardship had to be endured. Your Committee are, however, of the opinion that this amount of unavoidable suffering [was] mainly to be attributed to dilatory and inefficient arrangements for the supply of this army with necessaries indispensable to its healthy and effective condition.[15]

Two serious shortcomings of Roebuck's initiative were the impossibility of cross-examining personnel with the Army, and all the information they considered was necessarily out of date. Incidentally, Herbert made pertinent observations with respect to the AMD: '[The Committee's] acceptance of gossip and hearsay evidence, [...] the bullying Old Bailey tone to Dr Menzies and the small fry contrasted with the civility to Newcastle [and] the condemnation of Dr Hall, who is unheard.'[16] Similarly, Maxwell opined that too: 'great importance was given to statements made by civilians who had gone out without medical authorization and or official sanction and whose criticisms, made in ignorance of the facts, were proved to be exaggerated, and in some instances and inaccurate in others.'[17]

The Committee made no specific recommendations. An omission perhaps, though by June 1855 most of the problems would have been addressed, either wholly or in part.

Dr Hall's rejoinder: Hall was obviously upset by criticisms that he and the AMD received in the report on matters which were either outside his control or for which he had no executive responsibility. This prompted him to write a letter to *The Times* on 9 July 1855 setting the record straight:

> [In] the report of the Committee [I] notice the following statement: 'With this confirmation by Dr Dumbreck [...] of the whole testimony relating to this painful subject, your Committee are totally at a loss to comprehend the report of Dr Hall [regarding] the Barrack Hospital, the scene of so much misery and suffering. The Duke of Newcastle states that the disgraceful condition of the hospitals was first brought under his notice in the middle of October. *Dr Hall was at Scutari from the 3rd to the 23rd of October. Dr Hall's report seems to have misled both Lord Raglan and the government at home, and to have occasioned much delay in measures taken afterwards for the remedy of evils which might have been arrested earlier in their progress.*'[18]

---

15 Select Committee, 5th Report, p.3.
16 Herbert to Gladstone, 9 July 1855; Lord Stanmore, *Sidney Herbert. Lord Herbert of Lea* (London: John Murray, 1906), 2, p.451.
17 See Anon [Maxwell], *Whom Shall We Hang?*, pp.272–83 for further discussion on this vexing issue. Maxwell was particularly critical of the evidence given by 'three gentleman who visited the hospitals at Scutari as amateurs,' viz. Messers Stafford, Macdonald and Osborne.
18 The text in italics was transcribed in Nightingale, *Notes;* McDonald, *Florence Nightingale. The Crimean War,* p.642.

You pronounce these observations [...] to be 'a just rebuke for my false report,' without [...] knowing anything of the circumstances under which it was written. [...] so far from my report being a false one, *I reiterate and adhere to every syllable I then wrote, and I consider I am quite as good a judge of the subject, and quite as worthy of credit, as the Duke of Newcastle's informants, whose reports may, perhaps, refer to an earlier or a later period than mine.*

Dr Dumbreck's evidence [...] refers to a later period than [...] my report. [As] he was [...] in the Crimea [...] until the 17th of November. Now, my report refers to a period not later than the 21st of October [when] I left Scutari, and [when] every man in hospital had new and clean bedding, and all his substantial wants were [...] attended to. With ordinary capacity on the part of the principal medical officer [...] and [...] purveyor, this condition of things ought to have been maintained, if not improved. [...] The Barrack Hospital [had been] temporarily and hurriedly converted into a hospital for the reception of sick and wounded brought in suddenly in great numbers, there was, necessarily, considerable confusion for the first few days; [...] and I have no hesitation in saying that 2,000 wounded men would derange the economy of any hospital in London for some days, notwithstanding all the resources of means and medical attendance. [...] When I was at Scutari there was ample accommodation for the sick and wounded then in hospital, and for half as many more, but the battles of Balaklava and Inkermann (*sic*) [which took place after Hall had return to the Crimea] filled this at once.[19]

It would seem that the confusion arose because those in London failed to appreciate what was happening at the front because of the time it took for news to reach them from the Crimea. As a consequence Newcastle's criticism of Hall was unfounded because he must have been referring to events at Scutari which took place shortly after the battle of the Alma when things were indeed extremely disorganized. By the time Hall arrived matters had settled down and this was confirmed by several commentators (see next paragraph). Nightingale later changed her mind by saying that Raglan could have 'corrected' the 'wrongs' if he had not been misled by Hall's report of 'flourishing' conditions in Scutari.[20] However, this was a misinterpretation of events on her part as it was some weeks after Hall's departure when the hospitals were overwhelmed by the large number of seriously ill and wounded patients from the Crimea; something nobody could have predicted at the time.[21]

The Commander-in-Chief (Hardinge) also censured Hall and suggested that Raglan should have taken action against him.[22] However, there was never a need for

19 *The Times*, 27 July and *The Lancet*, 4 August 1855.
20 McDonald, *Florence Nightingale. The Crimean War*, p.20.
21 Over 12,000 patients were admitted to the hospitals on the Bosphorus during the three months from November 1854; *Medical and Surgical History*, 2, General Hospital Returns I.
22 Select Committee, 4th Report, pp.243–4.

an enquiry on Raglan's part as he would have been satisfied with Hall's assessment since it had been confirmed to him by the British ambassador,[23] his senior ADC, Lord Burghersh,[24] and Paulet (Commandant on the Bosphorus).[25] This suggests that it was unreasonable of Nightingale to agree months later with the opinion expressed by Hardinge at that time.[26] Matters continued to improve so that by the end of 1854 Herbert reported to Smith that he had heard from both Cumming and Maxwell that: 'Scutari is fast getting into order'[27] while a despatch dated 1 January 1855 reported that Sir George Brown and HRH the Duke of Cambridge had visited the hospitals and had been: 'highly gratified by the notice thus taken of [the] suffering [of the men of their divisions.]'[28]

9.3 Supplies Commission

The Commissioners, Sir John McNeill and Colonel A.M. Tulloch, arrived in Constantinople on 6 March 1855, too late to have much impact as by then abundant supplies of food, clothing and other necessaries were being received, huts were being erected, a railway was under construction, and the roads were under improvement so wheeled transport could be used again. The Commissioners subsequently reported their retrospective assessment to Panmure on 10 June:

> The sick from the Crimea were nearly all suffering from diseases chiefly attributable to diet [...] supplied [...] during the winter, consisting principally of salt meat and biscuit with [...] insufficient [...] vegetables, [which] was calculated [...] to produce those diseases. [...] Dr Sutherland, of the Sanitary Commission [...] entirely concurred in the necessity of substituting fresh meat for salt, and fresh bread for biscuit, as well as increasing the supply of fresh or preserved vegetables.[29]

The commissioners also made some additional observations in their official report:

> The medical evidence appears [...] against [...] anything peculiarly unfavourable in the climate, and all the officers [...] examined, referred to overwork, improper diet, exposure to cold and moisture, with deficient shelter, inadequate clothing, and defective boots, as the causes of disease. [...] there can be no doubt that the

---

23 Stratford Canning to Clarendon, 25 October 1854: TNA: FO 78/1004.
24 Raglan to Newcastle, 18 November 1854; TNA: WO 1/170/ff.109–12.
25 Paulet to Raglan, 1 December 1854; National Army Museum: 6807–293–8.
26 McDonald, *Florence Nightingale. The Crimean War*, p.84.
27 Herbert to Smith, 24 December 1854; Select Committee, 4th Report, pp.343–4.
28 *The Times*, 15 January 1855.
29 Supplies Commission Report, p.1.

mortality was really the effect, not of any one cause apart from the others, but of a combination of the whole. [...] this enquiry [has] demonstrated how indispensable it is to the soldier's efficiency, especially in the field, that he shall be supplied with [sufficient] wholesome food.[30]

As with the Hospital Commission, no formal recommendations were made and hence the report represents little more than a source of historical information. This was published after the war and the response of the Army was to convene a 'Board of General Officers Appointed to Enquire into the Statements Contained in the Reports of Sir John M'Neill and Colonel Tulloch;' now usually referred to as the Chelsea Board.[31] Their report proved controversial as it exonerated the QMG and AG from any blame for the events of the winter of 1854–55, although Filder, the commissary general, did come in for some criticism, and he responded to this by publishing a pamphlet as a defence.[32]

Several contemporary commentators considered the Chelsea Board report a whitewash; and by implication an animadversion of the Commissioners. McNeill chose to make no response publicly,[33] but Tulloch published a rejoinder in which he emphasized that in his opinion the losses from disease would have been substantially less if supplies had been adequate, and, on this basis he could not accept the conclusion of the General Officers that nobody in the Crimea was blameless, as more should have been done to source food and other necessaries locally.[34]

No specific comments were made in the Supplies Commissioners' report about the functioning of the AMD, and there was little on health matters with the exception of an apparent misunderstanding about the availability of quinine and the supply and distribution of lime juice to prevent scurvy. Later Smith asked Hall for his opinion and his reply of 28 April 1856 included comments on marquees and other equipment, the provision of transport, the issue of warm clothing (Figure 9.1), and the availability and supply of medicines. He also suggested corrections on matters of detail.[35]

30   Supplies Commission Report, pp.37 & 47.
31   HCPP 1856 (2119) XXI.1: *Report of the Board of General Officers Appointed to Enquire into the Statements Contained in the Reports of Sir John M'Neill and Colonel Tulloch* and HCPP 1856 (422) XXI.651: *Index to the Report of the Board of General Officers Appointed to Enquire into the Statements Contained in the Reports of Sir John M'Neill and Colonel Tulloch.*
32   Commissary General Filder, *The Commissariat in the Crimea: being Remarks on those Parts of the Report of the Commission of Enquiry into the Supplies of the British Army which Relate to the Duties of the Commissariat* (London: W. Clowes, 1856) and also as HCPP 1856 (2042) IX.377.
33   McNeill subsequently provided a foreword to the 2nd edition of Colonel Tulloch, *The Crimean Commission and the Chelsea Board Being a Review of the Proceedings and Report of the Board* (London: Harrison, 1857) published during 1880. In this he was critical of both Kinglake and the Chelsea Board.
34   Tulloch, *The Crimean Commission*, pp.149–69.
35   Mitra, *Life and Letters*, pp.479–503.

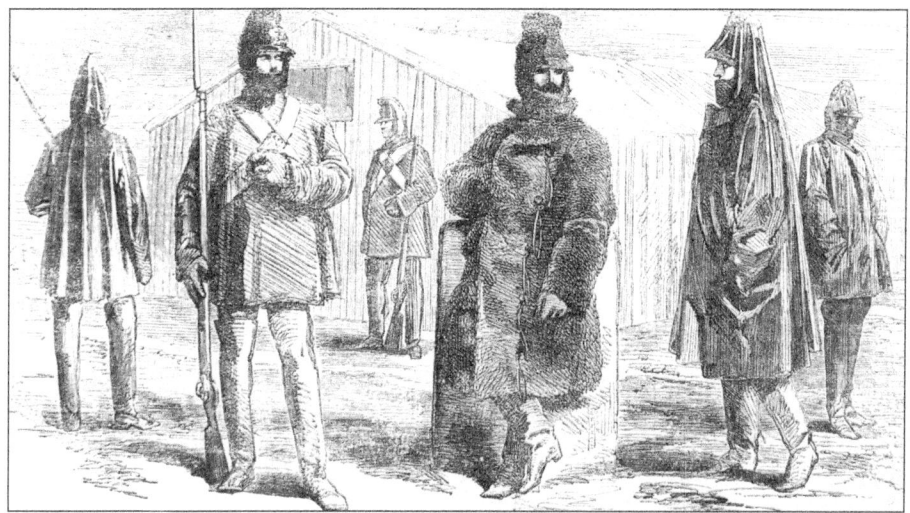

Figure 9.1 Winter clothing for the British troops in the Crimea. (*Illustrated London News*, 23 December 1854, p.649)

9.4 Sanitary Commission

Palmerston appreciated that that the health problems in the Army were not dissimilar to those faced by the public health authorities in Britain and shortly after he became Prime Minister he sent a Sanitary Commission to the East with a view to establishing civilian standards of hygiene in the camps and hospitals.[36]

The Commissioners, Dr J. Sutherland, Mr R. Rawlinson, a civil engineer, and Dr H. Gavin, received their instructions from Panmure on 19 February 1855, and they, with a small staff,[37] arrived at Constantinople on 3 March tasked with dealing with 'the hospitals, but not with the sick, and the camp, but not with the troops.'[38] Their brief was to attend principally to environmental matters, and it is clear from their report there were opportunities for this in and around the various general hospitals and the town and harbour of Balaklava, and much effort was subsequently expended in attempting to put these matters to rights.

Palmerston, who had been a supporter of Edwin Chadwick, adopted a bellicose attitude over the sanitary issue before the Commissioners arrived in Turkey.[39] He assumed they would be: 'opposed and thwarted by the medical officers, by the men

---

36 Palmerston to Panmure, 13 February 1855; Douglas and Ramsey, *Panmure Papers*, 1, p.63.
37 Gavin died following a shooting accident. He was replaced by Dr G. Milroy who arrived in the Crimea on 22 July 1855.
38 Sanitary Commission Report, p.4.
39 Chadwick is remembered for his championing of the need for the improvement on sanitation and public health, particularly in the poorer areas of cities.

who have charge of the port arrangements, and by those who [clean] the camp. Their mission will be ridiculed and their recommendations and directions set aside unless enforced by the peremptory exercise of [Raglan's] authority.'[40]

This extreme view proved unwarranted as the Commissioners told the Commandant at Scutari that they 'cannot but express their gratification at the zealous cooperation they have received not only from your Lordship, but from the officers [...] at Scutari and Kulali.'[41] In like manner, Raglan instructed that every facility should be given to the Commissioners 'in the execution of the duties confided to them.'[42] Hall collaborated with them by providing 'much information respecting the health of the Army, and for facilities in examining the camps and hospitals.'[43] At the end of May, Hall informed Raglan that: 'Every precaution is being taken to remove nuisances from the camps [...] and to improve their sanitary condition [...] and in this the Sanitary Commissioners [...] afford cordial assistance;'[44]though, as the editor of the *Association Medical Journal* surmised, progress was probably not as rapid as it might have been because: 'The mismanagement of medical matters in the East [had] arisen rather from the want of fuller power and authority in the heads of the AMD, than from any absence of ability or deficiency of skill, is a sufficient proof of the necessity there is for entrusting all purely sanitary arrangements to properly qualified medical men.'[45]

It is appropriate to add that the active support of the Commander-in-Chief was essential to achieve progress and it has been suggested that in this respect Raglan should not escape censure. For example, he: 'had it within his power to beat cholera [when in Bulgaria as his] medical staff had already pointed out the need to construct latrines [and] filter the drinking water;'[46] while after the invasion he tried unfairly to blame the medical department for the inadequate treatment of the sick and wounded, when in fact the it was members of the Army staff who should have been held responsible.[47]

9.4.1 Scutari

The military barrack at Scutari was far from ideal as a hospital, yet in February 1855 Panmure seemed content with the arrangements that Paulet had made for the sick,[48] while the resident engineer reported favourably on a visit paid by the Commissioners on 6 March: 'On their inspection of the various buildings in British occupation [...] they expressed themselves as agreeably surprised at the cleanliness and comfort of the

---

40 Palmerston to Raglan, 22 February 1855; National Army Museum: 1968-07-290-1.
41 TNO: WO 33/1/24/55, p.4.
42 General Order, 26 March 1855.
43 Sanitary Commission Report, p.79.
44 Hall to Raglan, 14 May 1855; RAMC: 397/F/CO/1/2/2086.
45 *Association Medical Journal*, 4 May 1855.
46 Small, *Crimean War*, pp.40-3.
47 Ponting, *Crimean War*, pp.192-3.
48 Panmure to Paulet, 23 February 1855; TNA: WO 6/70 & 28/199/1.

different establishments,' and 'there was little or nothing left for them to point out, by way of amelioration.'⁴⁹ The Commissioners themselves told Paulet on 10 March that they had found that: 'The wards of the Barrack Hospital are lofty, and not over crowded. [In our opinion] the Barrack Hospital bears marks of much having been done to improve its sanitary condition; [...] The General Hospital [...] is the best of all the Scutari hospitals, as its structure admits of adequate ventilation, and the greater part of it is scrupulously clean.'⁵⁰

Paulet subsequently reported to Panmure: 'Drs Sutherland and Gavin [...] who have made a cursory inspection of the hospitals, have expressed themselves agreeably surprised at their cleanliness and comfort, and state that there will be very little for them to point out here.'⁵¹ It was certainly not: 'as filthy as the vilest slums in London' as has been suggested by a recent commentator.⁵² The Commissioners initial reaction was confirmed later in their final report when they recorded that 'there was abundant evidence that the military authorities had been actively engaged before our arrival, in improving this hospital, and much had evidently been done with that object.'⁵³

That there was scope for improvement in the various hospitals is not at issue and the Commissioners set to work in clearing animal carcasses and filth from the vicinity, and suggested modifications for the hospital building. Nightingale appeared to be satisfied by their industry though the PMO, resident engineer, and Charles Bracebridge, Nightingale's companion, seemed less impressed:

> Nightingale: The Sanitary Commission is doing something, and has set to work burying dead dogs and whitewashing infected walls, two prolific causes of fever.⁵⁴
>
> PMO: The Sanitary Commission [...] went mooning about here telling us what every one with eyes and nose could not fail to detect and have left the place much in the same state they found it.⁵⁵ [...] The graveyard has been inspected by the Sanitary Commissioners who have made some suggestions. There never appeared to me any injurious consequences to be apprehended from it. The smell is from the sewer.⁵⁶

49 Elphinstone, *Journal*, Appendix 53, pp.292–3.
50 TNA: WO 33/1/55/24, pp.1–2. This point was repeated in the official report; Sanitary Commission Report, p.18.
51 Paulet to Panmure, 8 March 1855; Reports on Hospitals in Turkey, p.1.
52 H. Small, 'The Impact of the Crimean War on Public Health' in Wellcome Collection,: Deutsches-Hygiene Museum Dresden, *War and Medicine* (London: Black Dog, 2008), p.31.
53 Sanitary Commission Report, p.14.
54 Nightingale to Herbert, 18 March 1855; British Library: Add Ms 43,393.
55 Cumming to Hall, 10 April 1855; National Army Museum: 2007-07-16-19.
56 Reports on Hospitals in Turkey, p.37 and Royal Commission Report, Appendix LXXIX, pp.46 & 132.

> Resident engineer: One of their few recommendations, (with respect to the ventilation of the privies built in the angle of the Barrack yard), was at variance with the expressed opinion of the Engineer officer, and ordered the compliance with which was the cause of subsequent complaint on the part of the medical authorities. [...] In March the Commissioners ordered some slight alterations to some of the privy drains, and the reconstruction of one of the main sewers, the results of which were of a very dubious character and were the cause of constant complaint by the medical authorities.[57]

> Bracebridge: The Commissioners were 'incompetent' and that 'these patchings are of little use.'[58]

An anonymous contemporary commentator, who called himself a 'Non-Commissioner' also questioned the effectiveness of the Commissioners in a well-researched pamphlet printed after the publication of the Royal Commission's report:

> The Eastern Sanitary Commission [...] after ten days spent in examining, and maturing their plans [...] commenced their works [but by] the beginning of July, they say, 'after all that could be done in the way of temporary improvement, cleansing, and flushing, the drains under and near the hospitals, from their inherent bad construction, were still nothing but cesspools, communicating, by open tubes, with the interior of the hospitals.'[59] Such miserable results, after four months of 'scientific labours,' appeared unsatisfactory even to the Commissioners, though they in no degree retarded *the rapid decrease of the mortality* in the hospitals.[60]

It was not unreasonable for the Non-Commissioner to question why the Commissioners took so long to reach this conclusion and why they did not admit that the objectionable smells did not appear to have a detrimental effect on the health of the patients. The Non-Commissioner continued by quoting several more extracts from the report and concluded that their 'endeavours [...] were attended with no better success than those of the officer of the Royal Engineers during the winter [of 1854–55].' This is a reasonable opinion in the circumstances but it does not accord with suggestion made by Chadwick's biographer who wrote that the influence of the 'famous Crimean Sanitary Commission [...] is incalculable in its importance;'

---

57 Elphinstone, *Journal*, Appendix LIII, pp.292–3.
58 Bracebridge to WEN, 18 March 1855; Claydon 273 quoted by Bostridge, *Florence Nightingale*, p.249.
59 Sanitary Commission Report, p.52.
60 A Non-Commissioner, *A Report on the Sanitary Condition of the Army Particularly during the Late War with Russia* (Undated pamphlet), pp.25–7; RAMC: 397/M/2.

but ducked the issue by noting that 'the story of that intervention is too well known to be repeated here.'[61] More recently McDonald stated erroneously that the Barrack Hospital at Scutari 'had to be re-engineered by a team of visiting experts before the death rate could be brought down.'[62]

Nearly all the British land forces were located in a relatively small area of the Crimean peninsula, and, as was demonstrated in Chapters 5 and 7, it was the high incidence of serious and potentially fatal diseases amongst them that strongly influenced the mortality rates in the hospitals at Scutari; a point made by Hall in his evidence to the Royal Commission on 19 June 1857: 'The sanitary commission claim credit for reducing the sickness at Scutari [...] but forgot that Scutari was supplied from the Crimea, and that the supply of sick had fallen off one half. [...] It was the character of disease that had changed.'[63]

It would appear that Nightingale agreed with Hall at that time when she told Herbert unequivocally that:

> Scutari was only a symptom of the army's malady, not a cause, and once things began to improve at Balaclava, things improved at Scutari. Once the men on the plains below Sevastopol began to get better food and the weather became warmer, their strength increased, they became more resistant to disease, the numbers arriving at Scutari went down, the wards became less crowded, and the medical personnel were under less pressure.[64]

Sutherland, nevertheless, questioned Hall's assertion by suggesting to the Royal Commission that the some of the improvements were due to the activities of the Sanitary Commissioners, though he did 'attribute part of the diminished mortality in the hospitals to the very cause to which Sir John Hall appears desirous of attributing the whole.'[65]

Clearly there was a conflict of interests as Sutherland would have been anxious for the Commissioners to get some credit, otherwise their mission might be perceived as pointless. Nightingale suggested, misleadingly, that their work was nearly complete by June 1855,[66] while Shepherd has proposed a more realistic scenario:

> [Kinglake's] suggestion that the mortality rates fell at the end of March because of the work of the Commission is scarcely tenable. It is inconceivable that the

---

61 S. E. Finer, *The Life and Times of Sir Edwin Chadwick* (London: Methuen, 1952), pp.483–5.
62 McDonald, *Florence Nightingale at First Hand*, p.72.
63 Royal Commission Report, p.181.
64 Undated reference; Gill, *Nightingales*, p.383.
65 Royal Commission Report, p.344.
66 McDonald, *Florence Nightingale. The Crimean War*, p.884 and McDonald, *Florence Nightingale at First Hand*, p.87.

work involved in relaying drains and other major improvements was completed in two weeks. More likely the mortality rate fell because the admission rate came down at this time, thus reducing the lethal effect of overcrowding, because the severity of the medical cases admitted from the Crimea lessened at this time, and because the climatic conditions improved.[67]

Another issue that affected peoples' judgment of the hospitals was their previous experience. For example, Assistant Surgeon E. Wrench, informed his father on 28 December 1854 that he had received two letters from Scutari. One was from somebody who had not been to the Crimea and thought that it was uncomfortable and horrid and the other from Assistant Surgeon H. Ludlow who thought it was a sort of Paradise,[68] while at the end of January Assistant Surgeon J.J. Scott, 57th Regiment, who, like Ludlow was at Scutari on sick leave from the Crimea, thought the Barrack hospital was 'as comfortable as can be expected' and 'well supplied in with good rations and warm dress.'[69]

9.4.2 Crimea

Work to improve the state of the camps commenced after the hardships of the winter were over and this was carried forward following the convening on the 10 March 1855 of a local Sanitary Committee which was chaired by Dr Hall and included a senior medical officer from each Division.[70]

The Sanitary Commissioners landed in the Crimea on 2 April 1855 and though they considered that the 'health of the army [...] was by no means good,' it was 'hardly below [...] the usual standard of armies in the field, and its health was better than that often experienced by armies similarly circumstanced.'[71] This was likely to have been due in part to Hall and several medical officers having visited the camps weekly to inquire 'into the state of the sick and the sanitary condition of the camp.'[72] Two weeks after the Commissioners arrival Simpson, the Chief of Staff, informed Panmure that: 'The state of our camps is another subject of misrepresentation at home. I know them all [...] and more cleanly encampments I never saw. I consider them quite healthy and wholesome in all respects.'[73]

---

67 Shepherd, *Crimean Doctors*, 2, p.400.
68 University of Nottingham: Wr/C/2/23. Acting Assistant Staff Surgeon Ludlow served in the Crimea until invalided to Scutari with a medical certificate where he died there on 4 April 1855.
69 Letter dated 26 January 1855 quoted by Dawson, *Letters*, p.156.
70 For the report of the Committees see *Medical and Surgical History*, 2, pp.53–4 and Smith, *Précis of Letters*, 1, Appendix No. 11, pp.712–4.
71 Sanitary Commission Report, p.79.
72 Special Correspondent, 19 March; *The Times*, 2 April 1855.
73 Douglas and Ramsey, *Panmure Papers*, 2, pp.151–3.

Balaklava: The town and harbour of Balaklava[74] were small and it was soon 'in a filthy and revolting state', and though Raglan issued orders for it to be cleansed there was no one to attend to it.[75] A board of inquiry into the sanitary state of the town was convened on 17 January 1855 with Sir Colin Campbell as President.[76] The report has not been found but despite any recommendations it may have made matters deteriorated further as a consequence of the excessive traffic passing to and from the port.[77] Towards the end of March things began to improve and the resident PMO informed Hall that 'attention was at last aroused and the town is in consequence improving in every way,' latrines 'much wanted here are about to be built' and a 'police has been established to prevent the committing of nuisances in the street, a practice much in vogue at one time.'[78]

Not surprisingly the Commissioners deemed the harbour unsatisfactory. The non-tidal water became congested with refuse including, carcasses, offal and dung, with the consequent 'evolution of large quantities of sulphuretted hydrogen gas.' However, they conceded that the Commandant and Port Admiral had used 'their best endeavours to improve the sanitary condition of the place' but they were hampered by a 'want of labour and means of transport;' a problem that, despite the activities of the Commissioners appeared to persist until the arrival of the Army Works Corps as native labourers were 'by no means efficient [...] and most expensive.'[79]

The Commissioners made several requests to Headquarters during the following weeks for assistance with labour and equipment, only to be informed that the demands of the siege frequently made this impossible. Raglan, though not unsympathetic, considered that the government should have provided the Commissioners with the wherewithal to obtain the resources they needed and not to have to rely on the Army to provide them. Incidentally, this was a potential problem anticipated earlier by the Earl of Shaftsbury when he wrote to Panmure on 18 February 1855: 'The Commissioners should have the power of hiring, on their account, such numbers of workmen as they may find necessary. The entire success of this undertaking will depend on instructions given to Lord Raglan, Lord W. Paulet, and other authorities, *to carry into execution without delay* whatever the Commissioners may declare to be essential to health and safety.'[80]

---

74 The management of shipping in the harbour is explained in Gordon, *Balaklava*.
75 Russell, 4 October; *The Times*, 23 October 1854.
76 The board members included three Medical Officers, two chaplains (presumably one Anglican and one Roman Catholic), a captain, RN, if possible, and the Commandant; TNA: WO 28/108. This was about a month before Panmure issued the Sanitary Commissioners with their instructions on 19 February 1855.
77 For example, see a letter dated 26 February in the *Illustrated London News*, 24 March 1855.
78 RAMC: 397/F/RT/1/1.
79 Sanitary Commission Report, pp.89–91.
80 E. Hodder, *The Life and Work of the Seventh Earl of Shaftsbury, K.G.* (London: Cassell, 1898), p.504.

Sutherland later acknowledged that improvements occurred only gradually so that by 'several months before the evacuation' Balaklava had 'became as clean and healthy a little sea-port as one would wish to see' and that 'it required little or no interference on [the Sanitary Commissioners] part.' He also pointed out that this satisfactory state of affairs was only achieved after 'a great expenditure of labour and money.'[81] This improvement was confirmed by Major R. Barnston who wrote on 7 January 1856 that Balaklava: 'is a most astonishing place now; and nothing could be cleaner or more regular. The harbour is quite black with cormorants; they have turned out such excellent scavengers that any one shooting at them is immediately flogged [...] and his gun seized.'[82]

Harbour police: This unit comprised ten men. They wore a distinctive uniform resembling that of the Thames Police and was responsible for maintaining the sanitary condition in the port.[83] However, despite unambiguous harbour regulations, the masters of the cattle transports ignored these instructions on occasions and threw carcasses and dung over board while in harbour instead of waiting until after they put to sea.[84] The disposal of general filth and the offal from the animals slaughtered in the town presented a continual logistical challenge and, like the carcasses, most had to be taken out to sea in a 'dirt barge' and disposed of well away from land.[85]

On the matter of carcasses the QMG [Airey] requested the Port Admiral [Boxer] to 'devise some means for preventing the dead carcasses towed out to drift again into harbour.' He responded by stating the captains of steam tugs had strict instructions 'to tow cattle and offal well out to sea and to the lee of the harbour's entrance. Every practicable means are made to keep the harbour [clear] and great praise is due to the water police for their vigilance.'[86] On occasions the carcasses did not sink and those 'floating off the rocks beneath the Genoese Castle and Sanatorium' represented a 'serious detriment [to] the inmates and [was] in direct violation of the port and harbour regulations, with respect to dead cattle and the like.'[87] To obviate this problem it was recommended that 'before being let go their sides and entrails should be freely slashed, so as to cause the carcass to sink.'[88]

---

81 J. Sutherland, *Reply to Sir John Hall's 'Observations' on the Report of Sanitary Commission Despatched to the Seat of War in the East, 1855–56* (London: Harrison, 1857), p.23.
82 Trevor-Barnston, *Letters*, pp.138–9.
83 Boxer to Admiral Lyons, 1 June 1855; Correspondence of Balaklava Harbour, p.2. For an illustration see *Illustrated Times*, 9 June 1855.
84 The regulations were dated 6 March 1855 and reproduced in *Correspondence on Balaklava Harbour*, pp.10–1. They were reissued on 1 January 1856; TNA: WO 28/194.
85 There are several references to this matter in the Sanitary Commissioners' report.
86 QMG to Boxer, 27 April 1855 and his reply; TNA: WO 28/123 & 183.
87 Sanitary Commission to Captain Hamilton, RN, 14 June 1855; TNA: WO 32/7580. See also Staff Surgeon Matthew to Sanitary Commission, 30 October 1855; Royal Commission Report, Appendix LXXIX, p.193.
88 Sanitary Commission to Port Admiral, Balaklava, 30 October 1855; TNA: WO 32/7580.

Camps before Sevastopol: The impression given by some commentators is that Hall and his colleagues were remiss in not ensuring that the camps, including the latrines, were kept in a satisfactory hygienic state. Hall was well aware of these problems and reported incidents to HQ from time to time, but it was the Queen's Regulations that placed the responsibility for camp cleanliness with the military authorities, and not the AMD.[89] For example, a General Order of 12 May 1854 required the privies to be examined daily by a QM and medical officer, and to report weekly on their cleanliness.

The issue was the subject of several General Orders issued during the summer of 1854, with one of 11 November requiring that burials: 'take place at a sufficient distance from the sources of water supply, from the camps of any troops.'[90] The topic apparently ceased to be a priority following the hurricane of 14 November until the spring of 1855 when a proactive interest was taken once again by Headquarters. For example, the GOC of Divisions were reminded that their AQMG was required to ensure that: 'all dead animals are buried at least three feet deep; latrine trenches are dug sufficiently deep and earth thrown on the soil every morning, and [...] the most stringent measures are taken to prevent men answering the calls of nature except in the latrines; all offal, dirty clothes, rags, broken bottles etc. are burned or buried every morning; and particular attention is paid to the cleanliness of that part of the camp near the commissariat, ambulance, hospital and reserve ammunition.'[91] These instructions do not appear to have been followed implicitly on occasions and a divisional commander had to be reminded of his responsibilities: 'I am desired by Lord Raglan to call your attention to the sanitary condition of the camp under your command, and to beg that dead horses may be buried, the latrines attended to, and the collections of the refuse, rags and rubbish either buried or burnt. In the latter case, care must be taken to prevent accidents.'[92]

Hall wrote in strong terms to the AG on the subject of 'camp nuisance' on 24 January 1855:

> Proper latrines should be dug in all camps, and the soil covered over daily with earth, all dead animals ought to be buried [...] The pioneers [should be] directed to clean round the hospital marquees and men's tents daily, collect all offal, dirty and condemned cloths, and rags which are merely thrown outside the tents and allowed to rot. The trenches [...] should be deepened to carry off surface water [...] the matter will have to be enforced by authority, because no regiment can be so pressed for duty men, as not be able to spare a party for a short time daily to perform the essential offices of camp economy.[93]

---

89   See McDonald, *Florence Nightingale. The Crimean War*, pp.655–7.
90   On 12 May, 27 June, 1 August, and November 1854.TNA: WO 28/51.
91   AG to GOC, 2nd Division, 8 February 1855; TNA: WO 28/72, and a memorandum issued by the QMG on the same day; TNA: WO 28/159.
92   AG to GOC, Cavalry Division, 31 January 1855; TNA: WO 28/192.
93   Royal Commission Report, Appendix LXXIX, p.113.

Shepherd considered that the need for Hall to remind the AG: 'of such elementary rules of hygiene at this stage of the campaign was a considerable reflection on all concerned.' Shepherd did not exclude the regimental doctors from criticism. He considered that they should have done more to get matters better organized, though he conceded that this reflected in part: 'the complete lack of executive power of even the most senior medical officers.'[94]

The QMG subsequently requested that a general of the day be appointed to: 'supervise the regularity and cleanliness [of the camp] in every particular' in accordance with the Queen's Regulations.[95] This was not acceded to by Raglan although he convened a board of senior medical officers with Hall as President to investigate the sanitary condition of the Army, though this may have been a response to the impending arrival of the Sanitary Commissioners in the Crimea. The Board reported on 10 March with recommendations on diet and water, clothing, camps, and duties.[96] The attention of the COs was then drawn to the subject by the AG:[97] 'General Officers commanding Divisions, and the Officers Commanding in the camps of the siege trains, and of the R. Sappers and Miners, will send daily [...] a report that the cleanliness of their camps has been attended to, that dead animals have been buried, and rubbish and broken glass removed and destroyed.'[98]

These instructions resulted in improvements and by the end of March 1855 Hall was able to report to Raglan:

> The rations are abundant, the men are well clothed, and due attention is paid to the sanitary condition of the different camps. The supply of water is ample at present, and means are being adopted to insure it in future, by constructing new tanks, cleaning out those already in use, and digging fresh wells. [...] The hospitals are on a respectable footing, and amply provided [...] for [...] the sick.[99]

It was as a consequence of these developments that the Sanitary Commissioners found: 'the camp [before Sevastopol was] remarkably clean and the external sanitary arrangements [...] well attended to,' in spite of 'the pressing nature of the siege duties' and, although there were some defects, there were 'some regimental camps to which it would have been difficult to have suggested improvements.'[100] This state of affairs was reported to the QMG following an unannounced tour of the camps by the Commissioners towards the end of April. They expressed themselves:

---

94 Shepherd, *Crimean Doctors*, 1, p.313.
95 QMG to Military Secretary, 5 March 1855; TNA: WO 28/192.
96 Royal Commission Report, Appendix LXXIX, pp.118–20.
97 Hall to Smith, 12 March 1855; RAMC: 397/F/CO/1/2/1630.
98 Circular Memorandum, No. 299, 9 March 1855; TNA: WO 28/122
99 Hall to Raglan, 3 April 1855; RAMC: /F/CO/1/2/1743; *London Gazette*, 20 April 1855; and Sayer, *Despatches*, p.131.
100 Sanitary Commission Report, p.121.

much surprised and gratified with the appearance of the camp and of the hospitals, and said that were it were not for Balaklava, they might at once return to England, as no sanitary recommendations were required from them for the upper camp. One of them (Mr Sutherland) said 'It would be an insult to the Army if we were to offer any suggestion.' [while] Mr Rawlinson said 'There can be no sanitary measure we could recommend which I have not seen carried out today in some phase or other, varying, of course, in different regiments according to the ability and zeal of the commanding officers and surgeons.'[101]

The improved state of affairs was also confirmed independently by Philip Rathbone, a Quaker philanthropist from Liverpool, who visited the Crimea at the beginning of April 1855. He was 'expecting the worst' but 'was pleasantly surprised to discover that most of the muddle had been countered,' and 'on the plain before Sevastopol he waxed lyrical about the scene that stretched before him.' He also found the harbour of Balaklava in a 'good state' and that 'no pains had been spared to keep it clean.'[102]

On 17 May 1855 the Commissioners sent Raglan a list of sensible recommendations, viz. refuse should be burnt, carcasses and offal should be buried at least three feet deep, waste food should be burnt or buried and not thrown into latrines, latrines should not be kept open for too long and the contents should be covered daily with earth and charcoal until the level is within two feet of the surface when the latrine should be closed, places where animal are picketed should be kept constantly clean and the dung and refuse burnt, and tents should be struck regularly and the ground exposed to the air and sunshine.[103] Simpson confirmed to the Commissioners on the 20 May 1855 that most if not all of these recommendations had already been introduced, and hence no further orders were needed; indeed the camps were 'well policed, and clean considering all things.'[104]

Good reports were received in London and Panmure was able to write to Simpson on 3 July 1855: 'I have received from Mr Newlands the most satisfactory accounts of the sanitary condition of the camp and I am convinced that you cannot benefit the Army more or maintain the efficiency better than by strict attention to every provision which concerns the health of the men.'[105] The need for continued watchfulness proved necessary; however, when an inspection revealed that, unlike the infantry regiments, some cavalry camps were not in a 'good sanitary condition.'[106] Shortly afterwards it

---

101 AQMG to QMG, 26 April 1855; TNA: WO 33/1/49/55, Inclosure 12 and TNA: WO 28/192.
102 P.H. Rathbone, *A Week in the Crimea* (Liverpool, 1855), pp.61–2 quoted by Royle, *Crimea*, p.343.
103 TNA: WO 33/1/49/55, Inclosure 9, and Sanitary Commission Report, pp.127–9.
104 CO, 14th Regiment to AG, Horse Guards, 11 June 1855; National Army Museum: 1962–10–94–2.
105 TNA: WO 6/71.
106 Sanitary Commission Report, pp.149–50.

was stressed that 'great attention' was being paid 'to cleanliness in the camps, and to prevent overcrowding in either tents or huts.'[107]

Hall agreed with the Commissioners' suggestions, though he begged 'to observe, that almost all points had been anticipated,'[108] while after the war he informed the Royal Commission that 'the recommendations made by the Sanitary Commission had been recommended before by the medical men and most of the things had been put into effect, more or less.'[109] When he gave evidence to the Royal Commission on 17 July 1857 Sutherland claimed that he had not seen the recommendations made by Hall's Board, which in the circumstances seems rather unlikely, and he objected to Hall's statement as it implied that the Commission did not have much impact on events.[110] Sutherland was then requested to clarify the contents of a letter he wrote on 19 July 1855 to Lord Shaftsbury in which he had stated unequivocally 'that the sanitary recommendations made by [him] had been anticipated by the army medical officers on the spot.' In his reply Sutherland dodged the issue by stating that his comments referred only to the sanitary state of the camps, and not to either Scutari or Balaklava, and that the Commissioners 'had only wished the worst practices to be avoided and the best systematically adopted. [...] all depends on the commanding officers of regiments [but] we [...] found the medical officers thoroughly alive to the nature of the changes required [...] but without power to carry them out.' Sutherland also mentioned that they had 'endeavoured [...] to limit our requirements to what was barely necessity' and concluded by stressing that none of his comments should be construed as any criticism of the 'medical officers in the field', whom he held in 'high esteem.'[111]

In his unpublished account of the campaign Hall noted, with some justification, that 'if the same power had been granted to the medical officers of the Army that was conceded to the Sanitary Commissioners, there would have been no occasion to send the latter out to the seat of war,'[112] and, not unexpectedly, he considered that their contribution to the well-being of the troops in the Crimea was relatively limited, although he was mindful to add a caveat:

> So far as the labours of the Sanitary Commissioners came under my notice, I think their services might have been dispensed with without any detriment [...] as there was nothing [...] which had not been either suggested, or was not in actual operation before their arrival. I speak of what came under my own

---

107 Hall to Military Secretary, 14 August 1855. Forwarded to Panmure with Simpson's despatch of 17 August; TNA: WO 1/377/ff.859–60.
108 Hall to QMG, 27 May 1855; Royal Commission Report, Appendix LXXIX, p.124.
109 Sanitary Commission Report, p.181.
110 Royal Commission Report, pp.333–5.
111 Royal Commission Report, p.360. The letter was published in *The Times*, 22 August 1855.
112 Hall, *Observations*.

observation in the Crimea; but they may have furnished other reports and valuable information to the authorities at home.[113]

Hall was not alone in his views on the usefulness of the Commission as the following quotation from an anonymous letter, possibly a medical officer, attests:

> It makes me sick to read of people being sent out to investigate the cause of our great mortality. What else could any one expect under the circumstances? Starving men without clothes to their back, or shoes to their feet, exposed to inclement weather in a manner that beasts are never exposed; for the latter can run about, whereas the former were obliged to lie down.[114]

Trenches before Sevastopol: The conditions in the trenches clearly deteriorated during the autumn of 1854[115] and the men were exposed to 'an atmosphere, often unavoidably vitiated by the excretions of the masses engaged on such duty,'[116] and the poor conditions continued during the campaign. For example, a General Order of 11 May 1855 stated: 'The dirty state of some of the trenches [...] had been reported to the Commander of the Forces. Field Officers on duty will give directions that a party of the guard shall [supply] the places used as latrines with sufficient lime and soil. This work is to be continued daily,'[117] while on 1 July the AG informed the QM on duty in the trenches that: 'the caves on the left of the 3rd parallel are in a very dirty state and require immediate cleansing. The latrines in the 3rd parallel require more lime. In the Right Attack the privies and graves about the quarries are offensive and a coating of charcoal would prove useful.'[118]

William Simpson, the artist, inferred that the Sanitary Commissioners were unwilling to risk going close to the front line.[119] It is perhaps not surprising that, apart from a recommendation for burying the dead, there was only one specific reference to the trench system in their report when Sutherland wrote to Simpson on 18 July 1855 about the 'bad sanitary conditions in the trenches' and the 'offensive emanations' that arose following the disturbance of graves, and recommended the area should covered with peat charcoal.[120]

---

113 Hall, *Observations*, and Mitra, *Life and Letters*, pp.375–6.
114 *Medical Times and Gazette*, 19 May 1855.
115 See G. Eyre-Todd (ed.), *The Autobiography of William Simpson, R.I. (Crimean Simpson)* (London: T. Fisher Unwin, 1903), p.25.
116 *Medical and Surgical History*, 2, pp.75–6.
117 TNA: WO 28/130.
118 TNA: WO 28/110.
119 Eyre-Todd, *William Simpson*, p.53.
120 Sanitary Commission Report, pp.148–9 and TNA: WO 32/7580. Incidentally, there is no mention of the unsanitary conditions in the trenches in the reports of the Hospitals Commission and Royal Commission.

Personal cleanliness: The Sanitary Commission seemingly did not consider the troops' personal cleanliness part of their brief, as soap was not mentioned in their report. The shortage of soap became an issue within weeks of the invasion. For example, the surgeon in the 77th Regiment noted during November 1854 that there was none for washing 'hospital blankets and other things, as the patients are very filthy.'[121] This situation caused Smith to complain to Horse Guards that there was a 'great want of the means of securing personal cleanliness in the Army [arising] from the impossibility of obtaining soap.'[122] Hall was informed shortly afterwards that 'thirty tons of soap have been shipped for the use of the troops; ten of which were forwarded at the close of November.'[123]

There is no doubt that the personal cleanliness was an important issue as evinced by a memorandum issued by the AG following representations from medical officers. It was undated but the context suggests that it was written during the spring of 1855 and was directed at divisional commanders:

> Greater attention is necessary to the ventilation of the tents, and the cleanliness of the persons of soldiers. These are points [that should] be looked to by the Commanding Officers of regiments [...] They are subjects for their own care and vigilance. [...] The men must also be encouraged to wash their clothes and their persons thoroughly, and means should be taken to enforce this necessary duty of cleanliness upon those whose habits may less incline them to the exertion to do so.[124]

Hall also issued a memorandum to divisional PMOs informing them he was sorry to find that:

> itch, scurvy and ulcers and great personal filth prevail amongst the men [...] for want of [...] regimental medical officers in making periodic inspections [as] required by the Regulations of Service. He [Hall] therefore requests [...] that this duty is performed weekly. [...] government has provided soap, and there is no excuse for the men going about from one week's end to another without either washing their person or changing their flannels and shirts.[125]

---

121 *Medical and Surgical History*, 1, p.375.
122 Smith to Military Undersecretary, 21 December 1854; Smith, *Précis of Letters* and Royal Commission Report, Appendix LXXIX, p.24.
123 Smith to Hall, 2 January 1855; Smith, *Précis of Letters* and Royal Commission Report, Appendix LXXIX, p.25.
124 TNA: WO 28/195.
125 Medical Department Memorandum, 17 February 1855; RAMC: 397/F/CO/1/3 and Royal Commission Report, Appendix LXXIX, p.116.

Not surprisingly this terse memo provoked a defensive reaction from some medical officers. For example Surgeon W.G. Watt, 23rd Regiment, responded: 'The tents are frequently visited by the Assistant Surgeons or himself during the week and he is perfectly aware of the filthy state of the men and from the amount of duty this is almost unavoidable [...] and the extreme difficulty of procuring wood and water even for cooking has been pointed out by me more than once;'[126] while a letter from another surgeon was published in the *Daily News*:

> Dr Hall [...] accuses the regimental surgeons of inflicting scurvy and all kinds of disease and abominations on the men by their neglect. [...] Recrimination has always been held to be a bad arrangement, and to place those who have recourse to it in a very suspicious position. [...] Regimental surgeons have been well aware of the uncleanly state of their men [...] I have [...] tried with my commanding officer to devise a plan for the personal ablution of the men. But [...] hardly able to get sufficient water [...] with no means of heating water but open fires [...] no vessels for purposes of washing, no soap, [...] no change of underclothing etc. [...] it becomes impossible [...] to carry out a system of proper cleanliness. [...] the regimental surgeon has no power for forcing a system among men on duty in a regiment; his control extends only over the sick in hospital. He may recommend, but his power stops there.[127]

The anonymous surgeon clearly did not hold Hall in high regard as he then accused him unreasonably of negligence: 'Let the country judge between the regimental surgeons and Dr Hall whose name has become so familiar in connexion with the neglect at Alma, neglect in camp, neglect on sick transports, and neglect in the hospitals at Scutari.'

9.4.3 Responses to the report
During a debate in the House of Commons on the role of the Supplies Commissioners held on 12 March 1857 Palmerston made a passing reference to the Sanitary Commission: 'Dr Sutherland and his associates took the medical arrangements of the hospitals and of the camp into immediate consideration and suggested improvements which were of the utmost consequence to the troops [and] the sick and wounded.'[128] This seemingly innocuous remark provoked a riposte from Hall dated 14 March 1857:

> It was with astonishment that I read in the report of that part of Lord Palmerston's speech [...] that the excellent condition of the military hospitals in the Crimea was attributable to the advice and suggestions of Dr Sutherland

---

126 Watt to PMO, Light Division, 17 February 1855; RAMC: 397/F/CO/31/13.
127 *Daily News*, 10 March 1855.
128 *Hansard* and *The Times*, 13 March 1857.

and other Sanitary Commissioners. His Lordship has been misinformed on this matter, and I owe it to my reputation to state that neither Dr Sutherland nor any member of the Sanitary Commission had anything whatever to do with either the organization or management of the military hospitals in the Crimea, and I believe them all to be gentlemen of too much honour and probity to take credit of anything of the kind.

What valuable information they have furnished to the government at home I am unable to say; but as far as their suggestions on sanitary matters in the Crimea are concerned it is admitted by themselves that almost everything they could think of was either in actual operation, or had been recommended by the Medical Department before their arrival; but as they were invested by government with greater power than was accorded to the principal medical officer of the Army, they thought they might assist in getting useful measures carried out.

I should have allowed this report to remain unnoticed, as I have done many others, did it not proceed from an authority which stamps it in the public estimation as a denial, on that part of government, of all credit, due either to myself or the medical department, for months of anxiety, toil, and privation in the Crimea; and it is disheartening to medical officers to find that the need for praise which is so justly their due has been given to civilians who arrived after the difficulties of the army had been surmounted.[129]

In his reply Sutherland confirmed in part what Hall had enunciated but by summarizing the terms of the Sanitary Commissions responsibilities he attempted to imply that the Commissioners had achieved more than Hall was prepared to credit them with:

It is quite true as stated by Dr (*sic*: Sir John) Hall that the Commission had nothing whatever to do 'with either the organization or management of the military hospitals.' We were, in fact, precluded by our instructions with these matters. But we were required to see that the sanitary condition of the hospitals, as to ventilation, water supply, number of sick etc., was such as to give scope to medical treatment. We also had to see to the removal of all sanitary defects in the Crimea and at the hospitals on the Bosphorus.[130]

Two additional letters from A.M.D. and Pars Parva published in *The Times* applauded Hall's 'spirited and courageous' stance,[131] while he was also supported by J.M. [probably Dr Mouat] who served in the Crimea and made the point to the editor of the

---

129 Hall to Editor, 14 March; *The Times*, 17 March 1857.
130 Sutherland to Editor, 17 March; *The Times*, 18 March 1857.
131 A.M.D. to Editor, 17 March; *The Times*, 19 March 1857 and Pars Pava to Editor, undated; *The Times*, 19 March 1857.

Medical Times and Gazette that: 'The so-called Sanitary Commission only arrived in the Crimea in the month of April, when we had emerged from our difficulties, and "the sun of our prosperity had begun to shine," to use an Oriental proverb,' and that some of their ideas would have been 'amusing' if they had not been 'presumptuous and insulting.'[132]

The Commissioners' report contained no personal criticism of Hall though he responded to it by issuing a pamphlet, presumably because he thought there was necessity to defend his reputation.[133] This prompted Sutherland, to publish a reply,[134] following which Hall published a rejoinder.[135] Thereafter the debate ceased, in public at least.

The three pamphlets contain considerable detail and are valuable historical documents. Together they comprise over 40,000 words and there is evidence of the authors trying to score points off each other. In his response Sutherland pointed out that there had been no advanced planning with respect to the sanitary condition of the camps and hospitals, and suggested that if this may have contributed to the high mortality during the first winter. However, as was stressed in the Preface, a long siege had not been envisaged and so there would have been little incentive to spend time and money on such matters, and by the time the calamity of the first winter became apparent it was too late to do anything until camp life became better organized in the spring. Action was then taken to improve the environment generally from a sanitary viewpoint and for this Hall claimed some credit and not unreasonably stressed that in his opinion the contribution of the Commissioners was much less than they asserted.

9.5 Select Committee on the Army Medical Department

The proceedings of the Stafford Committee were published on the 3 July 1856 and the recommendations they made for the reform of the AMD were clearly influenced by what took place in the Crimea.[136] The committee members obviously appreciated the contribution made by the medical officers as they had been told of: 'the admirable manner in which the army and civil surgeons have performed their duties in the

---

132 *Medical Times and Gazette*, 4 April 1857. J.M. was probably James Mouat, MD, who was awarded the VC for his bravery during the battle of Balaklava.
133 Hall, *Observations*.
134 Sutherland, *Reply*. The Commissioners submitted a preliminary report to Panmure on 17 March 1855. A version was 'printed solely for the use of the Cabinet' on 14 April 1855; TNA: WO 33/1/24/55 & 33/1/25/55.
135 Sir J. Hall, *Sir John Hall's Rejoinder to Dr. Sutherland's Reply to his Observations on the Report of the Sanitary Commissioners, at the Seat of War in the East in 1855 and 1856* (London: W. Clowes, 1858).
136 *Select Committee on the Medical Department*. For a commentary on this topic, and a list of the recommendations, see Cantlie, *History*, pp.198–200.

East, and [the] Committee are glad to [acknowledge] the high opinion they entertain of their merits,'[137] while later in the report they recorded their praise for the 'zeal, energy, and courage' displayed by the medical officers and civil surgeons 'under the most trying circumstances.' The report contained only one specific reference to the health of the troops in the Crimea, viz. Colonel Lord West, 21st Regiment, opined on 30 May 1856 that this had been affected by overwork and want of proper food, and that the medical officers were not responsible for this or the 'great sickness that prevailed in the Crimea;' which was exacerbated by a 'deficiency of all proper appliances, medical comforts, and medicines.'[138] Incidentally, many years later Lord Wolseley, then a captain, wrote in a similar vein: 'What killed our men the most was the want of firewood. [ ] The consequence [...] was, that we all began to eat our salt pork and red navy-junk in a partially uncooked state, and this brought on diarrhoea which too frequently ended in dysentery, the scourge of which nearly all suffered, and which killed so many.'[139]

9.6 Royal Commission

Cantlie concluded that Herbert was the 'first Minister who ever set himself the task of saving the life of the soldier' and though out of office when the war ended he played a leading role in the most high profile post-war initiative, as President of the Royal Commission convened to enquire into the *'Regulations Affecting the Sanitary Conditions of the Army'*. The Commission took evidence between May and July 1857 and their report published in February 1858 was directed towards future reorganization rather than a retrospective analysis of what occurred in the Crimea. There was no attempt to apportion blame for any failures that occurred during that time. The Commission's recommendations included the reorganization of the AMD, the institution of an Army Medical School and a Statistical Branch, and the improvement in the construction of barrack and hospital accommodation; four topics addressed subsequently in greater detail by dedicated sub-commissions.[140] These developments suggest that the Crimean experience had awakened the national conscience to the reality that soldiers deserved to be treated with care and consideration during both peace and war. In addition, a Royal Warrant promulgated in October 1858 'brought about new and advantageous prospects for medical officers.'[141]

---

137 *Select Committee on the Medical Department*, p.iv and *The Lancet*, 26 July 1856.
138 *Select Committee on the Medical Department*, p.124.
139 Wolseley, *Soldier's Life*, 1, pp.140–1.
140 Incidentally this recommendation was not a new idea since the need for an army medical school, which had been 'strongly advocated [...] by such reformers as Richard Brocklesby [d.1777] and Robert Jackson [retired in 1819],' and was one of McGrigor's 'most cherished ambitions,' that never materialized; see Cantlie, *A History*, 1, p.439.
141 Cantlie, *A History*, 2, p.196.

The Commissioners did, however, consider it their 'duty not to neglect the lessons that may be drawn from [the late war].' For example, they emphasized the contrast between the two winters of the campaign thereby agreeing with other commentators that during the first winter the troops suffered from: 'work altogether disproportioned to their strength, from broken rest, insufficient clothing and shelter, unwholesome food, and want of cleanliness.'[142] The report continued: 'As the spring advanced, to these causes of disease and mortality were added others, arising from want of drainage and ventilation, and the nuisances resulting from the lengthened occupation of the same ground without sufficient countervailing precautions.' This opinion, which reflected the views of Nightingale, is at variance with that of the Sanitary Commissioners who had observed that during this time the camps were generally well managed from a sanitary standpoint. However, there can be little doubt that the improvements in the living conditions of the troops made during 1855 contributed to the good health that they enjoyed during 1856 and so it comes as no surprise that the Commissioners stressed that the provision wholesome food and huts that were well drained and ventilated, together with ensuring the camps were thoroughly cleansed, were all factors contributing to this success.

The Commissioners also analyzed data on mortality among home-based British troops during the 1840s and up to 1853, and were alarmed when they appreciated the mortality rate was higher than in the civilian population. The assessment of their recommendations demands care, however, since it can be demonstrated that the decrease in mortality rate which continued up to the beginning of the First World War seemingly started at the beginning of the 1850s and not after 1858, albeit for reasons which are likely to be complex and which are outside the scope of this monograph (Figure 9.1).[143]

9.7 Concluding remarks

The Hospital Commission had an opportunity for making an immediate difference as one of the Commissioners assumed medical charge at Scutari early in 1855, but the conflicting reports emanating from the hospitals during the following weeks makes it difficult to ascertain how much was actually achieved. Nightingale considered the Commission a 'lame duck', but given the Sanitary Commissioners found that

---

142 Royal Commission Report, p.xxxi.
143 For reviews of the work of the Royal Commission and the collection of army medical statistics during the century that followed see S. Rosenbaum, 'Report of the Royal Sanitary Commission (1858)', *Journal of the Royal Army Medical Corps*, 105:4 (1959), pp.1–11 and S. Rosenbaum, 'More than a Century of Army Medical Statistics', *Journal of the Royal Society of Medicine*, 83 (1990), pp.456–63.

288 Victory Over Disease

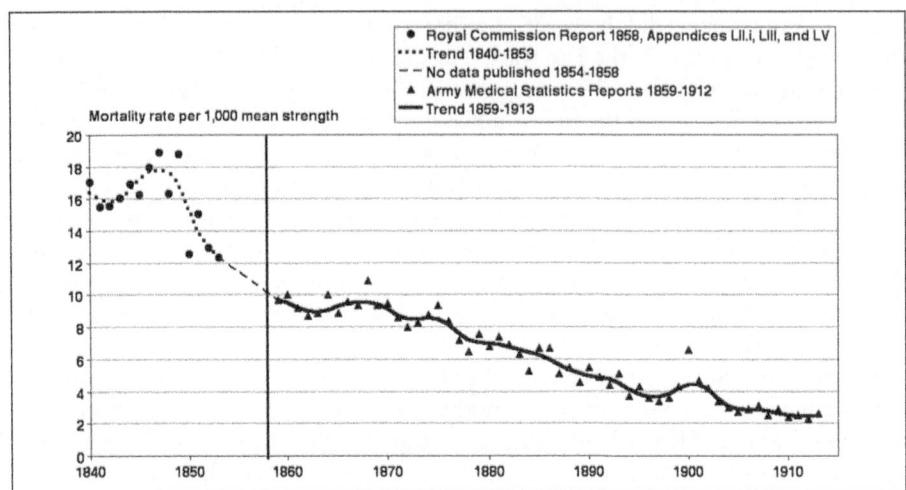

Figure 9.1 Mortality in British troops in the United Kingdom, 1840–1913.

conditions were not as bad as they expected some weeks later implies that improvements had been made in line with the Hospital Commissioners' suggestions.[144]

The reports of the Roebuck's Select Committee and the Supplies and Sanitary Commissions provide an insight into what went wrong during the winter of 1854–55 but their deliberations started too late to have any worthwhile impact on the health and well-being of the troops at the front. With respect to the Roebuck Committee Maxwell was of the opinion that too 'great importance was given to statements made by civilians who had gone out without medical authorization and or official sanction and whose criticisms, made in ignorance of the facts, were proved to be exaggerated, and in some instances, and inaccurate in others.'[145] Incidentally, Maxwell was critical of the way that the Committee had harassed Smith in the manner of their questioning though 'after hearing all the facts, [they] ended by acknowledging the administrative handicaps under which under which [Smith] was forced to work and the inattention and rebuffs of so many of his proposals' and thus 'their final report contained no word of censure.'[146]

Hall took steps to protect his reputation, and that of the AMD, when he appreciated that the Sanitary Commissioners were granted credit officially for merely enunciating what he and his colleagues knew what was required; and which could have been

144 Bostridge, *Florence Nightingale*, p.129.
145 See Anon [Maxwell], *Whom Shall We Hang?*, pp.272–83 for further discussion on this vexing issue. Maxwell was particularly critical of the evidence given by 'three gentleman who visited the hospitals at Scutari as amateurs,' viz. Messrs Stafford, Macdonald, and Osborne.
146 Cantlie, *A History*, 2, p.166.

rectified if the AMD had been accorded the necessary power and resources so to do. To suggest that his reactions were sour grapes, as suggested by some commentators, is unreasonable since most of the Commissioners' recommendations were little more than common sense. However, to be fair, Sutherland did appreciate that there was 'really nothing to learn' in 'sanitary methods or procedure [...] but much to avoid,' and there was undoubtedly 'the supreme necessity of greater vigilance in preventing the occurrence of sanitary defects.'[147] The Sanitary Commission remained in the Crimea until the end of the campaign and this would have assisted Hall as they had the power to insist on corrective measures being taken as required. A view supported by one of Hall's colleagues, J.M. [probably Dr Mouat], who suggested that the Commissioners were there merely 'to assist us in forcing on the military authorities more immediate and prompt attention to [the medical officers] recommendations, being invested in more power than [...] the principal medical officers of the Army'.[148]

Exchanges between Hall and Sutherland after the war reveal that both sought to justify their actions, and preserve their reputations. Hall was probably in a stronger position in that he had previously identified the problems, and that these could have been rectified by the AMD if provided with suitable resources. The relative weakness of Sutherland's position was illustrated by his responses to the Royal Commission in which he attempted to talk up the Commissioners successes. He had no alternative but to concede that the improvement in the 'health of all the hospitals' on the Bosphorus was due in part to 'the less severe character of the cases sent from the Crimea' but he was at pains to point out that this 'favourable change' had 'advanced simultaneously with the progress of the sanitary works.'[149]

The sustained improvement in health was acknowledged by Panmure in spring of 1856 when he informed Codrington that he was 'easy [...] as long as I see Dr Hall's columns in the Morning State as they are,' and then again in the House of Lords on 8 May 1856 when proposing a vote of thanks to the armed forces:[150]

> A comparison between [the Armies'] health and that of troops at home are truly remarkable [...] for the week ending April 21 [...] admissions to the hospitals were 1.56 percent in proportion to the strength; the deaths 0.02, and proportion of sick to well 3.72 percent. [...] During the above period the admissions [in the camp at Aldershot] were 2.71 percent; deaths 0.006, and the proportion of sick to well 3.59. It is very gratifying.[151]

---

147 Sutherland, *Reply*, pp.35–6.
148 J.M., 'The Crimean Sanitary Commission and the Army Medical Officers', *Medical Times and Gazette*, 4 April 1857.
149 Sanitary Commission Report, pp.48–9.
150 Panmure to Codrington, 21 December 1855; Wiltshire and Swindon History Centre: 2057/F8/III/C/43 & 47 and Douglas and Ramsey, *Panmure Papers, 2*, p.28.
151 *Hansard*, 8 May 1856.

Panmure's sentiments were reiterated by Nightingale who wrote in 1858 that: 'history does not afford its equal – of any army after a great disaster arising from neglect, having been brought into the highest state of health and efficiency.'[152] Nevertheless, by this time it suited the political agenda of Panmure, Nightingale, and the sanitarians to ascribe the Victory over Disease to environmental and other improvements recommended by the Sanitary Commissioners. However, in reality it was almost certainly due to the enhancement in living standards and primary health care, which involved, inter alia, segregation of patients and minimizing overcrowding, coupled with the ending of duty in unsanitary trenches that accounted for what was recorded.

After the war Nightingale and her associates reconsidered the medical statistics and chose to conclude that the fall in the mortality rate at Scutari was a direct result of the arrival of the Sanitary Commissioners. By doing this, they failed to acknowledge that improvements were already in hand, and that the majority of patients were from the Crimea where the health of the troops in the camps had improved during the spring without any input from the Commissioners and as a result by May 1855 1,750 of 3,000 beds at Scutari were unoccupied, and that nearly all patients were suffering from a 'fever of a rather peculiar form from which few die.'[153]

On the other hand, Martineau adopted a different approach when she prepared her well considered commentary on the reports of the various commissions and Nightingale's *'A Contribution to the Sanitary History of the British Army.'* She avoided 'all censure and praise' and attempted 'to be as impersonal as possible.' She stressed that civil and military hygiene 'are different things in a practical sense' with the latter science being: 'applied to the prevention of disease and mortality under conditions far more varied, more threatening to health, and [...] more sudden [...] than those which affect [civilians]' and is thus 'special, and must be provided for accordingly.' She also appreciated that at the time 'civil hygiene was a new art to us' and hence the 'more special art of military hygiene seems to have been unthought of, except in a desultory and ineffectual way.'[...] and thus when an 'artificial city [was set up] before Sebastopol [...] no arrangements like those of Birkenhead were in question at all.'[154]

Martineau considered that it made sense to separate clinical practice from community health care. She proposed that the 'personal hygiene' of the troops should 'be left to the medical officers to look after,' while 'The organisation which [controls] the social health of cities or camps [...] keeps the site dry and clean, provides water [...] and prevents the air being vitiated [...] cannot look after the personal habits of individuals.' The medical officers undertake 'the charge of the sick [and] look to the health of the men under them individually. The care of the health of the Army was

---

152 Cantlie, *History*, p.201 and McDonald, *Florence Nightingale. The Crimean War*, p.864.
153 *The Lancet*, 2 June 1855.
154 Incidentally, the first MOH appointed in England was W.H. Duncan at Liverpool. He took up the post during 1847. J. Simon was appointed the MOH for London a year later and became the first Chief Medical Officer of HM's Government in 1855.

not in their line. That it was in nobody's line [during the recent campaign] was due to everybody's ignorance.'

The 'medical *chef*' had 'no authority' and thus 'the health of the Army could not be provided for' and she favoured a Sanitary Officer being attached to the QMG's department as, 'the head of a sanitary police, to recommend measures as are needed to make the men's abode safe, and their food and clothing appropriate to their wants.' However, to make this workable 'the concert which is necessary between the Military and Medical Departments, and between these and the Sanitary must be secured by express arrangement and regulations [and] the same concert must be secured between military and medical officers of the regiment. (see Chapter 11 for further discussion.)

Martineau favoured the proposal that the AMD should be reorganized and that the Director General should be supported by a council comprising three members 'selected for their eminence on medical, sanitary and statistical knowledge, and appointed by the Secretary for War.' The long-term aim was to minimize losses from disease so that fewer soldiers need to be recruited to sustain military strength. This was certainly an objective that made good sense from a financial, military, and humane point of view.[155]

155 The paragraphs on Martineau's commentary were selected from Martineau, *England and Her Soldiers*, pp.v, 23–4, 104–5, 112, 151–3, 155, 271, & 274–5.

10

Reflections on the War

From the moment that General Codrington and the last elements of the British Army sailed for home from Balaklava Harbour on 12 July 1856 the campaign became a part of history. From then on heed must be taken of Anthony Beevor's dictum: 'History is a question of cause and effect. You need to take events in order to make sense of them.'[1] It is prudent, indeed essential, to avoid assessments using hindsight.

From an official point of view the convening of the Royal Commission was probably the most significant immediate outcome of the war (see Section 9.6). However, the conflict was also notable for the increasingly exploitation of modern technology; the institution of the Victoria Cross; reforms in the way in which the Army was administered; the development of charitable funds;[2] the increasing power of the press, the impact of visual arts; and the interest in providing memorials for those who died of illness and wounds in the service of their country.

10.1 Technology and medicine

Technological advances were a marked feature of the 19th century, and their utilization has justified several commentators to consider that the Crimean conflict was the first modern war. However, with the possible exception of Brunel's design for a prefabricated pavilion hospital, a concept which proved of value in future wars; there is little evidence that the conflict acted as a catalyst for specific developments. In contrast, the First and Second World Wars, which both lasted longer and involved large numbers of civilians in the war effort, stimulated many influential innovations

---

1 *The Guardian*, 31 May 2010.
2 For a review see: S. Fowler, '"Pass the Hat for your Credit's Sake and Pay-Pay-Pay" Philanthropy and Victorian Military Campaigns,' *Soldiers of the Queen*, No. 105 (2001), pp.2–5.

including advances in reconstructive surgery, and the development of medicinal drugs and equipment.

Steam battleships gave the Anglo-French coalition a critical advantage in the confined waters off Russia's Baltic and Black Sea coasts.[3] Likewise, extensive use was made of steam-powered ships to bring supplies from distant ports to harbours near the front, and to provide a regular shuttle service to from the Crimea to Turkey for the sick and wounded. The development of a railway network facilitated their distribution after their arrival. In contrast, the Russians had no alternative but to convey supplies over long distances overland using carts and pack animals.[4] Notwithstanding technological advances in firearms and ordnance, such as the rifled musket, other benefits of industrialization included the employment of a floating bakery (*Abundance*) and flour mill (*Bruiser*), steam-powered saw mills, steam distilling vessels, and an engineering factory ship; while the electric telegraph improved communications between London and the front and could have be used to facilitate the supply of essential items if necessary.

Victorian inventiveness resulted in various items of medical equipment being sent to the Crimea for assessment.[5] As early as July 1854 Hall noted in his diary that he had been sent several 'new inventions to report on, as if we have nothing else to think about but the jims of quacks and speculators.' These included electro-magnetic coils for stimulating weakly patients, Barton's collapsible baths, washing machines, soda-water makers, vapour baths, waterproof beds, Liston splints, chloroform inhalers, and patent cooking stoves. Hall's comment suggested that that some of this equipment probably proved of little or no value, although he reported that vulcanized India rubber cloth was better than oiled cloth,[6] and Ritchie's cork mattresses proved: 'A good and really useful invention for field service and in the event of the war continuing they will come into universal use.'[7]

Today people cannot imagine a world without anaesthetic agents but the application of Beevor's dictum to the mid-1850s would indicate that apart from a relatively small number of patients virtually everybody else in the population would have been unable to conceive a world in which these drugs were in general use. The anaesthetic age was less than a decade old when hostilities commenced, and though chloroform was used towards the end of the Cape Frontier Wars of 1846–1852, few if any of the surgeons who landed in the Crimea would have had experience of its administration under battlefield conditions.

---

3   A. Lambert, *The Crimean War*. p.5.
4   Though an important development, it is an exaggeration to suggest that 'the railway, a symbol of the industrial power commanded by the middle class, was the sole unqualified success of the Crimean War,' as proposed by Lalumia, *Realism*, p.52.
5   Cantlie, *History*, 2, p.136.
6   Hall to Smith, 24 April 1855; RAMC: 397/F/CO/1/2/1908.
7   Hall to Smith, 22 February 1856; RAMC: 397/F/CO/1/3/4287.

In the days preceding the invasion of the Crimea, Hall issued a comprehensive memorandum to medical officers. This was welcomed by Russell of *The Times* who wrote: 'Great care has been taken by the medical authorities to make the department as efficient as possible, and Dr Hall has issued a circular containing directions and suggestions as to surgical practice, which is highly spoken of.'[8] Within the document Hall offered the following advice on the use of chloroform on the battlefield:

> Dr. Hall takes this opportunity of cautioning Medical Officers against the use of chloroform in the severe shock of serious gunshot wounds, as he thinks few will survive where it is used. But as public opinion, founded, perhaps, on mistaken philanthropy, he knows is against him, he can only caution Medical Officers, and entreat they will narrowly watch its effects; for, however barbarous it may appear, the smart of the knife is a powerful stimulant, and it is much better to hear a man bawl lustily than to see him sink silently into the grave.[9]

Chloroform is toxic in excess and hence 'there was some justification [for Hall's] warning, for in civilian practice there had been an increasing recognition of the risks attending [its] use.'[10] The topic was a matter of debate among the highest echelons of the medical profession. Professor James Syme of Edinburgh University was critical of Hall's advice,[11] while others seemingly were not. For example, Dr Dumbreck, who deputized for Hall when he visited Scutari during October 1854 on Raglan's orders, pointed out in evidence to the Select Committee on the Army before Sebastopol that: 'Dr Guthrie [the President of the Royal College of Surgeons] entertains opinions approximating to those of Dr Hall; [...] Dr Hall never meant it to be an imperative upon the officers of the army to follow his suggestion, and they all did, even in his presence, as they pleased.'[12]

Hall also received support from Maxwell, one of the hospital commissioners and a barrister, when he clarified the interpretation of Hall's words in a commentary on the Sevastopol enquiry: 'As to chloroform, it was universally used, not withstanding its supposed prohibition. [...] the instructions [...] turn out, when calmly weighed, to be but suggestions of a humane caution. [...] His [Hall's] language clearly points [to the non-use of chloroform in] those cases [of serious gun-shot wounds] only.'[13]

8   *The Times*, 21 September 1854.
9   The text was reproduced in several newspapers including *The Times*, 20 September and *Illustrated London News*, 23 September 1854. A printed version can be found in the Royal Army Medical Corps (hereafter: RAMC) archives located at the Army Medical Services Museum, Keogh Barracks, GU12 5RQ, namely RAMC: 397/F/CO/6/13.
10 Shepherd, *Crimean Doctors*, 1, p.144, and confirmed by reference to contemporary medical journals. It is now known to be due to the induction of fatal cardiac and respiratory arrhythmias.
11 *The Times*, 12 October 1854.
12 Select Committee, 2nd Report, p.610.
13 Anon [Maxwell], *Whom Shall We Hang?*, p.197.

Some modern authors have accepted this view. For example, Nixon concluded that though Hall's advice might appear barbaric: 'it was based on the honest belief that if the patient was conscious and screaming then he would be more likely to survive.'[14] However, there are others who have chosen not to appreciate a barrister's interpretation and perpetuate the notion that Hall was a villain. These include Small and Taylor who wrote (respectively) that Hall 'was notorious for instructing surgeons not to use anaesthetic for amputations,'[15] and that he 'positively did not believe in chloroform to ease pain and terror in amputations. Pompously he would assert that it was preferable for a man to "bawl lustily" [...] than to "sink silently into the grave."'[16]

Perusal of reviews on the use of chloroform during the Crimean campaign by Shepherd, Connor, Kaufman, and Metcalfe, gives an insight into the difficulty faced by Hall.[17] Most of the surgeons would have had little or no experience of performing 'capital' operations during or shortly after a battle, when they who would be expected to work fast and without a professional assistant to administer and monitor the patient. With hindsight Hall's approach may appear to be over-cautious but at the time chloroform, which was known to be potentially toxic, was untested under combat conditions. In the event, the agent was used widely and there is no evidence that Hall tried to interfere with its use during surgical procedures. After the cessation of hostilities Hall confided in Smith: 'But as I have already incurred much public odium for a well intentioned, but carelessly worded caution, [...] only I feel authorized in saying that I have seen much to confirm the propriety of that caution, and all candid and unprejudiced men, I rather think, will admit the same.'[18]

The crucial role of water in the epidemiology of cholera was not generally accepted during the mid-1850s. Because the germ theory was a development for the future, the management of what are now classed as infectious diseases was along the traditional lines current at the time, and do not necessarily resonate with 21st-century clinical medical practice. In contrast, attention to basic hygiene, including the separation of wounded convalescents from medical cases and reducing overcrowding, clearly paid dividends; the mass administration of lime juice successfully prevented scurvy;[19] simple casualty-clearing stations utilized during the assaults of 18 June and 9 September 1855 permitted patient selection, now termed 'triage'. The advantage of

---

14 K. Nixon, *The World of Florence Nightingale* (Pitkin Publishing, 2011), p.14.
15 Small, *Florence Nightingale: Avenging Angel*, p.49.
16 Taylor, *Wartime Nurse*, p.26.
17 J.H. Shepherd, 'The Smart of the Knife – Early Anaesthesia in the Services', *Journal of the Royal Army Medical Corps*, 132 (1985), pp.109–15; H. Connor, The Use of Chloroform by British Army Surgeons during the Crimean War', *Medical History*, 40 (1998), pp.161–93; Kaufman, *Surgeons at War*, pp.140–2; and N.H. Metcalf, 'The Influence of the Military on the Civilian Uncertainty about Modern Anaesthesia between its Origins in 1846 and the End of the Crimean War in 1856', *Anaesthesia*, 40 (2005), pp.594–601.
18 Hall to Smith, 15 March 1856; *Medical and Surgical History*, 2, pp.268–9.
19 Incidentally, scurvy, which may retard the healing of fractures, proved a problem during the American Civil War and some theatres in the First World War; G.H. Bourne,

treating of battlefield injuries close to the front, amply demonstrated during the First World War, was also recognized by Hall and his colleagues.[20]

Surprisingly little was published on clinical topics during or after the war. From this Shepherd concluded that: 'It was not easy to judge to what extent the intensive clinical experience in medicine and surgery gained [...] was assimilated [and] influenced practice in either service or civilian life.'[21] Macleod and Fraser published on the surgical treatment of gunshot wounds, but it was not until the New Zealand Wars that the benefits of avoiding interference with wounds, burning all foul dressings, employing an effective disinfectant based on potassium permanganate, and the insistence on frequent hand-washing were recognized.[22] As a result, conditions such as erysipelas, gangrene, and secondary haemorrhage became less of a problem, while starving a fever and blood-letting both become a 'thing of the past.'[23]

The need to keep the troops healthy and to protect them from threats to their health and well-being became evident shortly after the formation of the camps before Sevastopol. This prompted the sending of a Sanitary Commission to the East in the spring of 1855 to investigate matters. That they arrived too late to have a major impact on events has been discussed (see Section 9.4) but the need for a Sanitary Officer to advise the GOC on matters of what is now termed 'public health' became abundantly clear and these were employed with benefit in subsequent campaigns. For example, Staff Surgeon Rutherford, a veteran of the Crimean War, acted as the Sanitary Officer during the China Wars (1857–60). This 'provided a handsome dividend, and disease prevention was regarded as of the highest importance and carefully practised.' His duties included the 'sanitation of the camps and buildings and the supervision of water supplies [and] advice on food and clothing.' Similarly, the campaigns in New Zealand (1860–67) also 'benefited from the presence of a Sanitary Officer on the staff of the Commander-in-Chief. [although] it was not long before he [Surgeon Major MacKinnon] discovered that [his proposals] were largely ineffective because of his lack of executive power [...] and he had to fall back on the support which the GOC offered by ordering all Commanding Officers to co-operate.' Good results were also obtained during the Abyssinian War (1867–68) when the 'Sanitary Officer focused attention on the importance of sanitary precautions which on the whole were faithfully observed. General Napier was a keen sanitarian and appears to have appreciated the work of his medical staff' and the war proved 'an excellent example of good hygiene in the field.' It would seem, however, that not every campaign was necessarily attended with such good results since Lord Wolseley opined that 'in the numerous

'Records of Older Literature of Tissue Changes in Scurvy', *Proceedings of the Royal Society of Medicine*, 37 (1944), pp.512–6.
20   Harrison, *Medical War*, p.297.
21   Shepherd, *Crimean Doctors*, 2, p.597.
22   Macleod, *Notes* and P. Fraser, *A Treatise upon Gunshot Wounds of the Chest* (London: John Churchill, 1859).
23   Cantlie, *A History*, 2, p.257.

campaigns where I have served with a Sanitary Officer, I can conscientiously state I have never known him make any useful suggestions, whereas I have known him make many silly ones.'[24] Good efforts in one army may come to naught if the other belligerents fail to prevent problems.[25]

10.2 Victoria Cross, orders and medals

A lasting legacy of the war was the institution of the Victoria Cross by a Royal Warrant dated 29 January 1856.[26] The names of the 111 selected for the award were published in eight editions of the *London Gazette* between the 24 February 1857 and 6 May 1858. Three medical officers were included in the 2nd, 5th, and 6th lists, namely, Assistant Surgeons T.E Hale, 7th Regiment,[27] and H.T. Sylvester, 23rd Regiment,[28] for their bravery on 8 September 1855, and Surgeon J. Mouat, 6th Dragoons, who saved the life of Captain Morris, 17th Lancers, during the battle of Balaklava.[29] All three surgeons had been assisted by an NCO, and in the cases of Mouat and Sylvester, they also received the VC, namely, Corporal R. Shields, 23rd Regiment, and Sergeant Major C. Wooden, 17th Lancers.[30] When the draft citation for Hale's VC was submitted to Panmure on 28 April 1857 he queried if the sergeant (C. Fisher, 7th Regiment) had been recommended. The Military Secretary confirmed that he had not, although his name appeared in Hale's citation.[31] On the other hand, Lieutenant W. Hope, 7th Regiment, who assisted in saving the wounded Lieutenant Hobson during the same action, did receive the medal.[32]

Of the 83 VCs won by Army personnel 49 (59 percent) were awarded during six days of engagement in battle with the remainder during the year-long siege. A surprisingly large number 34 (41 percent) of the deeds involved assisting a wounded comrade, either wholly or in part. This included all three surgeons and over half (56 percent) of the NCOs.[33]

---

24 This paragraph is based on Cantlie, *A History*, 2, pp.253, 258, 265, & 286.
25 Prinzing, *Epidemics*, pp.1–10.
26 *London Gazette*, 5 February 1856.
27 *London Gazette*, 5 May 1857 and *Medical Times and Gazette, The Lancet.* & *British Medical Journal*, 9 May 1857.
28 *London Gazette*, 20 November 1857; *The Lancet* & *Medical Times and Gazette*, 28 November; and *British Medical Journal*, 5 December 1857.
29 For an account of Mouat's gallantry in New Zealand see M. Hinton and P.H. Starling, 'A Possible Third Double Victoria Cross for the Army Medical Services?', *Journal of the Royal Army Medical Corps*, 158 (2011), pp.191–2.
30 *London Gazette*, 26 October 1858 & 24 February 1857.
31 TNA: WO 32/7303.
32 *London Gazette*, 5 May 1857.
33 Based on the synopses in M. Arthur, *Symbol of Courage. The Men Behind the Medal* (London: Pan Books, 2005).

It was stipulated in the Royal Warrant that the VC could be awarded to any member of the armed services irrespective of rank. However, there was a strong bias against the rank and file. medical officers, military officers, NCOs, and men comprised approximately less than 1, 4, 14, and 82 percent of the army strength yet they were awarded 3.5, 31.5, 32.5, and 32.5 percent respectively of the 83 VCs.[34]

Crimea medal: Medical officers, other members of the AMD, and civilian surgeons who served in the Crimea between 18 September 1854 and the fall of Sevastopol were entitled to the Crimea medal and where appropriate the clasps for Alma, Inkermann (*sic*), Balaklava, and Sebastopol (*sic*).[35] Personnel who arrived after 8 September 1855 or, who served only in Turkey did not qualify for the medal, although some commentators held the opinion that those stationed in the base hospitals in Turkey merited the medal, given the risks they took to their health attending the sick, and to a lesser extent, the wounded.

Order of the Bath: Several senior medical officers were awarded the Order of the Bath.[36] The distribution did not entirely satisfy the editor of the *Medical Times and Gazette* who pointed out that only one naval surgeon (Dr D. Deas) received the CB, in contrast to one KCB (Hall) and nine CBs awarded to military surgeons.[37] The naval hospitals appear to have functioned better than those of the Army, and, although Deas deserved credit for that, the comparison is hardly fair since the soldiers generally suffered more hardship than the sailors, even those manning the batteries, as they did not have the benefit of assistance from the fleet for supplies and means of respite.

Incidentally, of the military surgeons, Drs Gibson and Linton were advanced to KCB in 1865. Drs Dumbreck and Mouat were similarly honoured in 1871 and 1894 while Deas, who died in 1876, received the KCB in 1867.[38]

Awards by Britain's allies: The recipients of the Legion of Honour were published in the *London Gazette* on 4 August 1856 (449 individuals) and 1 May 1857 (102).[39] Of 551 awards, five recipients participated in the siege of Kars while 30 of those who served in the Crimea were medical officers, of whom 23 were staff surgeons. The Legion of

---

34 This disparity illustrates the divisive aspect of any system of awards; a topic discussed *in extenso* with respect to the VC by G. Mead, *Victoria's Cross. The Untold Story of Britain's Highest Award for Bravery* (London: Atlantic Books, 2015).
35 The medal rolls from the Crimean campaign are TNA: WO 100/22–34.
36 *London Gazette*, 5 February 1855 with two further awards of the CB being gazetted on 2 January 1857.
37 *Medical Times and Gazette*, 29 March 1856.
38 *Annual Register Chronicle*, 1876, pp.129–30.
39 *London Gazette*, 4 August 1856. A decree issued by the Emperor of France on 3 April 1857 authorized the award of the Legion of Honour (5th class) to a further 12 medical officers printed in the *London Gazette*, 1 May 1857 as well as in the *Medical Times and Gazette* and *The Lancet*.

Honour was not awarded for bravery but five of ten medical staff officers awarded the 5th Class had been noticed for conspicuous bravery, namely, DIGH J. Mouat, CB; 2nd Class Staff Surgeon H.T. Sylvester, MD; Assistant Staff Surgeon T.C. Brady; and Acting Assistant Surgeons G. Fair, MD, and C. O'Callaghan. Similarly, two of the three regimental surgeons similarly honoured were mentioned in despatches for their courage, namely, Assistant Surgeons W.Y. Jeeves and J. Gibbons. The overall ratio of medical officers to Army Officers to NCOs and men in the Army was about 1:4:95 while the comparable ratios for those decorated were 1:19:5 thus indicating bias in favour of the military officers. In addition, a number of NCOs and men were selected to receive the French Military War Medal.[40]

Dr H. Sandwith was the first member of the medical profession to receive the Order of the Medjidie for special services rendered during the siege of Kars,[41] The award of the various classes of the Order to 66 medical officers who served in the Crimea were published during 1858.[42] Of these 30 and 36 were staff and regimental surgeons respectively.

Victor Emmanuel II, King of Sardinia, authorized the issue of 400 *'Al Valore Militaire'* medals to officers, NCOs, and men of the British Army. Seven medals were awarded to regimental surgeons, but none to staff surgeons.[43]

10.3 Administrative reform

This topic was considered in a monograph by Sweetman to which reference has been made, and the final chapter forms the basis of the following summary.[44]

Discussions on the reform of the Army during the decades prior to the war evinced little enthusiasm for change, and it needed the declaration of war to provide an impetus for reorganization, albeit limited in extent. Briefly, the administration was simplified with the responsibilities for War and Colonies being separated into two departments (June 1854); the transfer of the Commissariat from the Treasury to the War Office (December 1854); the discontinuation of Herbert's post of Secretary at War (February 1855); and the abolition of the Board of Ordnance (May 1855). The war thus ended with the Secretary for War having political control over the 'Commissariat, Ordnance Department, Reserve and Line troops together with the legal and financial duties of the War Office.

---

40 HCPP 1856 (2120) XL.233: *Names of Non-Commissioned Officers and Men Selected for* [...] *the French Military Medal*, with a supplement, viz. 1857 Session 1 (0.54) IX.221
41 *London Gazette*, 8 February 1856.
42 *London Gazette*, 2 March & 8 June 1856.
43 HCPP 1857 Session 2 [2259] XXVII.215: *List of Officers, Non-Commissioned Officers, and Men Selected to Receive the 400 War Medals for Military Valour, Presented by His Majesty the King of Sardinia to the British Army Engaged in the Late War in the East.*
44 Sweetman, *War and Administration*, pp.128–33.

Several senior politicians clearly considered that the Commander-in-Chief of the Army [Lord Hardinge] was not a 'powerful military voice' and the failure to appoint a dynamic successor [HRH Duke of Cambridge] meant that the Army had little impact on departmental changes, and hence 'tighter political control [was] achieved over the Army, and outstanding problems of civil-military relations [...] had moved decisively in favour of the politicians.' The result was that 'the relevant victories and defeats in the field of army administration occurred not on the Heights of Sevastopol, but in the Palace of Westminster.'[45]

Despite these positive developments the 'relative positions of the Minister for War and the Commander-in-Chief [were not] as clearly defined as desirable' and when the '[War] Department concentrated in Pall Mall [...] Horse Guards [was left] utterly isolated in Whitehall.' Whether this physical separation contributed to the lack of progress in reform is a matter of speculation. Nevertheless, it required Bismarck and Napoleon III later in the century 'to goad the British national conscience into military reform once more.' Furthermore, the Army remained largely amateur, with promotion by purchase remaining in place until 1871. This was consistent with British concerns about militarism but it limited the scope for effective reform.

At the level of practical administration the Crimean War reinforced 'the oft-repeated cries for military supply services,' and this resulted in belated the formation of several 'quasi-military' units, viz. the Medical Staff Corps, Land Transport Corps, Mounted Staff Corps, Army Works Corps and Civil Engineering Corps.' Of these, two 'survived the war to be fully militarised and reorganised as the Army Hospital Corps and the Military Train. Making use of able-bodied soldiers and ultimately commanded by Horse Guards, they became part of the Army.' The short comings of the army staff was also appreciated and as a consequence the experience of the Crimean War prompted the creation of a British staff college in 1858.[46]

10.4 Royal Patriotic Fund and other charities

The Royal Patriotic Fund was a legacy of the Crimean War that persisted for over 150 years.[47] It has the distinction of being the 'first Service charity to be created as a result of national demand' and its objectives were set out in a Royal Warrant dated 7 October 1854. Its principal aim was to provide a 'just and generous benevolence towards widows and orphans of those of our soldiers, sailors, and marines who have

---

45 Sweetman, *War and Administration*, p.133.
46 Melvin, *Sevastopol's Wars*, pp.142–4.
47 For the history of the Royal Patriotic Fund, upon which this paragraph is based, see D. Blomfield-Smith, *Heritage of Help. The Story of the Royal Patriotic Fund* (London: Robert Hale, 1992).

been killed, or who may hereafter die amidst the ravages and casualties of war.'[48] The original members of the commission, which first met on 18 December 1854 under the chairmanship of Prince Albert, included several who had achieved a high profile during the war, viz. the Duke of Newcastle, the Earl of Aberdeen, Viscount Palmerston, Lord Hardinge, Lord Raglan, Sir John Burgoyne, Lord Rokeby, Lord Panmure, Sidney Herbert, Sir James Graham, and Samuel Peto. 'Commissioners in Aid' were soon appointed and a 'formidable network' was set up in order to 'tap the generous flow of public contributions to the Fund.' This eventually amounted to an impressive £1,471,375. By the 1990s the Fund had assisted almost 135,000 widows and about 150,000 orphans. It was merged with the Soldiers, Sailors, Airmen and Families Association (SSAFA) in 2011.

The Royal Patriotic Fund must not be confused with the 'Central Association for the Benefit of Widows and Orphans of the Army in the East', which seemingly did not prosper; the Crimea Army Fund, whose impressive committee was chaired by the Earl of Ellesmere;[49] or *The Times* 'Sick and Wounded Fund', whose local agent John MacDonald was an employee of the paper. The second and third charities contributed to the welfare of the troops in the Crimea and at Scutari but their activities seemingly came to an end with the cessation of the conflict.

10.5 The British and the French

Few references to the French have been made in this monograph owing to a paucity of published data, though a comparison of the British and French Armies published by Longmore made the French the winners during the first winter from a medical point of view; and the British during the second:

> The situation of the French and British armies [...] was so similar in respect to soil and locality, the climatic influences [...] and the nature of the work [...] that practically the two armies might almost be regarded as parts of [...] the same force. [...] there was no similarity between them in respect to their conditions of health. [...] the British [were] remarkably unhealthy during the first period of the siege, and as remarkably healthy during the second period [...] while a precisely opposite state of things existed in the French part [...] which was in a generally

---

48 The orphans of Army and Navy personnel supported by the Fund up to 1859 are listed in HCPP 1860 (51) XL.219: *Return of Name of Every Child Maintained at Charge of Patriotic Fund*.
49 For details of the Fund's activities and a list of the subscribers see the *Report of the Committee of the Crimean Army Fund, September 1855* (London: Richard Clay, 1855). The honorary agents in the Crimea were the Hon. Algernon Egerton, St Leger Glyn, Jervoise Smith, and Thomas Tower, and the principal depot was located in Kadikoi.

good condition of health during the first period, but in an extremely unhealthy condition during the second period.[50]

The mortality rate from disease increased considerably in the French Army during 1856 and Dr Baudens, a senior French medical officer, drew the following conclusion about the difference between the two armies:

> [The British] medical service, directed by the skilful and learned Sir John Hall, left nothing to be desired to the end of the campaign. [...] The field hospitals of the English were extremely clean, which cannot be said of [the French]. The difference was in part due to the higher and more independent position of the English military surgeons, who exercise more authority in the enforcement of hygienic measures.[51]

This was perhaps an unexpected turn of events, for only a year before several prominent critics of the British Army had been fulsome in their praise for the efficiency of the French. Longmore, however, did not agree that all the credit for this improvement should be accorded to the AMD. He conceded that the medical officers knew what was required but they had insufficient 'sanitary influence and authority' at that time to 'restore the well being and efficiency of the army' on their own volition, and that the 'generous impulse of the whole nation, from highest to lowest' had been required to achieve this objective.[52] Longmore continued by summarizing the reasons that M. Scrive, the French PMO, considered the cause of the French 'tragedy' in 1855/56, viz. the harshness of winter without sufficient shelter (the French were still under canvas); excessive work; infection of camps; inadequate rations; decay of the constitutions of the older soldiers; and the feebleness of the new contingents. Exactly those reasons were considered the cause of the Sanitary Disaster in the British Army during the previous winter.[53] This prompted Bryce to opine: 'Peace with Russia was obligatory on France in the spring of 1856 because of the sanitary state of her Crimean army.'[54]

---

50 T. Longmore, *The Sanitary Contrasts of the French and British Armies during the Crimean War* (London: Charles Griffin & Co., 1883), pp.5–6.
51 L. Baudens (Translated by F.B. Hough), *On the Military and Camp Hospitals and the Health of Troops in the Field Being the Result of a Commission to Inspect the Sanitary Arrangements of the French Army, and Incidentally Other Armies in the Crimean War* (New York: Baillière Brothers, 1862), pp.73–4.
52 Longmore, *Sanitary Contrasts*, pp.25–6.
53 For a review see Barham, 'A Tragic Second Winter'.
54 Bryce, *England and France before Sebastopol*, p.195.

10.6 Civilian disasters

War is necessarily an unpleasant and uncertain undertaking, but disasters involving civilians can be extremely catastrophic, and it is instructive to keep matters in perspective. For example, an editorial entitled 'Lives Wasted and Lives Spent' pointed out that the loss of life during the battle of the Alma could be more than matched by both outbreaks of epidemic disease and tragic accidents. For example, the collision that took place on the other side of the Atlantic between two steam ships, the *Arctic*, which sailed from Liverpool on the day of the battle, and the *Vesta*:

> Nearly at the same moment that between 300 and 400 fellow-countrymen gave up their last breath on the field of the Alma for a just cause, and with a glorious result nearly the same number perished off the American coast for no cause, and with no result at all. A collision in fog at sea between two steamers [*Arctic* and *Vesta*] cost in an hour as many lives as a desperate conflict between two hostile armies. Our annals teem with similar startling comparisons. The loss of the *Arctic* is only one of many such cases which have occurred within two years in which the victims have to be reckoned by hundreds. Single ship wrecks of late have been more fatal than the most famous battles; three, four, five, even eight hundred fellow creatures have found by a single casualty, a sudden and futile grave. [...] We are shocked, we are compassionate, we subscribe – and we forget. Nor is this all. In six weeks cholera has swept away in the Metropolis *alone* ten times as many English lives as were sacrificed in the great Crimean victory. During the twenty-two years of our Napoleonic wars – we lost in actual *killed* only 12,796, or 900 per annum. In the two years of 1848 and 1849, London lost a nearly equal number (18,036) by cholera, and choleraic diarrhoea alone. The number we lose by drowning each year is calculated at about 2,600; – the number we lost in war, even a bloody war, scarcely, as we have seen exceeded one-third of that figure.[55]

These words were penned before the disastrous events of the first Crimean winter but nevertheless losses in London from disease in a single cholera epidemic resulted in the deaths of nearly as many individuals who lost their life to disease during the two years of the Eastern campaign. A sobering thought.

10.7 Power of the press and official publications

The war, and in particular the campaign in the Black Sea theatre, was notable for the press coverage it received from war correspondents such as W.H. Russell and T.

---

55 Reprinted from the *Economist* in the *Cheshire Observer*, 4 November 1854.

Chenery of *The Times* and E.L. Godkin of the *London Daily News*.[56] The reports in the main newspapers were frequently reproduced in regional and international journals. The abolition of the newspaper tax in 1855 resulted in the growing, and increasingly important, middle classes being able to obtain information on the progress of the war more readily than hitherto; both the successes and failures.

Unlike the situation in France, there was little or no censorship and thus the Duke of Newcastle was minded to write to newspaper editors requesting them to take care not to publish information that might prove of value to the Russians, who, through their agents in the United Kingdom, would have ready access to the newspapers.[57] However, this did not preclude the government from publishing a range of Blue Books during the course of the war and thereby providing an insight into the activities of both the government and the armed forces.[58]

Incidentally, Surgeon Maclean speculated, with hindsight, that if newspaper correspondents had covered the China War of 1839–1842, which was 'one of the most disgraceful episodes in military history [and] which cost so many lives', it is probable that 'public opinion would have been so effectively called to the defects in our military and sanitary organization, as to have led to reforms in both that would have gone far to prevent the miserable breakdown in the Crimea.'[59]

10.8 Visual arts

Up until the Napoleonic wars, oil paintings, tapestries, and murals 'espoused Georgian England' by depicting heroic military exploits 'as the ultimate stage for the highborn',[60] but in general these works of art were available only to upper class families, their visitors, and households. However, by the mid-19th century it was possible to reproduce images such as lithographs and woodcuts relatively cheaply, and in large numbers. This resulted in 'picture journalism' in the 'illustrated press.' These images provided a more realistic presentation of the campaign, than hitherto; as many featured the 'rank and file as the principal actors' rather than the 'aristocratic martial

---

56 See for example: A. Hankinson, *Man of Wars. William Howard Russell of* The Times (London: Heinemann Educational Books, 1982); C. Chapman, *Russell of* The Times. *War Despatches and Diaries* (London: Bell & Hyman, 1984); N. Bentley (ed.) *Despatches from the Crimea* (London: Frontline Books, 2008); T. Coates, *Delane's War* (London: Biteback Publishing, 2009); and B. Best, *The Luckless Tribe. The Golden Age of British War Reporters* (Peterborough: FastPrint Publishing, 2012).
57 HCPP 1854–55 (135) XXXII.393: *Letter from the Duke of Newcastle, dated 6th day of December 1854, and addressed to certain newspapers respecting the publication of the intelligence from the seat of war in the Crimea.*
58 See reference list.
59 W.C. Maclean, *Memories of a Long Life* (Edinburgh: Constable, 1895), pp.96–7.
60 Lalumia, *Realism*, p.150.

caste;' a topic considered *in extenso* by Lalumia[61] and Keller.[62] In addition, invaluable illustrated catalogues of Crimean War artifacts of different artistic genre have also been published more recently.[63]

Prints and lithographs: Images based on sketches provided by professional artists, such as J.A. Crowe, C. Guys, and E. Goodall, and talented military officers,[64] were published in journals such as the *Illustrated London News*[65] and *Illustrated Times*, or as collections in albums, and in these formats reached a wide audience, particularly the increasingly influential and vociferous middle class.[66]

The depictions of the battles are not particularly informative from the point of view of this monograph as they did not include the activities of the surgeons during the action. On the other hand, illustrations of the burying the dead and the conveyance of invalids from the camps to the ports provided an indication of conditions near the front.[67] The appearance of the Crimea during the first winter portrayed by William Simpson, when conditions proved so difficult for the Army, tend to understate the situation as his scenes would not have been dissimilar to those experienced during a hard winter in the British Isles.

Similarly, the portrayal of the military hospitals failed to support the harrowing accounts of the conditions reported in private letters and by the press. An issue upon which Keller opined:

61 Lalumia, *Realism*.
62 Keller, *Ultimate Spectacle*.
63 For example, A. Massie (ed.), *A Most Desperate Undertaking. The British Army in the Crimea, 1854–56* (London: National Army Museum, 2003); O.M. Koç (ed.), *150th Anniversary of the Crimean War* (Istanbul: Sadberk Hanim Museum, 2006); and W. Hutchinson, M. Vice, and B.J. Small, *Crimean Memories. Artefacts of the Crimean War* (Atglen, PA: Schiffer Publishing, 2009).
64 Several military officers were gifted artists and some of their watercolours were particularly graphic; though the majority would have been for private consumption and not for the general public. For reproductions of the paintings by Colonel the Hon. G. Cadogan, Grenadier Guards, Major the Hon. H.H. Clifford, Rifle Brigade, and for other artists see Calthorpe, *Cadogan's Crimea*; P. Kerr, G. Pye, T. Cherfas, M. Gold, and M. Mulvihill, *The Crimean War* (London: Boxtree, 1997); and Massie, *Desperate Undertaking*.
65 The *Illustrated London News* sent its own artists in the Crimea, such as Crowe and Guys. As a consequence: 'In 1855 *Punch* had quipped that the Crimean War was undertaken for the benefit of the *Illustrated London News*;' Keller, *Ultimate Spectacle*, pp.77 & 252. For details on the artists employed by the journal see pp.71–106.
66 Incidentally, the circulation of newspapers would have been boosted during 1855 by the repeal of the 1712 Stamp Act.
67 For paintings of the evacuation of an officer on a stretcher and the French ambulance by Captain Wilkinson and Colonel Cadogan respectively see Massie *Desperate Undertaking*, pp.295 & 277.

Remarkably, in the contemporary arts spectrum from press illustration to academic painting [...] save for an indifferent view of a ward at Scutari and a somewhat mythologizing image devoted to the 'Lady with the Lamp', the great *Illustrated London News* showed no interest in how the sick and wounded were housed – and this was not for lack of evidence. The Crimea and Bosphorus were littered with hospitals which [...] accommodated a large percentage of the British expedition forces.[68]

Keller suggested that this omission may have occurred because: 'At a certain threshold of horror, it seems, art stopped serving eyewitness functions, considering itself bound to contemporary standards of propriety;'[69] and although scenes, 'some fictitious', were circulated as lithographs, they were bereft of anything likely to cause revulsion and tended to emphasize the beneficial involvement of female nurses in the wards.[70] This is in contrast to the disarray found in a Russian hospital in Sevastopol after the evacuation of the city,[71] though even this image fell well short of reality given Assistant Surgeon Wrenchs' report: 'The scenes in the [Russian] hospitals were awful, quite too disgusting to narrate [...] some of the dead are supposed to have been so for a few days if not weeks. Many of our men fainted who were employed removing them;'[72] while the QMG [Airey] noted in his diary on 12 September that he had visited the Russian barracks: 'whence they were bringing out the dead, which were lying in some of the large rooms [...] the effluvia from the bodies was dreadful and the appearance of some of the bodies defies description.'[73]

Photography: Roger Fenton, who was sent to the Crimea by Thomas Agnew and Sons, 'consistently *avoided* all controversial subjects from hospital to trench conditions' which meant that none proved specifically relevant to this monograph; except perhaps the 'studio style' contrived photograph of a cantinière treating a wounded zouave. Fenton also failed to 'document the numerous improvements which, according to all accounts, including his own letters, had began to make themselves felt by March 1855,' and thus, when all things are considered, he 'missed the very war that had drawn him to the Crimea,' principally because he 'had [seemingly] come to photograph heroes [principally officers] not places.'[74] In addition it was also necessary for the

---

68 Keller, *Ultimate Spectacle*, p.106.
69 Keller, *Ultimate Spectacle*, p.107.
70 For analysis of these images see Keller, *Ultimate Spectacle*, pp.109–12.
71 For the original watercolour painting by E.A. Goodall see Massie *Desperate Undertaking*, p.315. An engraving was reproduced in *The Illustrated London News*, 6 October 1855.
72 Wrench to his sister Sara, 14 September 1855; Nottingham University: Wr C/152/2 (Copy of original).
73 Herefordshire Record Office: BY/53/2.
74 See Keller, *Ultimate Spectacle*, pp.123–50.

images to be 'commercially appealing' and not 'embarrass the sitting ministry' while Agnew would regard 'photographs of the battle dead unmarketable.'[75]

James Robertson and his collaborator Felice Beato generally 'eschewed individual and group portraiture for subjects that better revealed the destructive forces of war' and the 'unaltered reality of the siege' and hence 'achieved the most faithful version of the Crimean War with the camera,'[76] though the images were not taken until evidence of the carnage had been removed.

The impact of images captured by Fenton, Robertson, and others would have been limited because the large scale reproduction of the photographs was not then possible. Only a relatively small number of copies would have been available for exhibition and purchase 'unless [they were] translated into line engraving' for mass distribution though this would inevitably result in the image being 'robbed of its specific character.'[77] This is exemplified by the images of Sergeant Thomas Dawson, Grenadier Guards; an amputee who received the Crimea medal from the Queen on 16 May 1855.[78] The photograph taken at Chatham by J.J.E. Mayall[79] is particularly striking while the subsequent augmentation to include his wife and the medal resulted in the distinctly less impressive engraving published in the *Illustrated Times* on 9 June 1855 (Figure 10.1).

Public art: There is no statue to Lord Raglan though he is commemorated, together with other former pupils of Westminster School who died in the Crimean War and Indian Mutiny on an impressive memorial located near the Abbey in Broad Sanctuary. It was designed by George Gilbert Scott.[80]

Other monuments in central London include statues of those who survived the war, namely, Field Marshal Burgoyne, Lord Clyde, Sidney Herbert, and Florence Nightingale in Waterloo Place, together with a memorial to the Guards. The Duke of Cambridge, Viscount Wolesley, and Viscount Palmerston can be found in Whitehall, on Horse Guards Parade, and in Parliament Square respectively while there are

---

75 Lalumia, *Realism*, p.118. For examples of Fenton's *oeuvre* see G. Baldwin, M. Daniel, and S. Greenough, *All the Mighty World. The Photographs of Roger Fenton, 1852–1860* (New Haven: Yale University Press, 2004); D.R. Jones, *In the Footsteps of Roger Fenton Crimean War Photographer* (Lulu Publishing, 2012); and S. Gordon, *Shadows of War, Roger Fenton's Photographs of the Crimean, 1855* (London: Royal Collection Trust, 2017).
76 Lalumia, *Realism*, pp.123–4. For a selection of photographs taken in the Crimea and in and around Constantinople see respectively D.R. Jones, *In the Footsteps of James Robertson and Felice Beato, Crimean War Photographers* (Lulu Publishing, 2013).and B. Öztuncay, *Robertson, Photographer and Engraver in the Ottoman Empire* (Istanbul: Vehbi Koç Foundation, 2013).
77 Keller, *Ultimate Spectacle*, p.171.
78 *The Times*, 17 May 1855.
79 Royal Collection Trust: RCIN 2500126.
80 For details on memorials to Raglan, including a blue plaque at his residence at 5 Stanhope Gate, Mayfair, London, see M. Hinton, 'Memorials to Lord Raglan in England and Wales', *The War Correspondent* 35:2 (2017), pp.8–11.

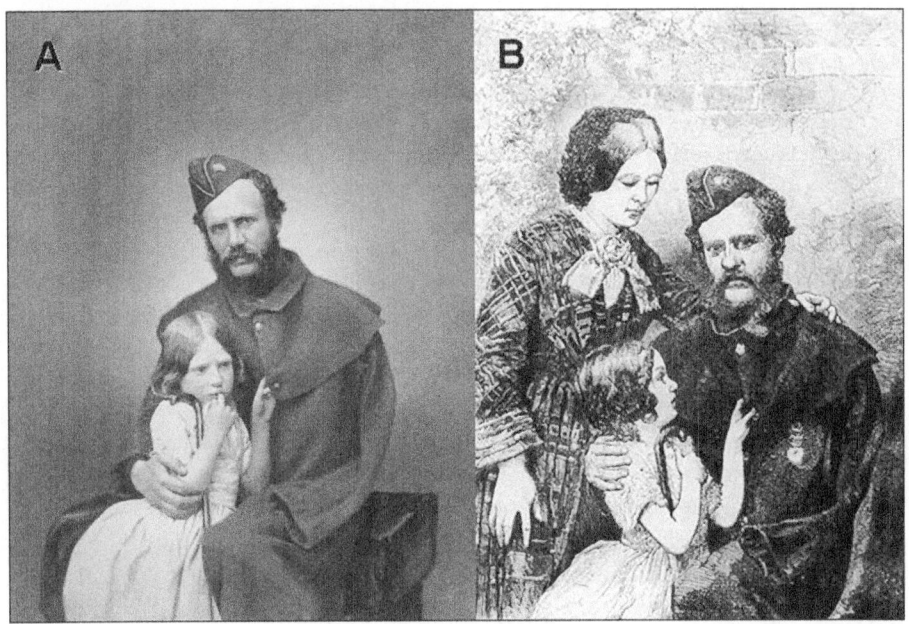

Figure 10.1
A Sergeant Dawson and his daughter at Chatham by J.J.E. Mayall. (Royal Collection Trust/© Her Majesty Queen Elizabeth II, 2019)
B A convalescent from Inkerman. (*Illustrated Times*, 9 June 1855, p.5)

statues of Isambard Kingdom Brunel in Temple Place and Paddington station, and Mary Seacole in the grounds of St Thomas' Hospital.

The general public's engagement in the Crimean War was influenced by the considerable amount of uncensored information published in the press; and in some instances these accounts were enhanced by including illustrations based on paintings and sketches sent home by people on the spot. However, there was clearly a limit on how far the publishers were prepared to go in terms of realism and this unofficial censorship clearly limited the value of the majority of the images entering the public domain as historical documents, although they did go some way to indicating how things were in the camps and trenches before Sevastopol, especially when dealing with scenes of a more peaceable or non-military nature.

10.9 Memorials to the fallen

Inevitably after the battles and other major engagements it would have been necessary to bury the fallen in mass graves; a task that must have been a gruesome and harrowing for the survivors (Figures 10.2. and 10.3); while at other times it would have been more usual to bury the dead in individual graves (Figures 10.4 and 10.5). The sector

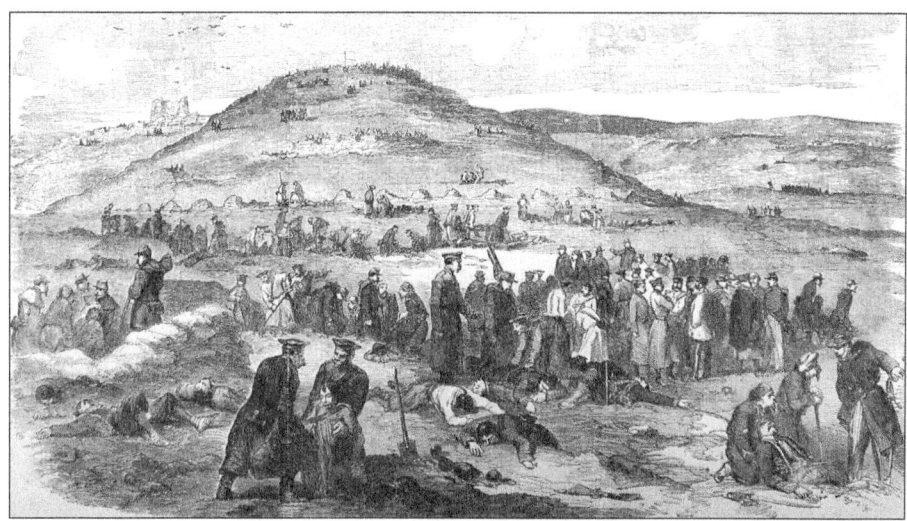

Figure 10.2 The siege of Sebastopol – Burial of the dead in front of the Malakoff Tower. (*Illustrated London News*, 21 April 1855, p.384)

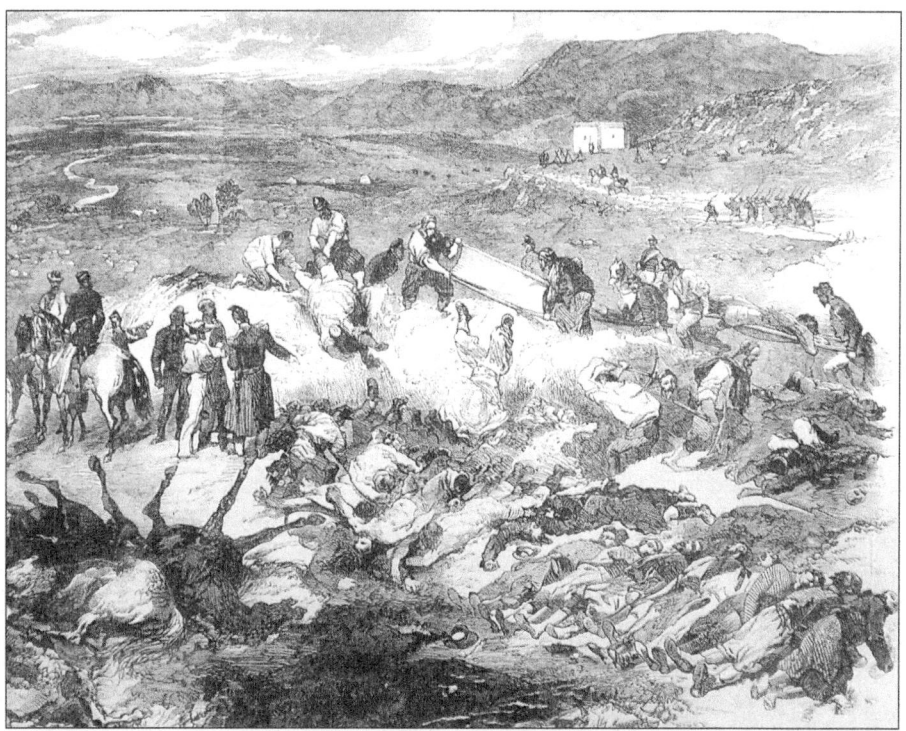

Figure 10.3 The battle-field of the Tchernaya – Burying the dead. (Sketched by Julian Portch, *Illustrated Times*, 15 September 1855, p.237)

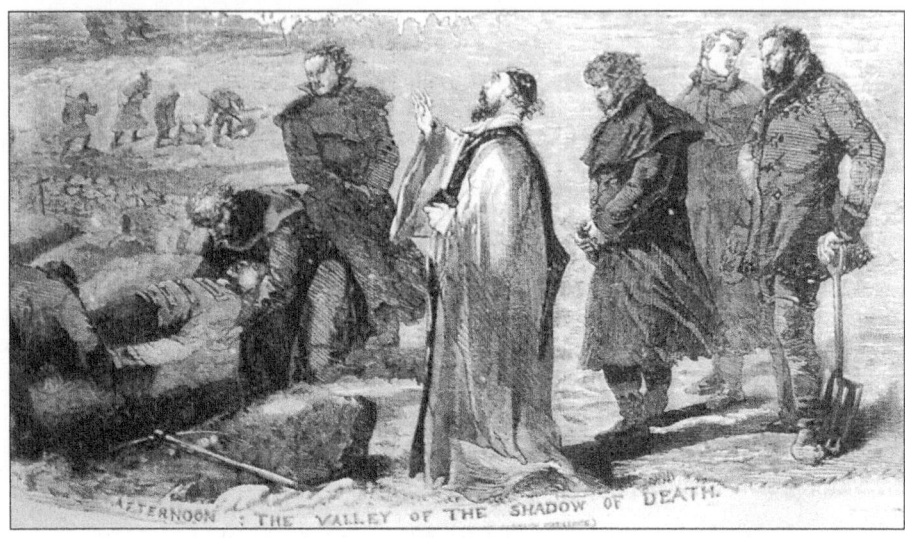

Figure 10.4 Afternoon: The valley of the shadow of death. (*Illustrated Times*, 14 July 1855, p.89)

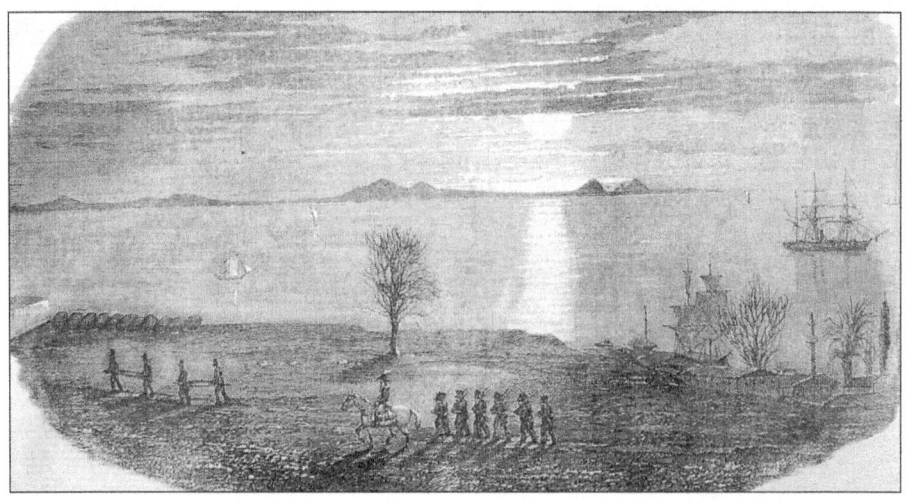

Figure 10.5 Graves at Scutari. (*Illustrated London News*, 24 March 1855, p.288)

occupied by the British forces during the campaign contained over 130 cemeteries of varying sizes; with the one on Cathcart's Hill being the most important. Before the final evacuation of the Crimea Captain the Hon. J. Colborne, 77th Regiment, and Captain Frederic Brine, RE, carried out an inventory of the tombstones, wooden grave markers, and other memorials (Figures 10.6 and 10.7). The inscriptions were recorded in full and these, together with lithographs of the principle cemeteries by E. Walker, were published in book form during the following year.[81]

The cemeteries were surveyed in 1872 by Brigadier J.M. Ayde and Colonel C.J. Gordon[82] and during the 1880s many of the surviving monuments, but not the mortal remains, were moved to Cathcart's Hill, which had been enlarged for the purpose. The cemetery was almost totally destroyed during the Second World War and only a few tombstones were identified by the British Navy Liaison Officer, Black Sea on 18 December 1944.[83] Colborne and Brine's book thus forms an incomparable record, as only a fragment of the tombstone of Sir George Cathcart and that of Lieutenant Oliver Colt, 7th Regiment, have survived into the 21st century;[84] and these have been relocated at the British War Memorial erected at Dargachi by the Ukrainian Government.[85]

In contrast, the memorials located in the cemetery at Haidar Pasha (now Haydarpaşa) in Scutari (now Üskűdar) survive; and mostly in good condition. They are now in the care of the Commonwealth War Graves Commission as the cemetery contains the graves of members of the armed forces who died during the First and Second World Wars.

Discussions about the possibility of erecting war memorial in the cemetery commenced during the summer of 1855.[86] The design of Baron Carlo Marochetti proved controversial but the 'inauguration' of the model, which was initially termed

---

81 J. Colborne and F. Brine, *The Last of the Brave; or the Resting Place of our Fallen Heroes in the Crimea and Scutari* (London: Ackermann, 1857). A second edition published the next year was entitled *Memorials of the Brave*.
82 HCCP 1873 (C.719) XL.433, *Report on the Crimean Cemeteries*.
83 The memorials and tombstones identified included: Officers and men of the Royal Engineers; Officers and men of Rifle Brigade (original); Officers and men of Rifle Brigade (erected 1900); Lieut. Gen. Sir George Cathcart, KCB; Major Gen. Sir John Campbell; Major Gen. Bucknall, Adjutant General (*sic*); Colonel Cobbe, Kings Own Regt., Commander L.U. Hammet, HMS *Albion*; Lieut. Col. George Carpenter, 41st Regt.; Major J.B. Rose of Kilravock Castle, 55th Regt.; Captain W.H. Jesse Royal Engineers; Lieut. Lea Birch (?), Captain H.T. Butler, Surg. Lt. J.J. Harris, 55th Regt.; Lieut. Henry Tryon, Rifle Brigade; Lieut. Cockerell, R.A.; Sergt. Edward Walsh, Fifth Batt. R.A.; Commonwealth War Graves Commission Archive: WG 1500/1/19 Part 4.
84 Colborne and Brine, *The Last of the Brave*, pp.10 & 47. Colt's tombstone had been moved to Cathcart's Hill from the cemetery of the 1st Brigade, Light Division.
85 For a photograph see D.R. Jones, *Forgotten Places of the Crimean War*. (Raleigh, USA: Lulu, 2015), p.110.
86 For example, Panmure and Marochetti, 30 July & 9 August 1855; TNA: WO 32/5999.

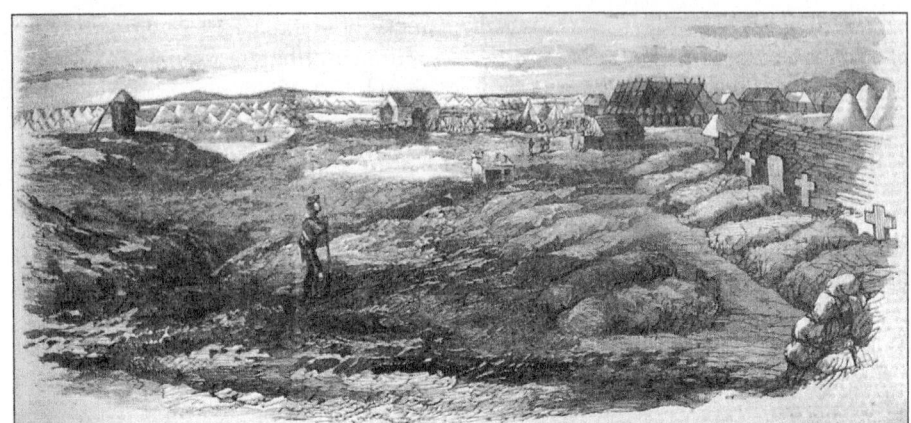

Figure 10.6 Inkerman Mill – The scene or the recent explosion. (*Illustrated London News*, 8 December 1855, p.673)

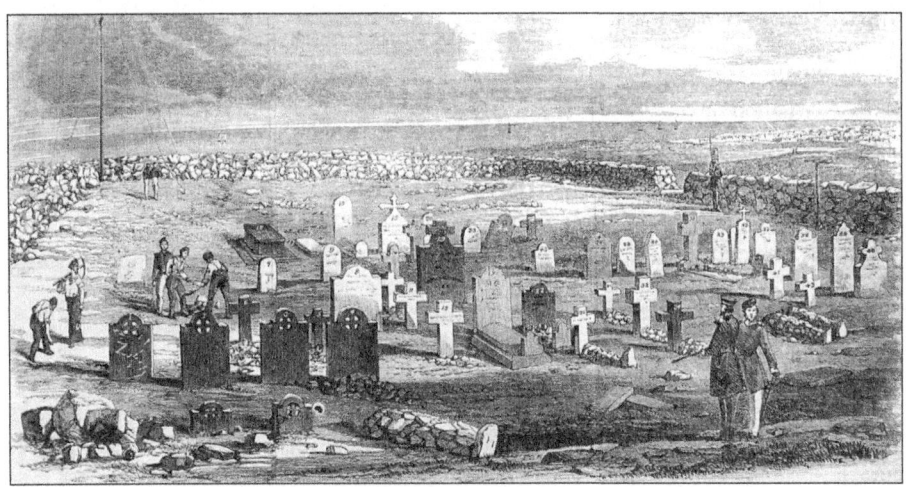

Figure 10.7 Burial ground on Cathcart's Hill in the Crimea. (*Illustrated London News*, 2 February 1856, p.129)

the 'Scutari monument', took place at the Crystal Palace on 9 May 1856 in the presence of Queen Victoria and the Royal Family.[87]

The ambassador in Constantinople reported to the Foreign Secretary, that a suitable site had been identified 'near the centre of the burial ground;'[88] and Panmure later

---

87 *The Times*, 7 & 10 May and the *Illustrated London News*, 17 May 1856.
88 Stratford to Clarendon, 4 May 1857; TNA: FO 78/1261.

confirmed that he was grateful for the trouble that had been taken with the selection of the site.[89]

The masonry was prepared in the British Isles and transported to Scutari. The size of the stone blocks (1,500 lbs-2½ tons) presented problems; both for unloading and for transporting them up the hill to the cemetery.[90] By the beginning of June 1858 the 'pedestal and the four angles' had arrived, but the obelisk was still in transit. 'English workmen' were employed with the construction, and the edifice was 'rising rapidly in spite of the want of mechanical contrivances.'[91] When the project was completed the total cost, which was defrayed by public funds, amounted to £17,500.[92]

W.H. Russell visited the cemetery with the Prince and Princess of Wales on 4 April 1869, and he was unimpressed by the monument:

> The most remarkable object in the cemetery is the monument to the dead who fell 'fighting for their country on the war against Russia in 1854, 1855, and 1856,' [...] Admirers of the works of Marochetti will point to the fine expression and beauty of the four female figures at the angles of the quadrilateral which support the simple obelisk above – a copy in petto of the Luxor column; but it must be admitted that the general effect of the whole work is rather paltry. The total cost, including transport, etc., was, we learn with wonder, £17,500, which is assuredly a good deal of money. There are eight-six graves marked by tombstones or tablets, but the nameless dead lie in solemn rank and file under the sward from end to end of the place, with not a line to mark their resting-places quia carent vate sacro [since they are without a divine poet]. [93]

The memorial inscription on the plinth, which are in French, Italian, and Turkish on the other three panels reads: 'To the Memory of the Officers and Men of the British Army and Navy who in the War against Russia in 1854, 1855, and 1856, Died for their Country. This monument was raised by Queen Victoria and her People, 1857.' Russell pointed out that at the time of his visit the gold lettering had become faded on three of the panels – but not the one in French on the West – and the need for refurbishment was confirmed a couple of years later by Ayde and Gordon.[94]

A plaque to the memory of Florence Nightingale was affixed to the plinth nearly a hundred years after the completion of the monument. It is below the main inscription

---

89   Clarendon to Stratford, 22 May 1857; TNA: FO 195/542.
90   *The Times*, 27 March 1858.
91   Special correspondent, 2 June; *The Times*, 12 June 1858.
92   G.A. Hamilton, Treasury, to Benjamin Hawes, Deputy Secretary for War, 5 May, 1859; TNA: WO 32/5999.
93   W.H. Russell, *A Diary in the East during the Tour of the Prince and Princess of Wales*. (London: George Routledge, 1869), pp.494–5.
94   HCCP 1873 (C.719) XL.433, p.29. Incidentally, when the author visited the cemetery in 2013 the gold lettering appeared in good condition.

that faces the Bosphorus; and was unveiled by the British Ambassador, Sir James Bowker, on 24 May 1854.[95] The text reads: 'To Florence Nightingale, whose work near the cemetery a century ago relieved much human suffering and laid the foundations for the nursing profession.'

10.10 A lasting legacy?

The historian G.M. Trevelyan identified two unexpected legacies of the Crimean War. One of which, the growing of beards, has merited a contemporary monograph in its own right[96] while the other continues to have serious implications for human health the world over to this day:

> In imitation of our heroes [...] smoking became fashionable again after having been banished from polite circles for eighty years. For the same reason beards returned after an absence from well-bred society of two centuries. The typical mid-Victorian of all classes was a man with a beard and a pipe.[97]

---

95 *The Times*, 25 May 1854.
96 T.S. Gowing, *The Philosophy of Beards* (London: T.T. Lemare, 1875).
97 G.M. Trevelyan, *English Social History* (London: The Reprint Society, 1948), p.554; originally published by Longmans, Green and Co, 1944.

11

Afterword

When compared with other British campaigns prior the First World War the Crimean War was not particularly exceptional from a medical point of view, though it proved challenging for several reasons: dysfunctional management systems in the Army as a whole, especially during the early months; long lines of communication and the total reliance on shipping for supplies; the need to evacuate large numbers of sick and wounded during the first winter; epidemics of cholera in 1854 and 1855; and the appearance of scurvy and other medical conditions associated with malnutrition, and excessive hardship during the winter of 1854–55. The last two factors proved crucial in precipitating the catastrophic deterioration in the health of the troops; rather than a primary breakdown in hygiene or the presence of the cholera bacillus. An opinion ventured by Captain G.F. Dallas, 46th Regiment, in a letter written two days after the hurricane of the 14 November: 'A medical report has gone in to Lord Raglan to say that men cannot do the work imposed on them and that there will be none of them left if it goes on much more. It is signed by the Medical Officers of the [4th?] Division and the Colonels of Regiments.'[1]

The practical problems of attempting the invasion of the Crimea late in the season were set out in a memorandum prepared by Burgoyne on 29 August 1854:

> There are two causal circumstances that may prove great impediments to the success of this enterprise. One is the advance of the season. The equinoctial gales [...] may interrupt [...] the communications between the armies and the fleet. And the other is, that [...] the troops [...] enfeebled and much shaken in body, as well as [...] morale, by climate, disorder, and the want of excitement by engaging with the enemy.[2]

---

1   M.H. Mawson (ed.), *Eyewitness in the Crimea* (London: Greenhill Books, 2001) pp.49–50.
2   G. Wrottesley, *Life and Correspondence of Field Marshal Sir John Burgoyne, Bart* (London: Richard Bentley,1973), 2, p.72.

The overall consequences of landing in the Crimea under these circumstances were summarized subsequently in a private letter written by the AG [Estcourt] on 23 February 1855 to the AG [Wetherall] at Horse Guards:

> The cause of our difficulties and losses too is simply a want of preparation for such an enterprise as this. When the Government had determined to undertake for political reasons the invasion of the Crimea contrary to military advice, it would at least have been wise, in as much as the military discouragement arose from the lateness of the season, the want of time before winter, to prepare for a winter's siege. If they had done so: if they had prepared the huts, and warm clothing; and all had been waiting in the Bosphorus for our call, we should not have cared much about winter. If we had been successful and had marched into Sebastopol [...] the expense would have been added to the expense of the war. [...] Ah! If you had been listened to and each man had been supplied with a water proof sheet, I do believe we should have saved many lives. [...] we have lost many men because our men have been lying upon the ground.[3]

In the spring of 1855 the editor of the *Medical Times and Gazette* noted that Pringle had observed that 'winter expeditions, though severe in appearance, are attended by little sickness, if the men have good shoes, quarters, fuel and provisions.' However, these simply stated requirements were not met during the winter of 1854–55 and hence the 'mortality has been what might have been anticipated' and that the men 'died by thousands' from those diseases expected under these circumstances such as 'diarrhoea, dysentery, fever, rheumatism, thoracic inflammations, and frost-bites.'[4] This disaster necessitated the evacuation of large numbers of patients with a grave or hopeless prognosis and this factor largely determined the mortality rates recorded in the hospitals on the Bosphorus. Improvements in hospital facilities and primary health care in the Crimea, which were made difficult by the exigencies of the siege, eventually resulted in the capacity to treat seriously ill and wounded patients locally. The health of the troops in the Crimea improved slowly, but not uniformly, from the end of January 1855, nearly two months before the Sanitary Commissioners arrived in the Crimea. Given that most patients at Scutari came from the Crimea, the reduction in the mortality rates after their arrival would, at least in part, be attributable to this factor. Nightingale supported this opinion when she informed Panmure that: 'The men sent down to Scutari in the winter died because they were not sent down till half dead,'[5] while Cantlie considered, on the basis that many patients suffered untreatable conditions such as intestinal ulceration associated with dysentery or typhoid, and that

---

3 National Army Museum: 1962–10–95–2.
4 *Medical Times and Gazette*, 10 March 1855.
5 H. Small, *Florence Nightingale*, p.76.

Fortescue had implied incorrectly that it was bad hospital conditions that caused many deaths.⁶

Raglan appreciated both the reasons for the problems faced by the Army and also that conditions had began to improve after the turn of the year when he wrote to the Queen and the Newcastle on the 20 and 23 January 1855 respectively:

> To the Queen: Lord Raglan can [...] assure your Majesty that [...] all his thoughts are occupied in endeavouring to provide for [...] your Majesty's troops. It has not been [possible] to lighten [...] their duties. Those exacted [...] for the preservation of the trenches and batteries; and there are many other calls upon the men, [...] the roads are so bad that wheeled carriages [cannot] be used, and [...] horse transport is diminished by sickness and deaths and the Commissariat [...] cannot bring up the daily supplies without their assistance thereby adding [...] to their labour and fatigue. [...] the Allied Armies [...] can derive no resources from [the country] and consequently all [...] stores and provisions [...] must be imported. Such a necessity forms [...] a difficulty of vast magnitude [...] productive of the most serious consequences to the comfort of the Army.⁷

> To the Duke: The weather has become milder; but the country is still in a dreadful state from melted snow. The army is well supplied with warm clothing, and if the Commissariat were adequately provided with transports, and the huts could be at once brought up, there would be no other cause of suffering than the severity of a Crimean winter, and the duties imposed of carrying on a siege in such a climate at this season of the year.⁸

Improvements in the Crimea were also appreciated in Constantinople when the Ambassador reported on 8 February that 'a marked improvement has taken place in [the Crimea that] is of much consequence to the health of the Army.'⁹ A few days later a staff officer at Scutari was informed by an officer 'just come in from the Crimea' that 'matters are greatly improved in the last few days and it is really to be hoped they will continue improving.'¹⁰ On the same day, Paulet, the commandant on the Bosphorus, informed Herbert that 'Everything seems to be improving and the increased

---

6   Cantlie, *History*, 2, p.125.
7   A.C. Benson and Viscount Esher (eds), *The Letters of Queen Victoria* (London: John Murray, 1907), 3, pp.87–8.
8   *The Times* and *West Briton and Cornwall Advertiser*, 8 & 9 February 1855 respectively.
9   Stratford to Clarendon, 8 February 1855; TNA: FO 78/1072.
10 Captain Macdonald, 93rd Regiment, to his mother, 8–12 February 1855; M. Hinton, 'A Letter from Captain William Donald Macdonald, 93rd Regiment, together with a Commentary on Medical Matters', *The War Correspondent*, 28:3 (2010), pp.27–8.

accommodation [...] will enable us to thin the hospitals considerably.'[11] Panmure also heard of these developments from Raglan when he wrote on 24 February: 'There is certainly an improvement in the sick, and if the weather becomes moderate, I expect further amendment.'[12] Likewise, Sir Henry Ward, the Lord High Commissioner in the Ionian Islands, reported to Panmure privately on 4 March: 'Things are certainly improving in the Crimea. All letters today agree about that. The weather has been atrocious, but the camp is healthier, the warm clothing generally is in use, and the rations more regularly received.'[13] The QMG [Airey] informed the AG at Horse Guards on 15 March: 'the general health of the men is improving vastly; still we want one thing to put us right on our legs again, viz. rest.'[14]

These opinions were confirmed by the official report of the Hospital Commission:

> [...] our visit to the Crimea took place [during the first three weeks of January] when the condition of the sick and wounded and the state of the hospital accommodation [...] were at their worst. We believe that they have much improved since our departure. Signs of improvement were already perceptible before we sailed from Balaklava; for abundance of warm clothing was in course of distribution, and the materials for huts were being carried up to the camp. Since then, commodious huts have been [...] erected in the encampment of each regiment, for hospital, as well as other purposes and the sickness which prevailed among the troops in December and January has become both less general and less severe.[15]

This report provided independent confirmation of Hall's medical report for February 1855: 'Altho' much sickness, and mortality continued to prevail in the Army [...] there is evident improvement in the general health of the men; and from their increased comforts there is every reason to believe that this will continue.'[16] Hall's prediction proved correct as admission rates to the hospitals in the Crimea, and the mortality from disease in the Army, fell during the spring until late May 1855, when the illnesses frequently associated with summer campaigning made their appearance. If it had not been for a recrudescence of cholera in the Crimea during the summer, the overall mortality rate from disease would have been much reduced, although not to the low levels recorded following the fall of Sevastopol (see Figure 1.6).[17]

---

11 Wiltshire and Swindon History Centre: 2057/F8/III/C/21.
12 Douglas and Ramsey, *Panmure Papers*, 1, p.78.
13 National Archives of Scotland: GD45/8/200. NB: Letters received at Corfu would have been written at least seven to ten days previously.
14 Airey to AG, Horse Guards, 15 March 1855; National Army Museum: 1962-07-97-17.
15 Hospital Commission Report, p.14.
16 TNA: WO 17/1730, with a longer version in Hall's hand in RAMC: 397/FRT1/1.
17 Snow's conclusion that cholera was spread by water was published in 1855; too late to have an impact on the management of the epidemics in the Crimea; Snow, *On the Mode of Communication of Cholera*.

Most senior officers lacked the experience at the start to prosecute a campaign far from home; a position summarized by Harrison: 'It was not that generals were particularly callous, or that military doctors were incompetent, as some observers later claimed. Rather, the nations involved had not fought a large war for some time; war ministers, generals and senior medical officers were all largely inexperienced in planning the logistics of a major campaign.'[18] It is not surprising, therefore, that things went wrong during the months following an inadequately planned invasion late in the season by an inexperienced and relatively poorly equipped army, sent to face an enemy of uncertain strength in a country about which little was known, and which had extremely limited resources to provide for the needs of the armies such as harbour facilities, shelter, roads, and sources of forage and fuel.[19]

The majority of Medical Officers would have had little or no experience of active campaigning and working under battle field conditions. They had to learn on the job,[20] while to complicate matters the composition of the Army changed constantly.[21] Many new arrivals were young lads ill-equipped for camp life and trench warfare and had to learn the ropes after their arrival in camp. Fortunately, as time progressed there would have been an increasing number of experienced NCOs and men (many of whom would have replaced those in the original invading force) who could provide necessary discipline, assistance, and encouragement which would have been greatly to their benefit.

The senior Army staff came in for criticism for their apparent lack of efficiency, particularly during the first winter when they were faced with insuperable difficulties. In response to this Panmure sent General James Simpson in February to investigate matters on the spot as he was minded to have Airey [QMG] and Estcourt [AG] replaced.'[22] In the event, Simpson found no serious fault with the way the Army was administered and stayed on as the Chief-of-Staff until he unwillingly succeeded to the command of the Army following Raglan's death.

It would be wrong to assume that the likes of Airey, Estcourt, Filder, and Hall were not essentially effective men of business who were well aware of what was needed to rectify matters. A glance at their official and private correspondence will confirm that they were this from the start, while perusal of the General Orders demonstrates that

---

18 M. Harrison, 'War and Medicine in the Modern Era', in Wellcome Collection,: Deutsches Hygiene-Museum Dresden, *War and Medicine* (London: Black Dog, 2008), p.14.
19 Roger Fenton's photographs of the British camps attest to the barren nature of the countryside. See, for example, Gordon, *Shadows of War*.
20 For example, on 14 September 1854 Smith wrote to Hall; 'You will have [...] great difficulties for the first twelve months while the inexperienced get experienced;' National Army Museum: 2007-07-16-5.
21 For example, the Guards Brigade had seven COs during the campaign; M. Springman, *The Guards Brigade in the Crimea*, (Barnsley: Pen & Sword Military, 2008), pp.202–5.
22 Panmure to Ragan, 19 February 1855; Douglas and Ramsey, *The Panmure Papers*, 1, pp.69–70.

the Army was administered formally throughout the campaign irrespective of the trials and tribulations experienced.

The main problem was that these heads of department and their subordinates had to operate within a system which had been run down since 1815 and had not been reformed. It may have been sufficient to manage during peacetime but proved woefully inadequate for an army on campaign. In due course, and in a relatively short time, workable systems of management were developed locally which were satisfactory by the standards of the day and ultimately contributed to the Victory over Disease of 1856.

The signing of the peace treaty in March of that year resulted in a major change in priorities, and the rapid evacuation of the troops became the imperative. Fortunately the military authorities remained committed to maintaining sanitary discipline in the camps. For example, each regiment was required to leave its camp: 'perfectly clean, the huts empty, temporary stables and kitchens leveled, [...] tents and latrines filled up. General Officers will [...] turn their attention to this subject, which is of importance to the health of the troops who remain.'[23] It is not possible to determine the impact of this Order but the inevitable reduction in the impetus for further infrastructural improvements, coupled with the concomitant dismantling of the camps, did not have a detrimental effect on the men's health during the final weeks of occupation.

The historiography of the campaign has tended to concentrate on the disasters of the first winter and the perceived incompetence of the heads of department on the one hand, and to overemphasize the worthwhile and commendable contributions made by the talented and well connected Nightingale and the experienced government-sponsored Sanitary Commissioners on the other. Inevitably this has established an unbalanced view of what really took place. This view has been distorted further by commentators who have failed to consider events in strict order of occurrence and have indulged in the knowledge of hindsight. In consequence this aspect of the war has been inaccurately portrayed in both academic works and popular culture.

Smith and Hall both came in for considerable criticism, particularly during the first year of the campaign. However, they both remained in post throughout when there would have been ample opportunities to have had them replaced. Why was this? Could it be that they and their medical colleagues were good at their jobs and that the blame lay elsewhere?[24]

In the final analysis, the Army's health problems were not strictly medical as the spread of infections would have been facilitated by: 'the assembly of large numbers of people, lack of food, badly cooked food, sleeping out in the cold and rain, and fatiguing activities' coupled with the difficulty of keeping the camps 'unpolluted by

---

23 General Order, 22 May 1856.
24 It would seem that Hall was sufficiently well regarded by Panmure for him to support his application for an increase in his half-pay pension of £1/10/- a day given that he had served for 39 years and 11 months. An increase to £1/17/11d, backdated to 1 January 1857, was finally authorized; TNA: WO 43/519/ff.25–81.

the excrement of man and animals, and refuse of all kinds [since the army was] located in one place.'[25]

More recent analyses of 18th and 19th century medical records by McKeown and others have suggested that improvements in the health of civilian populations could take place in the absence of any significant developments in medical science as a consequence of improved nutrition, water supply, sewage management, and living accommodation; all objectives that were achievable in the camps before Sevastopol and elsewhere. This explanation is now sometimes referred to as the 'McKeown Hypothesis', and though still considered controversial, it does provide an explanation why the disease problems experienced during the winter of 1854–55 were ultimately defeated later in the campaign;[26] or, as Prinzing opined, the provision of: 'good food and shelter could prevent outbreaks of pestilences.'

The medical services in the two World Wars have been evaluated *in extenso* by Harrison. He concluded, inter alia, that an 'army in disarray [...] finds it extremely difficult to implement effective measures for the prevention of disease and treatment of the sick and wounded' and because 'such difficulties were never insurmountable' they could be overcome by 'efficient organization and sanitary discipline.' The 'medical failures were generally a failure of command, and that their [successful resolution] depended on the intelligent co-operation of the Army as a whole;'[27] hence 'epidemics are as much a consequence of military failure as their cause,'[28] though even 'ubiquitous' diseases such as dysentery could be controlled by introducing appropriate control measures and paying attention to detail.

Harrison's conclusions resonate with the events of 1854–56 when the British Army, initially thrown into 'disarray', subsequently proved that the 'difficulties were never insurmountable.' A systematic evaluation of archival and contemporary published sources have verified that the turning point in the Army's fortunes was achieved early in 1855 and that the foundations for the recovery of the troop's health were laid by personnel in all departments of the Army working under hazardous and trying conditions of siege warfare. The Sanitary Commissioners together with railway navvies and AWC, with the assistance of the LTC, were then able to build on these foundations, and their contribution, coupled with improvements in management and infrastructure generally, ensured that the 'plenty' referred to by Maxwell was brought to the camps, and that the hard-won Sanitary Success of 1855 continued throughout the final months of the campaign to give a Victory over Disease.

---

25   See Prinzing, *Epidemics*, pp.1–10 & 170–5.
26   For example, T. McKeown, and R. G. Record, 'Reasons for the Decline of Mortality in England and Wales during the Nineteenth Century', *Populations Studies* (1962), 16, pp 94–122 and T. McKeown, R. G. Brown, and R. G. Record 'An Interpretation of the Modern Rise of Population in Europe', *Population Studies* (1972), 26, pp.345–82.
27   Harrison, *Medicine and Victory*, pp.277 & 283.
28   Harrison, *Medical War*, p.292.

Appendix

Principal personalities

Name in the text	Full name*	Post(s)
Aberdeen	George Hamilton-Gordon, 5th Earl of Aberdeen	Prime Minister to January 1855.
Airey	Major General Sir Richard Airey, KCB	QMG, Army of the East, September 1854 to November 1855 when succeeded Sir James Freeth as QMG to the Forces.
Alexander	Dr Thomas Alexander, CB	PMO, Light Division. A member of the Royal Commission, he succeeded Sir Andrew Smith as Director General of the Army Medical Department during 1858, and died in 1860.
Boxer	Rear Admiral Edward Boxer	Sometime Port Admiral on the Bosphorus and then at Balaklava. He died of cholera on 4 June 1855.
Bracebridge	Charles Holte Bracebridge	He and his wife accompanied Miss Nightingale to the East.
Brunel	Isambard Kingdom Brunel	Brunel designed the ss *Great Britain,* which was employed as a troop ship, and the prefabricated hospital erected at Renkioi.
Burgoyne	Lieutenant General Sir John Burgoyne, RE	Served on the staff of the Army, but not as the CRE. An advocate of a formal siege, he was recalled during February 1855 to resume his duties as Inspector General of Fortifications.
Calvert	Frederick William Calvert	HM's consul on the Dardanelles.
Christie	Captain Peter Christie, RN	Agent of Transports, Balaklava. He died of disease on 1 May 1855.
Clarendon	George William Frederick Villiers, 4th Earl of Clarendon	Foreign Secretary, 1853–1858.
Codrington	General (LR) Sir William John Codrington, KCB	GOC, Light Division and then GOC Army of the East, 11. November 1855–July 1856.
Cumming	IGH Alexander Cumming	A Hospitals Commissioner and then PMO, Scutari, February–October 1855.

322

Name in the text	Full name*	Post(s)
Dumbreck	DIGH David Dumbreck	Acted as PMO when Dr Hall when was sent to Scutari by Raglan. He was invalided to England during November 1854.
Dundas	Vice Admiral Sir James Whitely Deans Dundas	C-in-C of the Mediterranean Fleet from 1852 until the was replaced by Admiral Lyons at the beginning of 1855.
Estcourt	Major General James Bucknall Bucknall Estcourt	Adjutant General, Army of the East, August 1854 until his death on 24 June 1855. He was succeeded by Brevet Colonel William Lygon Pakenham.
Fergusson	Lieutenant General Sir James Fergusson, KCB	GOC Malta and then Governor of Gibraltar.
Filder	William Filder	The Commissary General until recalled in July 1855. He was replaced by Sir George Maclean.
Fremantle	Rear Admiral Charles Howe Fremantle	Sometime Port Admiral on the Bosphorus and then at Balaklava. He succeeded Rear Admiral Boxer on both occasions.
Gavin	Dr Hector Gavin, MD	A Sanitary Commissioner. He died on 21 April 1855 as a result of a shooting accident and was replaced by Dr Gavin Milroy.
Hall	Sir John Hall, MD, KCB	PMO, Army of the East.
Hardinge	Field Marshal Viscount Henry Hardinge	C.-in-C. British Army 1852–1856.
Hawes	Benjamin Hawes	Hawes held an unelected position of Deputy Secretary for War, 1851–7. He was a brother-in-law of I.K. Brunel,
Herbert	Sidney Herbert, later Baron Herbert of Lea	Secretary at War to February 1855; Chairman of the Royal Commission, 1857; Minister of War 1859–1861.
Lawson	DIGH Robert Lawson	Sometime PMO at Balaklava. Transferred to Scutari after the *Avon* affair on the authority of a General Order.
Linton	IGH William Linton, CB, MD	Served in the Crimea until becoming the PMO at Scutari during October 1855 in succession to IGH Cumming.
Admiral Lyons	Admiral Sir Edmund Lyons	Lyons succeeded Admiral Dundas in command of the Mediterranean Fleet.
Dr Lyons	Robert D. Lyons	A civilian appointed by Panmure to investigate 'the nature of the diseases from which the troops were suffering.' He was assisted by Dr Aitken and their report was published as HCPP 1857 Session 2 [2229] XVIII.533: *Report of the Pathology of the Diseases of the Army of the East*.
McGrigor	Sir James	Sir Andrew Smith's predecessor as Director General of the Army Medical Department.
McNeill	Sir John	A Supplies Commissioner who collaborated with Miss Nightingale after the war.
McMurdo	Colonel (LR) William Montague Scott McMurdo	The Director General of the Land Transport Corps.

Name in the text	Full name*	Post(s)
Mapleton	Dr Henry Mapleton, MD	Sometime physician to Lord Raglan. His report 'relative to the sanitary condition of the Army of the East' was prepared for Smith in 1855 and published as HCPP 1857–58 (425) XXXVII.105: *A Report* [...] *Relative to the Sanitary Condition of the Army of the East* [...] *by Dr Mapleton*..
Maxwell	Peter Benson Maxwell	A barrister and Hospitals Commissioner. Author of the anonymously published pamphlet *Whom shall we hang?*
Menzies	DIGH Duncan Menzies	PMO, Scutari from June 1854 until invalided in January 1855.
Milroy	Dr Gavin Milroy	A Sanitary Commissioner from 22 July 1855. He replace Dr Hector Gavin who died as a result of a shooting accident.
Mundy	Colonel G.C. Mundy	Military Undersecretary at the War Office.
Newcastle	Henry Pelham Clinton, 5th Duke of Newcastle	Minister of War until February 1855 when he was succeeded by Lord Panmure.
Nightingale	Florence Nightingale	Superintendent of a party of nurses sent to Turkey by Sidney Herbert and remembered by many by the sobriquet 'the lady with the lamp.'
Osborne	The Hon. the Revd Sidney Godolphin Osborne	Visited Scutari in a private capacity for about six weeks, leaving on the 19 December 1854. He gave evidence to the Roebuck Committee and published *Scutari and its Hospitals* in 1855.
Pakenham	Brevet Colonel William Lygon Pakenham	Succeeded Major General Estcourt as AG.
Palmerston	Henry John Temple, 3rd Viscount Palmerston	Prime Minister from February 1855.
Panmure	Fox Maule, Lord Panmure	Minister of War from February 1855. His brother Colonel Lauderdale Maule died of cholera in Bulgaria on 1 August 1854.
Parkes	Dr Edmund Alexander Parkes, MD	A civilian who was the Superintendent at the Renkioi Hospital.
Paulet	Major General (LR) Lord William Paulet	Commandant on the Bosphorus from November 1854 until he assumed command of the Light Division, November 1855.
Peel	Frederick Peel	Liberal MP for Bury and Undersecretary for War under Lord Palmerston.
Raglan	Field Marshal Fitzroy Somerset, 1st Baron Raglan	C.-in-C., Army of the East, until his death on 28 June 1855.
Rawlinson	Robert Rawlinson	A Sanitary Commissioner who was a civil engineer by profession.
Roebuck	John Arthur Roebuck, MP	Liberal MP for Sheffield. He chaired the Select Committee of the House of Commons which was convened to investigate the 'Condition of the Army before Sebastopol'.

Appendix 325

Name in the text	Full name*	Post(s)
Romaine	William Govett Romaine	The Deputy Judge Advocate General for the Army of the East. A civilian appointed by the Government, and hence not part of the military establishment.
Russell	William Howard Russell	Special correspondent of *The Times*.
Sayer	Captain Frederic Sayer	Sayer served in the Crimea until invalided for wounds in October 1854. Published *Despatches and Papers relative to the Campaign in Turkey, Asia Minor and the Crimea during the War with Russia in 1854, 1855, 1856* in 1857.
Sillery	Major Charles Sillery	Commandant at Scutari, June-November 1854. He continued serving there on the staff of his successor, Brigadier Paulet.
Simpson	General Sir James Simpson, KCB	Chief of Staff from March 1855 until he succeeded Lord Raglan. He resigned on 10 November 1855
Smith	Dr, later Sir, Andrew Smith, MD, FRS	Succeeded Sir James McGrigor as Director General, Army Medical Department, in 1852. A member of the Royal Commission, he resigned in 1858 and was appointed KCB (Civil) in the same year.
Spence	DIGH Thomas Spence, MD	A member of the Hospitals Commission He drowned on *Prince* on 14 November 1854.
Stafford	Augustus Stafford	Conservative MP for Northamptonshire North who visited Scutari and the Crimea in a private capacity. He was a member of the Royal Commission.
Storks	Major General (LR) Henry Storks	Commandant at Smyrna from March 1855 until he succeeded Paulet as Commandant on the Bosphorus in November 1855. He was a member of the Royal Commission.
Stratford	Viscount Stratford de Redcliffe	British Ambassador in Constantinople.
Sutherland	Dr John Sutherland, MD	A Sanitary Commissioner, a member of the Royal Commission, and a collaborator of Miss Nightingale after the war.
Tulloch	Colonel Alexander Murray Tulloch	A Supplies Commissioner.
Wetherall	Major General Sir George Augustus Wetherall, KCB	Adjutant General of the Forces at Horse Guards, 1854–1860.

* The rank of military personnel is that they held when the Peace Treaty was ratified on 27 April 1856, or when they died. LR = Local Rank

Bibliography

The principal sources consulted during the preparation of this monograph have been summarized in Section 1.7. The unpublished archival material and newspaper reports are referred to in the footnotes while this section provides details of those that have been published, and are accessible, either in libraries or in digitized versions on line.

1 House of Commons Parliamentary Papers (HCPP)

The abbreviations for the individual documents are taken from Cockton's catalogue of the House of Commons parliamentary papers.[1] The reference comprises three components without punctuation marks, viz.: Session; Paper number in parenthesis or square brackets for Command Paper; Volume number in Roman numerals with the page number following the point.

The references are prefixed with HCPP in the footnotes with an abbreviated title being used for several documents that are referred to on several subsequent occasions. This is included where applicable in parenthesis following the main title, which is in italics.

1.1 Reports of Committees
1854–55 (156) IX.Pt.I.7; (218) IX.Pt.II.1; (247) IX.Pt.III.1; & (318, 318–I) IX.Pt.III.365, 431: *Second, Third, Fourth and Fifth Reports of the Select Committee on the Army before Sebastopol.* (Select Committee, 2nd, 3rd, 4th, & 5th Reports respectively).

1.2 Reports of Commissions
1856 (2119) XXI.1: *Report of the Board of General Officers Appointed to Enquire into the Statements Contained in the Reports of Sir John M'Neill and Colonel Tulloch.*
1856 (331) XIII.359: *Report from the Select Committee on the Medical Department [Army].* (*Select Committee on the Medical Department*).

---

1 P. Cockton, *Subject Catalogue of the House of Commons Parliamentary Papers 1801–1900* (Cambridge: Chadwyck-Healey, 1988), Vol. 5.

1856 (422) XXI.651: *Index to the Report of the Board of General Officers Appointed to Enquire into the Statements Contained in the Reports of Sir John M'Neill and Colonel Tulloch.*

1856 [2007, 2007–I] XX.1.497: *Report of the Commission of Inquiry into the Supplies of the British Army in the Crimea* (Supplies Commission Report).

1857 Session 2 (2229) XVIII.533: *Report of the Pathology of the Diseases of the Army of the East* (Pathology Report).

1857–58 (2318) XVIII.1: *Report of the Commissioners Appointed to Inquire into the Regulations Affecting the Sanitary Condition of the Army, the Organization of Military Hospitals, and the Treatment of the Sick and Wounded* (Royal Commission Report).

1857–58 (2379) XIX.1: *Report of the Commissioners Appointed to Inquire into the Regulations Affecting the Sanitary Condition of the Army, the Organization of Military Hospitals, and the Treatment of the Sick and Wounded, Appendix LXXIX* (Royal Commission Report, Appendix LXXIX).

1.3 Accounts and papers

1854–55 (126) XXXII.431: *(Turkey). Return of the Medical Officers Attached to the Forces Serving in Turkey.*

1854–55 (135) XXXII.393: *Letter from the Duke of Newcastle, dated 6th day of December 1854, and addressed to certain newspapers respecting the publication of the intelligence from the seat of war in the Crimea.*

1854–55 (204) XXXII, 387: *Return of the Total Number of Officers and Men in the Army who have been Killed in the Crimea; and Like Return of the Number Wounded [...] up to 15th Match 1855*

1854–55 (212) XXXII.633: *Return of the Stores Sent to the East from 1st Day of January 1854 to 1st Day of January 1855, with the Totals of Each, the Dates when Sent, and when Arrived in the East.*

1854–55 (399) XXXII.307: *Number and Description of Articles of Clothing Supplied [...] since 1st Day of October 1854 for the Troops Serving in the Crimea.*

1854–55 [1901] XLV.41: *Report on the Results of Different Methods of Treatment Pursued in Epidemic Cholera throughout England and Scotland in 1854.*

1854–55 (4) XXXII.631: *Statement of Warm Clothing Lost on Board 'The Prince'.*

1854–55 (428) XXXII.421: *Medical Officers (Army and Navy).*

1854–55 (449) XXXIII.361: *Official Reports on the Hospitals at Scutari, Kululee, Abydos, and Smyrna, since February Last*, p.26. (Reports on Hospitals in Turkey).

1854–55 (512) XXXIV.107: *Correspondence Relative to the State of the Harbour of Balaklava.*

1854–55 [1893] XLV.69: *Letter of the President of the General Board of Health to Viscount Palmerston Accompanying a Report from Dr Sutherland on Cholera in the Metropolis in 1854.*

1854–55 [1920] XXXIII.1: *Report upon the State of the Hospitals on the British Army in the Crimea and Scutari* (Hospital Commission Report).

1856 (345) XLI.341: *Return of all ships engaged as regular transports, with the names (stating whether steam or sailing), from Jan 1st, 1855, to Apr 1st, 1856; the date of the engagement, with a list of ships in the service at the latter date, their registered tonnage, rates of freight, and mulets or deductions for the same, and why made; in steam ships, the horse power, the time occupied in their passages, and where information has been received, the quantity of coals or fuel consumed per hour.*

1856 (2042) IX.337: *Copy of a Letter from Commissary General Filder Covering Remarks of those Parts of the Report of Sir John M'Neill and Colonel Tulloch which Relate to the Commissariat Department.*

1856 [2103] LII.257: *Report of the Last Two Cholera-Epidemics of London as Affected by the Consumption of Impure Water.*

1856 (2120) XL.233: *Names of Non-Commissioned Officers and Men Selected for [...] the French Military Medal* with a supplement, viz. 1857 Session 1 (0.54) IX.221.

1857 Session 1 (0.51) IX.673: *Report on Smyrna by George Rolleston, Late Assistant Physician to the British Civil Hospital at Smyrna.*

1857 Session 1 (133) IX.11: *Return of the Names of Officers [...] of the Army* etc.

1857 Session 1 (71) IX.797: *Medical Statistical Returns of the Baltic and Black Sea Fleets, during the Years 1854 and 1855.*

1857 Session 1 [2196] LX.241: *Report to the Right Hon. Lord Panmure, G.C.B., etc. Minister at War, of the Proceedings of the Sanitary Commission Dispatched to the Seat of War in the East, 1855–56*, (Sanitary Commission Report).

1857 Session 2 (267) XXVII.155: *The Number of Huts Supplied to the Ordnance or War Departments during the Years 1854-5 and 1855-6.*

1857 Session 2 [2259] XXVII.215: *List of Officers, Non-Commissioned Officers, and Men Selected to Receive the 400 War Medals for Military Valour, Presented by His Majesty the King of Sardinia to the British Army Engaged in the Late War in the East.*

1857 Session I, (42) IX.1: *Return Concerning the Late Army of the East.*

1857, Session 1 (135) IX.211: *Report on the Organisation of the Russian Medical Department and the Sanitary State of their Crimean Hospitals.*

1857–58 (482) VIII.1: *Select Committee on Consular Services and Consular Appointments.*

1857–58 [2434] XXXVIII.Pt.I.1 & XXXVIII.Pt.II.1: *Medical and Surgical History of the British Army which Served in Turkey and the Crimea during the War against Russia in the Years 1854-55-56.* (*Medical and Surgical History*, 1 or 2).

1860 (51) XL.219: *Return of Name of Every Child Maintained at Charge of Patriotic Fund.*

1863 (3207) XIII.475: *Report of the Barrack and Hospital Improvement Commission on the Sanitary Condition and Improvement of Mediterranean Stations.*

1873 (C.719) XL.433: *Report on the Crimean Cemeteries.*

2 Published books, pamphlets, and articles in journals

2.1 Books published before the Crimean War

Gavin, H., *Sanitary Ramblings* (London: John Churchill, 1848).
Jackson, R., *Remarks on the Constitution of the Medical Department of the British Army* (London: Cadill & Davies, 1803).
Luscombe, E.T., *Practical Observations on the Means of Preserving the Health of Soldiers in Camp and in Quarters* (2nd edition) (Edinburgh: Archibald Constable, 1821).
Monro, D., *Observations on the Means of Preserving the Health of Soldiers, and of Conducting Military Hospitals* (2nd edition) (London: J. Murray, 1780), Vol. 1.
Pringle, J., *Observations on the Diseases of the Army in Camp and Garrison* (London: Miller and Wilson, 1752).

2.2 Diaries, letters, and autobiography

A Lady [Martha Nicol], *Ismeer, or Smyrna and its British Hospital in 1855* (London: James Madden, 1856).
A Lady Volunteer [Frances M. Taylor], *Eastern Hospitals and English Nurses* (London: Hunt and Blackett, 1856), Vol. 2.
An Officer on the Staff [S.J.G. Calthorpe], *Letters from Head-Quarters* (3rd edition) (London: John Murray, 1858).
Benson, A.C. and Esher, Viscount (eds), *The Letters of Queen Victoria* (London: John Murray, 1907), Vol. 3.
Bonham-Carter, V. M. and Lawson, M., *Surgeon in the Crimea* (London: Military Book Society, 1968), p.150.
Bostock, J.A., *Letters from India and the Crimea* (London: George Bell, 1897).
Bryce, C., *England and France before Sebastopol* (London: John Churchill, 1857).
Buzzard, T., *With the Turkish Army in the Crimea and Asia Minor* (London: John Murray, 1915).
Calthorpe, S.J.G., *Cadogan's Crimea* (London: Hamish Hamilton, 1979)
Douglas, G., and Ramsey, G.H. (eds), *The Panmure Papers* (London: Hodder and Stoughton, 1898), Vol. 1.
Eyre-Todd, G. (ed.), *The Autobiography of William Simpson, R.I. (Crimean Simpson)* (London: T. Fisher Unwin, 1903).
Fergusson, W., *Notes and Recollections of a Professional Life* (London: Longman & Co., 1846).
H.B. [Henry Blishen], *Letters from the Crimea during the Years 1854 and 1855* (London: Emily Faithfull, 1856).
Hamley, E.B., *The Story of the Campaign of Sebastopol Written in Camp* (Edinburgh: W. Blackwood and Sons, 1855).
Heath, L.G., *Letters from the Black Sea during the Crimean War, 1854–1855* (London: Richard Bentley, 1873).
Hill, D. (ed.), *Letters from the Crimea* (Dundee: Dundee UP, 2010).
Kelly, C. (ed.), *Mrs Duberly's War* (Oxford: University Press, 2007).

Lane-Poole, S., *Life of the Right Honourable Stratford Canning Viscount Stratford de Redcliffe* (London: Longman, Green, & Co., 1888), Vol. 2.
Lewis, G.F. (ed.) *Letters of Sir George Cornewall Lewis, Bart.* (London: Longman, Green & Co., 1870)
Maclean, W.C., *Memories of a Long Life* (Edinburgh: Constable, 1895).
Mawson, M.H. (ed.), *Eyewitness in the Crimea* (London: Greenhill Books, 2001).
Mitra, S.M., *The Life and Letters of Sir John Hall M.D., K.C.B., F.R.C.S.* (London: Longmans, Green, 1911).
Raymond, J (ed.), *Queen Victoria's Early Letters* (London: B.T. Batsford, 1963).
Robins, C. (ed.), *Romaine's Crimean War* (Stroud: Sutton Publishing, 2005).
Russell, W.H., *A Diary in the East during the Tour of the Prince and Princess of Wales.* (London: George Routledge, 1869).
Soyer, A., *Soyer's Culinary Campaign* (London: G. Routledge & Co., 1856)
Stanmore, Lord, *Sidney Herbert: Lord Herbert of Lea* (London: John Murray, 1906), Vol. 2.
Sterling, A., *The Highland Brigade in the Crimea* (Minneapolis: Absinthe Press, 1995, but first published in 1895 by Remington & Co., London).
Trevor-Barnston, M. (ed.), *Letters from the Crimea and India* (Whitchurch: Herald Printers, 1998).
Wolesley, Viscount *The Story of a Soldier's Life* (London: Archibald Constable, 1903), Vol. 1.
Wrottesley, G., *Life and Correspondence of Field Marshal Sir John Burgoyne, Bart.* (London: Richard Bentley, 1873), Vol. 2.

2.3 Published books and pamphlets by contemporary authors

A Non-Commissioner, *A Report on the Sanitary Condition of the Army Particularly during the Late War with Russia* (Undated pamphlet).
Anon [Peter Benson Maxwell], *Whom Shall We Hang? The Sebastopol Enquiry* (London: James Ridgeway, 1855).
Baudens, L. (Translated by Hough, F.B.), *On the Military and Camp Hospitals and the Health of Troops in the Field Being the Result of a Commission to Inspect the Sanitary Arrangements of the French Army, and Incidentally Other Armies in the Crimean War* (New York: Baillière Brothers, 1862).
Colborne, J. and Brine, F., *The Last of the Brave; or the Resting Place of our Fallen Heroes in the Crimea and Scutari* (London: Ackermann, 1857).
Elphinstone, H.C., *Journal of the Operations of the Corps of Royal Engineers*, Part 1 (London: Eyre and Spottiswoode, 1859).
Filder, Commissary General [W.], *The Commissariat in the Crimea: being Remarks on those Parts of the Report of the Commission of Enquiry into the Supplies of the British Army which Relate to the Duties of the Commissariat* (London: W. Clowes, 1856).
Fraser, P., *A Treatise upon Gunshot Wounds of the Chest* (London: John Churchill, 1859).
Gordon, W., *Balaclava and the Sebastopol Inquiry* (Dated December 1855; downloaded from Dracobooks, 5 May 2015).

Hall, Sir J., *Sir John Hall's Rejoinder to Dr. Sutherland's Reply to his Observations on the Report of the Sanitary Commissioners, at the Seat of War in the East in 1855 and 1856* (London: W. Clowes, 1858).
Kinglake, A.W., *The Invasion of the Crimea* (Edinburgh: Blackwood, 1891), Vol. 7.
Longmore, Deputy Inspector General T., *A Treatise on the Transport of Sick and Wounded Troops* (London: HMSO, 1869).
Longmore, Surgeon-General T., *The Sanitary Contrasts of the French and British Armies during the Crimean War* (London: Charles Griffin & Co., 1883).
Macleod, G.H.B., *Notes on the Surgery of the War in the Crimea with Remarks on the Gunshot Wounds* (London: John Churchill, 1858).
Martineau, H., *England and Her Soldiers* (London: Smith, Elder, & Co., 1859).
Nightingale, F., *A Contribution to the Sanitary History of the British Army during the Late War with Russia* (London: Harrison, 1859). [Published anonymously]
Nightingale, F., *Notes on Hospitals*, (3rd edition) (London: Longman, Green, Longman, Roberts, and Green, 1863).
Osborne, S.G., *Scutari and its Hospitals* (London: Dickinson Brothers, 1855).
Parkes, E.A., *Report on the Formation and General Management of Renkioi Hospital on the Dardanelles, Turkey*, (War Department, April 1857).
Rathbone, P.H., *A Week in the Crimea* (Liverpool, 1855).
Snow, J., *On the Mode of Communication of Cholera* (London: Churchill, 1855).
Sutherland, J., *Reply to Sir John Hall's 'Observations' on the Report of Sanitary Commission Despatched to the Seat of War in the East, 1855–56* (London: Harrison, 1857).
Tulloch, Colonel [A.M.], *The Crimean Commission and the Chelsea Board Being a Review of the Proceedings and Report of the Board* (London: Harrison, 1857).

2.4 Journal articles by contemporary authors

Hodge, W.B., 'On the mortality arising from military operations', *Journal of the Statistical Society of London*, 19 (1856), pp.219–71.
Milroy, G., 'On the Sickness and Mortality in the French Army in the East from 1854 to 1856', *British Medical Journal*, 17 April 1858 and *Medical Times and Gazette*, 1 May 1858.
Thomson, R.T., 'Mortality among Officers of the British Army in the Crimea', *Journal of the Statistical Society of London*, 20 (1857), pp.54–60.

2.5 Official and semi-official documents

Anon, *Instructions to Army Medical Officers for their Guidance on the Appearance of Spasmodic Cholera in the United Kingdom* (London: Eyre and Spottiswoode, 1856).
Gordon, A.H., *General Orders Issued to the Army of the East, from April 30, 1854 to December 31, 1855 Selected by the Hon Sir Alex H Gordon* (London: J.W. Parker, 1856).
Hart, H.G., *The New Annual Army List, and Militia List for 1856* (London: John Murray, 1856).

Report of Committee of the Crimean Army Fund, September 1855 (London: Richard Clay, 1855).

Sayer, Captain [F.], *Despatches and Papers Relative to the Campaign in Turkey, Asia Minor, and the Crimea during the War with Russia in 1854, 1855, 1856* (London: Harrison, 1857).

Sutherland, J., *Appendix (A) to the Report of the General Board of Health on the Epidemic of Cholera of 1848 and 1849* (London: HMSO, 1850).

The Queen's Regulations and Orders for the Army 1844 (3rd edition), (London: Parker, Furnivall, and Parker).

2.6 Later published books including biographies

Adkin, M, *The Charge. The Real Reason Why the Light Brigade was Lost* (London: Leo Cooper, 1996).

Arthur, M., *Symbol of Courage. The Men Behind the Medal* (London: Pan Books, 2005).

Ascherson, N., *Black Sea: Coast and Conquests: from Periciles to Putin* (London: Vintage Books, 2007).

Badem, C., *The Ottoman Crimean War (1853–1856)* (Leiden: Brill, 2010).

Baldwin, G., Daniel, M.and Greenough, S. *All the Mighty World. The Photographs of Roger Fenton, 1852–1860* (New Haven: Yale University Press, 2004).

Baring Pemberton, W., *Battles of the Crimean War* (London: Pan Books, 1968).

Barthorp, M., *Heroes of the Crimean War: The Battles of Balaklava and Inkerman* (London: Blandford, 1991).

Bartrip, P., *Themselves Writ Large: The British Medical Association 1832–1996* (London: BMJ Publishing Group, 1996).

Bentley, N. (ed.), *Despatches from the Crimea* (London: Frontline Books, 2008).

Best, B., *The Luckless Tribe: The Golden Age of British War Reporters* (Peterborough: FastPrint Publishing, 2012).

Blomfield-Smith, D., *Heritage of Help: The Story of the Royal Patriotic Fund* (London: Robert Hale, 1992).

Bodart, G., *Losses of Life in Modern Wars: Austria-Hungary: France* (Oxford: Clarendon Press, 1916).

Bostridge, M., *Florence Nightingale: The Woman and Her Legend* (London: Viking, 2008).

Bowler, R.A., *Logistics and the Failure of the British in the America 1775–1785* (Princeton: University Press, 1975).

Brandon, R., *The People's Chef: Alexis Soyer, a Life in Seven Courses* (Chichester: John Wiley, 2004).

Brighton, T., *Hell Riders: The Truth about the Charge of the Light Brigade* (London: Viking, 2004).

Buttery, D., *Messenger of Death. Captain Nolan and the Charge of the Light Brigade* (Barnsley: Pen & Sword Military, 2008).

Lloyd, C. and Coulter, J.L.S., *Medicine and the Navy 1200–1900, Volume 4, 1815–1900* (Edinburgh: E & S Livingstone, 1963).

Cantlie, N., *A History of the Army Medical Department* (Edinburgh: Churchill Livingstone, 1974), Vols 1 & 2.
Christopher, M., *Logistics and Supply Chain Management* (2nd edition) (London: Financial Times Management, 1998).
Coates, T., *Delane's War* (London: Biteback Publishing, 2009).
Conache, J.B., *Britain and the Crimea, 1855–56: Problems of War and Peace* (London: Macmillan, 1987).
Cook, E., *The Life of Florence Nightingale* (London: Macmillan, 1913).
Cooke, B., *The Grand Crimean Central Railway* (2nd edition) (Knutsford: Cavalier House, 1997).
Cowan, R., *Relish. The Extraordinary Life of Alexis Soyer* (London: Phoenix, 2007).
Curtiss, J.C., *Russia's Crimean War* (Durham, N.C.: Duke University Press, 1979).
Edgerton, R.B., *Death and Glory: The Legacy of the Crimean War* (Oxford: Westview Press, 1999)
ffrench Blake, R.L.V., *The Crimean War* (Barnsley: Pen & Sword Military, 2006).
Figes, O., *Crimea. The Last Crusade* (London: Allen Lane, 2010).
Finer, S.E., *The Life and Times of Sir Edwin Chadwick* (London: Methuen, 1952).
Fletcher, I., and Ishchenko, N., *The Battle of the Alma 1854* (Barnsley: Pen & Sword Military, 2008).
Fletcher, I., and Ishchenko, N., *The Crimean War: A Clash of Empires* (Staplehurst: Spellmount, 2004).
Flintham, D., *Civil War London* (Solihull: Helion, 2017).
Gill, G., *Nightingales: The Story of Florence Nightingale and her Remarkable Family* (London: Hodder and Stoughton, 2004).
Goldfrank, D.M., *The Origins of the Crimean War* (London: Longman, 1994).
Goldie, S.M., *Florence Nightingale: Letters from the Crimea 1854–1856* (Manchester: Mandolin, 1997).
Gordon, S., *Shadows of War, Roger Fenton's Photographs of the Crimean, 1855* (London: Royal Collection Trust, 2017).
Grehan, J., *Voices from the Past: The Charge of the Light Brigade* (Barnsley: Frontline Books, 2017).
Hankinson, A., *Man of Wars: William Howard Russell of* The Times (London: Heinemann Educational Books, 1982).
Harrison, M., *Medicine and Victory* (Oxford: University Press, 2004).
Harrison, M., *The Medical War. British Military Medicine in the First World War* (Oxford: University Press, 2010).
Hibbert, C., *The Destruction of Lord Raglan* (Ware: Wordsworth Editions, 1999; originally published by Longmans, 1961).
Hodder, E., *The Life and Work of the Seventh Earl of Shaftsbury, K.G.* (London: Cassell, 1898).
Howard, M.R., *Walcheren 1809: The Scandalous Destruction of a British Army* (Barnsley: Pen & Sword Military, 2012).

Hutchinson, W., Vice, M. and Small, B.J., *Crimean Memories: Artefacts of the Crimean War* (Atglen, PA: Schiffer Publishing, 2009).

Jones, D.R., *Forgotten Places of the Crimean War.* (Raleigh, USA: Lulu Publishing, 2015).

Jones, D.R., *In the Footsteps of James Robertson and Felice Beato, Crimean War Photographers* (Raleigh, USA: Lulu Publishing, 2013).

Jones, D.R., *In the Footsteps of Roger Fenton Crimean War Photographer* (Raleigh, USA: Lulu Publishing, 2012).

Kaufman, M.H., *Surgeons at War: Medical Arrangements for the Treatment of the Sick and Wounded in the British Army during the Late 18th and 19th Centuries* (London: Greenwood Press, 2000).

Keller, U., *The Ultimate Spectacle: A Visual History of the Crimean War* (Australia: Gordon and Breach, 2001).

Kent, N., *Crimea: A History* (London: C. Hurst & Co., 2016).

Kerr, P., Pye, G., Cherfas, T., Gold, M. and Mulvihill, M., *The Crimean War* (London: Boxtree, 1997).

Kirby, P.R., *Sir Andrew Smith, M.D., K.C.B.: His Life Letters and Works* (Cape Town: Balkena, 1965).

Koç, O.M. (ed.), *150th Anniversary of the Crimean War* (Istanbul: Sadberk Hanim Museum, 2006).

Lalumia M.P., *Realism and Politics in Victorian Art of the Crimean War* (Ann Arbour, Michigan: UMI Research Press, 1984).

Lambert, A.D., *The Crimean War: British Grand Strategy, 1853–1856* (2nd edition) (Farnham: Ashford, 2011).

MacMunn, G., *The Crimea in Perspective* (London: G. Bell & Sons, 1935).

Massie, A. (ed.), *A Most Desperate Undertaking: The British Army in the Crimea, 1854–56* (London: National Army Museum, 2003).

McDonald, L. (ed.), *Florence Nightingale. The Crimean War* (Waterloo, Ontario: Wilfred Laurier UP, 2010), Vol. 14.

McDonald, L., *Florence Nightingale at First Hand* (London: Continuum UK, 2010).

McGuigan, R., *Into Battle: British Orders of Battle for the Crimean War, 1854–56* (Bowdon: Withycut House, 2001).

Mead, G., *Victoria's Cross: The Untold Story of Britain's Highest Award for Bravery* (London: Atlantic Books, 2015).

Melvin, M., *Sevastopol's Wars: Crimea from Potemkin to Putin* (Oxford: Osprey Publishing, 1917).

Mercer, P., *Inkerman 1854: The Soldiers' Battle* (Westport, Ct: Praeger, 2008).

Miles, A.E.W., *The Accidental Birth of Military Medicine* (London: Civic Books, 2009).

Neuhauser, D. and Blanchard C.E., (eds), *Florence Nightingale: Measuring Hospital Care Outcomes* (Joint Commission on Accreditation of Healthcare Organizations, 1999), pp.229–46.

Nixon, K., *The World of Florence Nightingale* (Andover: Pitkin Publishing, 2011).

Öztuncay, B., *Robertson, Photographer and Engraver in the Ottoman Empire* (Istanbul: Vehbi Koç Foundation, 2013).
Ponting, C., *The Crimean War: The Truth Behind the Myth* (London: Chatto and Windus, 2004).
Porundominsky, V., *Pirogov in Sevastopol* (Moscow: Young Guard, 1965) Translated by A. Kennaway; Royal Society of Medicine Library, WZ 100 (Pir).
Prinzing, F., *Epidemics Resulting from Wars* (Oxford: The Clarendon Press, 1916).
Rappaport, H., *No Place for Ladies* (London: Arum Press, 2005).
Rich, N. *Why the Crimean War?* (Hanover & London: University Press of New England, 1985).
Robinson, J., *Mary Seacole: The Charismatic Black Nurse who became a Heroine of the Crimea* (London: Constable, 2005).
Royle, T., *Crimea: The Great Crimean War 1854–1856* (London: Little Brown and Company, 1999)
Scotland T. and Heys, S., *Wars, Pestilence and the Surgeon's Blade* (Solihull: Helion, 2013).
Shepherd, J., *The Crimean Doctors: A History of the Medical Services in the Crimean War* (Liverpool: University Press, 1991), Vols 1 & 2.
Silver, C., *Renkioi Brunel's Forgotten Crimean War Hospital* (Sevenoaks: Valonia Press, 2007).
Sinclair, J., *Arteries of War* (Shrewsbury: Airlife Publishing, 1992).
Small, H., *Florence Nightingale: Avenging Angel* (2nd edition) (London: Knowledge Leak, 2013).
Small, H., *The Crimean War: Queen Victoria's War with the Russian Tsars* (Stroud: Tempus, 2007)
Smallman-Raynor, M.R. and Cliff, A.D., *War Epidemics* (Oxford: University Press, 2004).
Springman, M., *Sharpshooter in the Crimea* (Barnsley: Pen & Sword Military, 2005).
Springman, M., *The Guards Brigade in the Crimea* (Barnsley: Pen & Sword Military, 2008).
Sweetman, J., *War and Administration: The Significance of the Crimean War for the British Army* (Edinburgh: Scottish Academic Press, 1984).
Sweetman, J., *Raglan from the Peninsula to the Crimea* (London; Arms and Armour Press, 1993).
Taylor, E., *Wartime Nurse: One hundred Years from the Crimea to Korea 1854–1954* (London: Robert Hale, 2001).
Troubetzkoy, A., *The Crimean War* (London: Robinson, 2006).
van Creveld, M., *Supplying War: Logistics from Wallenstein to Patton* (2nd edition) (Cambridge: University Press, 2004).
Vaughan, A., *Samuel Moreton Peto: A Victorian Entrepreneur* (Hersham: Ian Allen Publishing, 2009).
Watson, D., *Battlefield Detectives* (London: Grenada Publishing, 2003).

Wellcome Collection: Deutsches-Hygiene Museum Dresden, *War and Medicine* (London: Black Dog Publishing, 2008).
Woodham-Smith, C., *Florence Nightingale 1820–1910* (London: John Constable, 1950).

2.7 Later journal articles and book chapters
The *Soldiers of the Queen* and *The War Correspondent* and the journals of the Victorian Military Society and the Crimean War Research Society respectively.

Barham, J., 'A Tragic Second Winter for the French Army', *The War Correspondent*, 24:1 (2006), pp.23–6.
Barnsley, R.E., 'Sir John Hall', *Transactions of the Cumberland and Westmorland Antiquarian Society*, 64, (1966), pp.402–8.
Barnsley, R.E., 'Teeth and Tails in the Crimea', *Medical History*, 7 (1963), pp.75–9.
Bennett, J., 'The Medical Service in the Crimea', in *Redressing the Balance* (London: Florence Nightingale Museum Trust, 1991), pp.3–10.
Blanco, R., 'Sir James McGrigor and the Army Medical Corps', *History Today*, 21 (1971), pp.132–9.
Bourne, G.H., 'Records of Older Literature of Tissue Changes in Scurvy', *Proceedings of the Royal Society of Medicine*, 37 (1944), pp.512–6.
Boxall, M., 'Devotion to Duty at the Expense of Life: The Fire on the Troopship *Europa*', *The War Correspondent*, 34:2 (2017), pp.32–3.
Brebner, J.B., 'Joseph Howe and the Crimean War Enlistment Controversy between Great Britain and the United States', *Canadian Historical Review*, (1938), pp.300–27.
Connor, H., The Use of Chloroform by British Army Surgeons during the Crimean War', *Medical History*, 40 (1998), pp.161–93.
Cook, G.C., 'Influence of Diarrhoea Disease on Military and Naval Campaigns', *Journal of the Royal Society of Medicine*, 94 (2001), pp.95–7.
Cooter, R., 'Of War and Epidemics: Unnatural Couplings, Problematic Conceptions', *Journal of the Society of the Social History of Medicine*, 16:2 (2003), pp.283–302.
Dean, M.E. 'Selective Suppression by the Medical Establishment of Unwelcome Research Findings: the Cholera Treatment Evaluation by the General Board of Health', *Journal of the Royal Society of Medicine*, 109:5 (2016), pp.200–5.
Fisher, G., 'Doctor Dartnell's List', *The War Correspondent*, 30:4 (2013), pp.29–42.
Fisher, G., 'The Failure of the Ambulance Corps in the Crimean War', *Journal of the Society of Army Historical Research*, 91 (2013), pp.161–81.
Fisher, G., 'Treatment of the Crimean Wounded', *The War Correspondent*, 28:3 (2010), pp.33–44.
Fowler, S., '"Pass the Hat for your Credit's Sake and Pay-Pay-Pay" Philanthropy and Victorian Military Campaigns', *Soldiers of the Queen*, No. 105 (2001), pp.2–5.

Harrison, M., 'War and Medicine in the Modern Era', in Wellcome Collection,: Deutsches-Hygiene Museum Dresden, *War and Medicine* (London: Black Dog, 2008), pp.11–27.

Hendriks, I.F., Bovill, J.G., van Luijt, P.A. and Hogendoorn, P.C.W.,'Nikolay Ivanovich Pirogov (1810–1881): a Pioneering Russian Surgeon and Medical Scientist', *Journal of Medical Biography*, (2016) DOI: 10.1177/0967772016633399.

Hinton, M., 'A Letter from Captain William Donald Macdonald, 93rd Regiment, together with a Commentary on Medical Matters', *The War Correspondent*, 28:3 (2010), pp.27–8.

Hinton, M., 'A Recommendation that Maimed Men be Employed in the L.T.C.', *The War Correspondent*, 31:4 (2014), pp.31–2.

Hinton, M., 'A Short-lived Cholera Epidemic in Scutari during November 1855', *Soldiers of the Queen*, No. 171 (2018), pp.22–8.

Hinton, M., 'Capital Punishment in the Crimea', *The War Correspondent*, 29:1 (2011), p.38

Hinton, M., 'Cholera in the British Army and Navy during the Crimean War', in M. Holland, G, Gill, and S. Burrell (eds.), *Cholera in Conflict*, (Leeds: Medical Museum Publishing, 2009), pp.160–203.

Hinton, M., 'Death by Charcoal', *The War Correspondent*, 18:4 (2001), pp.33–7.

Hinton, M., 'Death by Drowning during the War with Russia', *The War Correspondent*, 34:3 (2014), pp.5–13.

M. Hinton, 'Memorials to Lord Raglan in England and Wales', *The War Correspondent* 35:2 (2017), pp.8–11.

Hinton, M., 'On the Watering of Horses', *Equine Veterinary Journal*, 10 (1978), pp.27–31.

Hinton, M., 'Reporting the Crimean War', *19: Interdisciplinary Studies in the Long Nineteenth Century*, 20 (2015), DOI: http://doi.org/10.16995/ntn.711.

Hinton, M., 'The Infamous Massacre at Sinope: a Turkish Perspective', *The War Correspondent*, 30:3 (2012), pp.19–22.

Hinton, M. and Starling, P.H., 'A Possible Third Double Victoria Cross for the Army Medical Services?', *Journal of the Royal Army Medical Corps*, 158 (2011), pp.191–2.

R. Huntsman, M. Bruin, and D. Holttum, 'The Naval Hospital at Therapia', *Journal of the Royal Naval Medical Service*, 88:1 (2002), pp.5–27.

Iezzoni, I.E., '100 Apples Divided by 15 Red Herrings: a Cautionary Tale from the Mid–19th Century on Comparing Hospital Mortality Rates', *Annals of Internal Medicine*, 124 (1996), pp.1079–85.

Littledale, S., 'Deptford's Navy Victualling Yard', *Magazine of the Friends of The National Archives*, 28:2 (2017), pp.7–10.

McKeown, T. and Record, R.G., 'Reasons for the Decline of Mortality in England and Wales during the Nineteenth Century', *Populations Studies*, (1962), 16, pp 94–122.

McKeown, T., Brown, R.G. and Record, R.G., 'An Interpretation of the Modern Rise of Population in Europe', *Population Studies*, (1972), 26, pp.345–82.

Metcalf, N.H., 'The Influence of the Military on the Civilian Uncertainty about Modern Anaesthesia between its Origins in 1846 and the End of the Crimean War in 1856', *Anaesthesia*, 40 (2005), pp.594–601.
Murray, C.K., Hinkle, M.K. and Yun, H.C., 'History of Infections Associated with Combat-Related Injuries', *Journal of Trauma*, 64 (2008), pp.S221–31.
Y. Naumova, 'Russian Medical Service during the Crimean War: New Perspectives', *19: Interdisciplinary Studies in the Long Nineteenth Century*, 20 (2015), DOI: http://doi.org/10.16995/ntn.712.
Robertson-Steel, I., 'Evolution of Triage Systems', *Emergency Medicine Journal*, 23:2 (2006), pp.154–8.
Rosenbaum, S., 'More than a Century of Army Medical Statistics', *Journal of the Royal Society of Medicine*, 83 (1990), pp.456–63.
Rosenbaum, S., 'Report of the Royal Sanitary Commission (1858)', *Journal of the Royal Army Medical Corps*, 105:4 (1959), pp.1–11.
Shepherd, J.H., 'The Smart of the Knife – Early Anaesthesia in the Services', *Journal of the Royal Army Medical Corps*, 132 (1985), pp.109–15.
Small, H., 'The Impact of the Crimean War on Public Health', in Wellcome Collection,: Deutsches-Hygiene Museum Dresden, *War and Medicine* (London: Black Dog, 2008), p.31.
Smallman-Raynor, M.R. and Cliff, A.D.,'The Geographical Spread of Cholera in the Crimean War: Epidemic Transmission in the Camp Systems in the British Army of the East, 1854–55', *Journal of Historical Geography*, 30 (2004), pp.32–69.
Starling, P., 'Sir John Pringle, 1707–1782: the Father of Modern Military Hygiene', *The War Correspondent*, 19:4 (2002), pp.48–9.
Stevenson, R., 'The Osmanli Irregular Cavalry: Organising Britain's Bashi-Bazouks', *The War Correspondent*, 33:1 (2015), pp.35–42.
Sweetman, J., '"Ad hoc" Support Services during the Crimean War, 1854–5', *Military Affairs*, 52 (1988), pp.135–40.
Sweetman, J., 'Military Transport in the Crimean War, 1854–1856', *English Historical Review*, 88 (1973), pp.81–91.
Sweetman, J., 'The Crimean War and the Formation of the Medical Staff Corps', *Journal of the Society of Army Historical Research*, 53 (1975), pp.113–9.
Toppin, D., 'The British Hospital at Renkioi 1855', *The Arup Journal*, 16:2 (1981), pp.3–20.
Wampler, P., 'Pick Sanitation Over Vaccination in Haiti', *Nature*, 470 (2011).

3 Unpublished documents

Hall, J., *Observations on the Difficulties Experienced by the Medical Department of the Army, During the Late War in Turkey, by Sir John Hall, M.D., K.C.B., Principal Medical Officer of that Army*. Unpublished versions in RAMC: 397F/RT/2 and TNA: WO 33/3B. (Hall, *Observations*.)

Köremezli, İ., Ottoman *War on the Danube. State, Subject, and Soldier, 1853–1856* (Unpublished PhD thesis, 2013: İhsan Doğramaci Bilkent University, Ankara).
Smith, K. (ed.) *Letters from Francis Beckford Ward*. (Unpublished typescript, 1994).

4 Miscellaneous publications

Browning, D.C., *Dictionary of Quotations and Proverbs* (London: Chancellor Press, 1988).
Cockton, P., *Subject Catalogue of the House of Commons Parliamentary Papers 1801–1900* (Cambridge: Chadwyck-Healey, 1988), Vol. 5.
Gowing, T.S., *The Philosophy of Beards* (London: T.T. Lemare, 1875).
Knowles E. (ed.), *The Oxford Dictionary of Phase and Fable* (Oxford: University Press, 2004).
Simpson, J., *The Concise Oxford Dictionary of Proverbs* (Oxford: OUP, 1981).
Trevelyan, G.M., *English Social History* (London: The Reprint Society, 1948).

Index

Aberdeen, George Hamilton-Gordon, 5th Earl of 25, 36, 72–73, 88, 108, 261, 301, 322
Abscesses 195, 197, 224, 251–252, 256–257
Abydos iv, x, 36, 98, 101, 104–105, 107, 115–116, 137, 155–156, 165, 190, 236, 327
Accidents 31, 50, 227, 277, 303
Adjutant General (AG), Army of the East xiv, 52, 58, 62–63, 65, 72, 78, 91, 100–101, 103, 122, 125, 139–142, 145, 148–151, 154–155, 162, 169, 171, 215, 268, 277–278, 281–282, 316, 319, 323–324
Adjutant General (AG), Horse Guards xiv, 32, 42, 45, 52, 55, 57, 60, 64–65, 72, 85, 90–91, 100, 151, 166, 172–173, 184, 187, 279, 316, 318, 325
Adjutant General's ledger v, 233, 238, 240
Admiralty xiv, 135, 151, 159, 169–170, 174–176, 179–180, 188
Advanced dressing stations 123, 231
Agent of Transports (AoT) xiv, 109, 139–140, 150–151, 169, 322
Airey, Major General Sir Richard xix, 45, 63, 79, 108, 137, 276, 306, 318–319, 322
Alma, Battle of the 25, 115, 136, 156–158, 225, 231, 233–234, 238–239, 242, 246, 266, 283, 298, 303, 333
Ambulance Corps iii, xiv, 66–67, 88, 132–133, 163, 190, 336
Ambulance, French xi, 66, 140, 145–146, 305
Ambulance/Hospital Waggons/Wagons xi 60, 66, 123, 133, 143–145, 147–148, 157, 231, 233, 317
Ammunition 85, 150, 277
Amputations 219, 243–244, 258, 295
Army Medical Department (AMD) iii, vi,
xiv, 23, 29, 35, 41, 43, 54–56, 59, 65–66, 68, 71, 75–76, 78, 136, 139–141, 151, 153, 161, 163–164, 191, 230, 261, 265, 268, 270, 277, 285–286, 288–289, 291, 298, 302, 323, 325, 333
Army of the East iii, vii, x, 25–26, 30, 35, 41–42, 50, 55, 77, 98, 165, 194, 196, 211, 233, 322–325, 327–328, 331, 338
Army Works Corps (AWC) xiv, 43, 84, 275, 300, 321
Assistant and Deputy Assistant Quarter Master General (AQMG/DAQMG) xiv, 19, 73, 86, 91, 94, 120, 137, 140, 142, 148, 150, 152, 157, 172, 277, 279
Association (later *British*) *Medical Journal* 27, 29, 64, 68–69, 73, 189, 270
Austria 24, 38, 332

Balaklava General Hospital x, 36, 98–99, 116–117, 130, 236
Balaklava, Battle of 285, 297,
Balaklava/Balaclava x–xi, iv, vii, 19, 25, 36, 52–54, 62–66, 79–80, 82–83, 86–88, 91–92, 94–95, 98, 106–107, 110, 115–119, 120–124, 130–131, 140–143, 145–146, 149–154, 156–158, 162–163, 167, 169, 171–172, 192, 210, 217, 231, 233–234, 236, 238–240, 244, 246, 253, 262, 266, 269, 273, 275–276, 279–280, 285, 292, 297–298, 318, 322–323, 327, 330, 332
Balkans 23
Baltic Sea and Region 24, 37, 135, 175, 188, 203, 293, 328
Barnston, Major Roger 82, 86, 276
Barrack Hospital, Scutari 31, 62, 101, 160, 247, 253, 263, 265–266, 271, 273–274
Bath, City of 179
Bath, Order of the 71, 298
Battlefield Casualties iv, 122, 240, 249–250

340

Black Sea iv, 21, 24–27, 37–38, 91, 93, 97, 106, 125, 137, 152, 163, 203, 227, 261, 293, 303, 311, 329, 332
Black Sea Fleet 37, 328
Blantyre, Charles Walter Stuart 12th Lord 72–73
Bosphorus Region v, viii, xi–xii, xviii, 21, 36, 60, 63, 67, 75, 101, 103–104, 109–111, 113, 121, 131, 137, 149, 159–160, 167, 202, 210, 215, 219–220, 223, 230, 235–236, 247–250, 253, 255, 266–267, 284, 289, 306, 314, 316–317, 322–325
Boxer, Rear Admiral Edward 86, 135, 209, 262, 276, 323
Bracebridge, Charles Holte 52, 89, 271–2, 322
Brighton 189
British Army/Army of the East iii, vii, xix, 22, 24–26, 30, 34–37, 39, 41–44, 47, 50–51, 53, 55, 68, 75, 77, 79, 85–86, 91, 95, 98, 101, 104, 112, 115, 124, 148, 165, 202, 210–211, 214, 233, 268, 290, 292, 295, 299, 302, 305, 313, 321–325, 327–331, 333–338
  1st Division 58, 114, 122, 264
  2nd Division 84, 91, 141, 264, 277
  3rd Division 60, 72, 83, 114, 141, 264
  4th Division 72, 123, 141, 144, 149
  Light Division xi, 68, 122, 124, 140, 145, 212, 245, 283, 311, 322
  Highland Brigade 79, 84, 208, 212, 217, 330
  Grenadier Guards 49, 305, 307
  Coldstream Guards 122, 225
  5th Dragoon Guards 206, 225
  6th Dragoons 71, 227, 297
  7th Hussars 70
  17th Lancers 297
  7th Regiment 71, 297, 311
  14th Regiment 279
  18th Regiment, 84
  20th Regiment 161
  21st Regiment 286
  23rd Regiment 71, 245, 283, 297
  30th Regiment 209
  31st Regiment 127
  33rd Regiment 138
  38th Regiment 264
  39th Regiment 84, 188
  46th Regiment 315
  50th Regiment 138
  55th Regiment 123
  57th Regiment 274
  66th Regiment 176
  77th Regiment 282, 311
  93rd Regiment Front cover, 312, 317, 337
  Rifle Brigade 41, 89, 144, 206, 215, 305, 311
British German Legion 42, 47, 194
British Italian Legion 47
British (previously *Association*) *Medical Journal* 29, 38, 297,331–332
British Swiss Legion 42, 47, 108
Brompton Barracks xi, 180–181, 183–184
Brunel, Isambard Kingdom 74, 93, 111, 292, 308, 322–323, 335
Bulgaria iii–iv, vii, xi, xiii, 24, 31, 36–37, 48, 56–57, 59, 66, 72, 77, 99, 113–115, 122, 130–132, 137, 199, 202, 207–208, 210–212, 228–229, 249, 270, 324
Burgoyne, Lieutenant General Sir John 87, 94, 301, 307, 315, 322, 330
Burnett, Sir William (Director General, Naval Medical Department) 189, 213
Burns 224, 234–235, 237, 245, 251–252, 258

Cacolets, French xi, 133, 142, 145, 147
Calthorpe, Major Somerset John Gough 87–88, 305, 329
Cambridge, HRH Duke of 70, 264, 267, 300, 307
Camp General Hospital 98–99, 119, 123, 130–131, 150, 236, 250
Campbell, Sir Colin 84, 122, 275
Cantlie, General Sir Neil 23, 30, 37, 52, 55, 58–60, 64–68, 71, 75, 79, 89, 97–98, 109–110, 114–115, 132–133, 135, 137, 139, 143, 188–189, 206, 219, 226, 230, 262–263, 285–286, 288, 290, 293, 296–297, 316–317, 333
Castle Hospital xi, 65, 98–99, 118–119, 121, 130–131, 192, 222, 236
Catarrh 195, 197, 222, 257–258
Cattle x, 79–80, 86, 144, 276
Cavalry vii–viii, x, 25–26, 31, 33, 35, 41–47, 66, 98, 104–105, 121, 123–124, 133, 141–142, 145, 149, 153, 190, 202, 208–209, 212, 217, 226–227, 237–238, 242–243, 245, 256, 277, 279, 338
Coal/Charcoal 81, 92, 153, 167, 227, 228, 279, 281, 328, 337

342 Victory Over Disease

Contusions 234–235, 245, 258
Chadwick, Edwin 269, 272–273, 333
Chatham xi–xii, 46, 60, 65–66, 132, 168, 170–175, 177–183, 186–187, 189–192, 222, 255–257, 259, 307–308
Chichester xii, 89, 165, 178–180, 186, 188–189, 257
Children 164, 169–170, 176–177, 179, 184–186
Chloroform 204, 293–295, 336
Cholera v, viii, xi, 22–23, 28, 31, 48–49, 54–55, 115, 127, 131–132, 163, 167, 176, 191, 194–197, 200–213, 220, 226–230, 249, 256–257, 270, 295, 303, 315, 318, 322, 324, 327–328, 331–332, 336–338
Clarendon, George William Frederick Villiers, 4th Earl of 26, 38, 87–88, 103, 105, 128, 162, 167–168, 260, 267, 312–313, 317, 322
Clothing/Clothes xii, xix, 23, 25, 43, 59, 82, 84, 88, 91–92, 126, 149–150, 177, 183, 190, 204, 206, 218, 263–264, 267–269, 277–278, 281–282, 287, 291, 296, 316–318, 327
Coal/Charcoal 81, 92, 153, 167, 227, 228, 279, 281, 328, 337
Codrington, General Sir William John 76, 84–85, 94, 108, 165, 223, 289, 292, 322
Colic 195, 197, 200, 224, 251–252
Commissariat iv, 41, 43, 53, 68, 78–79, 81, 84–86, 92, 96, 105, 129, 144, 227, 230, 268, 277, 299, 317, 328, 330
Commissary General 79, 81, 87, 152, 268, 323, 328, 330
Constantinople x, 26, 52–53, 72, 75, 81–82, 102, 107, 128, 151, 163, 165, 261–262, 267, 269, 307, 312, 317, 325
Contusions 234–235, 237, 245, 258
Convalescents xii, 32, 61, 63, 98, 100–101, 103–105, 107–110, 114, 116, 119–120, 122, 124–128, 130, 137, 150, 162, 164, 169–170, 182–183, 186–189, 192, 235–237, 246, 250, 295, 308
Corfu 82, 100, 125, 167, 318
Crimea Medal 298, 307

Daily News 34, 53, 68, 91, 161, 171, 174, 177, 185, 187, 190, 260, 283, 304
Dardanelles 23, 53, 60, 74, 104, 107, 111, 202, 322, 331
Dawson, Sergeant Thomas xii, 307–308

Deal 188–189
Debility 125, 218, 256–258
Deptford 95, 180, 337
Devonport 168, 172, 176, 179, 187–188
Diarrhoea v, xi–xii, 54, 107, 131, 168, 178, 195, 197, 200–203, 206–207, 212–213, 223–224, 227, 247–248, 251–252, 256–258, 286, 303, 316, 336
Discharge from the Army v–vi, viii–ix 36, 179, 182–183, 192–193, 222, 244–245, 255–260
Disease iii, v, vii–x, xix–xx, 21–22, 26, 31–32, 35, 38, 42, 47, 49–54, 64, 70, 74, 96, 105, 107, 110, 119, 124, 131–132, 152, 168, 184, 194–198, 200, 223, 226, 229–231, 247, 253, 255–260, 264, 267–268, 273, 283, 287, 290–291, 295–296, 302–303, 316, 318, 321–323, 327, 329, 336
Dispensers of medicines 57–59, 77, 158, 210
Drunkenness/Intemperance 66, 223–224
Dysentery v, xi–xii, 54, 107, 125, 131, 168, 195, 197, 200–201, 203, 206–207, 212–213, 217, 223–224, 227, 230, 247–248, 250–252, 257–258, 286, 316, 321
Dyspepsia 195, 200, 224, 251–252

Edinburgh 37, 190, 294
Erysipelas xii, 182, 195, 219–221, 228, 296
Estcourt, Major General James Bucknall Bucknall 52, 91, 100, 145, 151, 209, 316, 319, 323–4
Evacuation/Evacuees iv, vi, 18–19, 22, 25, 36, 52, 88, 93, 115, 117, 121, 127, 131, 132, 135–138, 149–153, 155–159, 163–166, 171–172, 189–190, 192, 203, 213, 230, 233, 235, 246, 249–250, 254, 256–258, 261, 276, 305–206, 311, 315–316, 320
Evans, Lieutenant General Sir de Lacy 83, 87, 264
Eye disease/Ophthalmia 116, 129, 172, 195–197, 222, 224, 251–252, 257, 258

Female nurses iv, 61, 74–76, 78, 103, 111, 165, 230, 306, 324, 329, 335
Fenton, Roger 306–307, 319, 332–334
Fever v, xi–xii, 22, 31, 34, 54, 107, 110, 125, 125, 128, 168, 189, 194, 196, 200–201, 206, 213–214, 218, 226–228, 256, 259, 271, 290, 296, 316

Common continued 12, 195, 197, 213–214, 223–224, 247–248, 250–252, 256–258
  Intermittent 195, 197, 213, 214
  Remittitant 197, 213–214
Filder, Commissary General William 79, 81, 84–85, 87, 92, 96, 268, 319, 323, 328, 330
First World War 21, 218, 230, 246, 287, 295–296, 315, 333
Flies 206, 225–226
Forage 81–82, 84–86, 143, 319
Fort Pitt xi, 179–183, 189
France 26–27, 38–39, 68, 230, 298, 302, 304, 329, 332
French Ambulance xi, 66, 140, 145–146, 305
French Army vii, x, 38–39, 93, 147, 211, 218, 220, 260, 301–302, 320, 331, 336
French Hospitals 113, 215, 301,
French, the vi, 25, 38, 88, 97, 104–105, 133, 143, 163, 202, 302, 330
French Military Medal 299, 328
Frostbite v, xii, 31, 107, 194, 196–197, 215–218, 228–229, 247, 249, 256–258
Fuel xix, 49, 79, 81, 84–85, 89–90, 92, 167, 316, 319, 328

Gavin, Dr Hector (Sanitary Commissioner) 27, 269, 271, 323–324, 329
Gallipoli vii, 21–23, 131, 171, 202
Gangrene xii, 195, 218–221, 228, 296
Gastrointestinal diseases viii, 194–196, 200, 202, 207, 224, 228, 251–252, 259
General Board of Health 204–205, 211, 327, 332, 336
General Hospital Returns viii, 74, 119–120, 130, 215, 219, 235–236, 252, 256–258, 266
General Hospitals iv, v, vii–viii, xi, xiii, 19, 34–35, 37, 57, 60, 62–64, 74–76, 88, 97–101, 104, 107, 114–117, 119–123, 130–131, 137, 140–141, 150, 159–160, 177, 179–180, 194, 196, 199–200, 215, 219, 222, 233, 235–236, 247, 250, 252, 256–258, 266, 269, 271
General Return A viii, 23,35–36, 52, 194–196, 200, 207, 210, 213, 217, 220, 222–225, 235, 237–238, 250–251, 256–258
General Return D 44, 46, 51,
Generosity vii, 177
Gibraltar 127, 164, 167, 172, 176, 323

Gozo 100, 125–127, 164, 192
Gravesend 164, 174, 190
Gunshot wounds v, viii, xii, 23, 120, 130–131, 179, 193, 219–220, 228, 234–237, 243–246, 249, 258, 294, 296, 330–331

Hall, Dr Sir John iii, 29–30, 37, 39, 46, 49–51, 54, 56–60, 62–67, 69–70, 72–74, 76, 78, 89–92, 98, 100–101, 103–105, 107–116, 119–121, 123–125, 127–129, 133, 136–145, 147–154, 157, 161–163, 167–169, 172, 190, 202, 204, 215, 217, 246, 262–263, 265–268, 270–271, 273–278, 280–285, 288–289, 293–296, 298, 302, 318–320, 323, 330–331, 336, 338
Hansard xix, 34, 37, 57, 68, 73, 92, 283, 289
Hardinge Field Marshal Viscount Henry 45–46, 60, 69, 98, 131–132, 135, 170, 173, 179, 186, 266–267, 300–301, 323
Harrison, Professor Mark 21, 24, 319, 321, 333
Haslar Hospital 180, 185, 188, 191
Hay 81, 89
Heath, Captain, RN, Leopold George 91, 109–110, 329
Herbert, Baron Sidney xix, 28, 46, 52, 59, 61, 63, 72–73, 80, 103, 107, 128, 131, 145, 253, 261–262, 265, 267, 271, 273, 286, 299, 301, 307, 317, 323–324, 330
Horse Guards 25, 32, 45, 52–53, 57–58, 60, 64–65, 70, 72, 85, 91, 96, 100, 135, 151, 170, 173, 217, 242, 279, 282, 300, 307, 316, 318, 325
Horses 66, 71, 84–85, 92, 116, 129, 133, 142–145, 147–148, 150, 166, 169, 172, 184, 206, 226, 277, 314, 317, 337
Hospital Commission/Commissioners vi, xviii, 36, 52, 55, 57, 61, 63, 80, 103, 116, 132–133, 138, 143, 145, 152–154, 159–160, 261, 268, 287–288, 294, 318, 327
Hospital Dressers 59, 77, 158
Hospital Orderlies iii, 60–66, 73–74, 100–101, 103, 113–114, 125–126, 132, 139–140, 151–155, 160, 165–166, 226, 261
Hospital Sergeants 63–64, 166

Hospital Ships/Transports iv, vii, xi, 35, 57, 64, 100–101, 103, 106–107, 123, 134–136, 138, 150–153, 155–156, 158, 160, 163–165, 167, 171, 172, 185, 187, 194, 196,

Hospitals iii–v vii—xiii, xviii–xix, 22, 28–32, 34–37, 39–40, 48–50, 52, 54, 57, 59–67, 72–78, 88–94, 97–131, 137, 140–142, 149–150, 156–157, 159–160, 163–170, 172–174, 176–197, 199–200, 203, 205, 207, 209–210, 213, 215, 218–228, 230, 233–236, 244, 246–253, 255–258, 261–263, 265–267, 269–274, 277–278, 281–289, 292, 298, 302, 305–306, 308, 316–318, 322, 324, 327–331, 334–335, 337–338

House of Commons vi, xiv, 36, 68, 71, 92, 189, 261, 263, 283, 325–326, 339

Huts 53–54, 81–82, 86, 92–94, 98, 101, 116–117, 119, 121, 123–124, 126–127, 130, 154, 220, 226–227, 267, 280, 287, 316–320, 328

Illustrated London News x–xii, 27, 34, 37, 40, 80, 83, 90, 93, 101–102, 105–106, 118–119, 133–134, 136, 143–144, 146–147, 169, 175, 181, 183–185, 188, 191, 232, 269, 275, 294, 305–306, 309–310, 312

Illustrated Times x–xii, 102, 106, 112, 117–118, 122, 134, 276, 305, 307–310

Incised wounds 23, 234, 237, 245, 258

India 30, 55, 77, 82, 128, 145, 293, 329–330

Infantry vii–viii, x, 25–26, 31, 33, 35, 41–48, 53, 57–58, 64, 98, 121, 133, 143, 159, 190, 202, 207, 209, 217, 222–223, 226–227, 237–238, 242–243, 245, 256, 279

Inkerman/Inkermann, Battle of xi–xii, 25, 70, 87, 134, 143–144, 156–158, 231, 233–234, 238–240, 242, 246, 266, 298,308, 312, 332, 334

Invalid Depot 114, 130, 172, 174–175, 177, 183

Isle of Wight 126, 164, 172, 176, 189–190

Kadikoi 53, 83, 124, 217, 301

Keller, Ulrich 38, 305–307, 334

Kinglake, Alexander William 50, 135, 268, 273, 331

Kuleli (also Kukeieh, Kulali and Kululee) iv, vii, x, 34, 47, 100–102, 103, 160, 192, 270, 327

Laing, Staff Surgeon Patrick Sinclair (Hospital Commissioner) 261

Lalumia, Matthew Paul 38, 293, 304–305, 307, 334

The Lancet 59, 63–64, 69–71, 73, 97, 106–107, 123, 129–130, 135, 141, 165, 189, 202, 266, 286, 290, 297–298

Land Transport Corps (LTC)/Land Transport iii–iv, x, xiv, 42–43, 50, 53–54, 67, 80–81, 84–85, 92, 96, 105, 129, 133, 148, 150, 194, 300, 321, 324

Latrines 94, 124, 206, 225, 262–263, 270, 275, 277, 279, 281, 321

Legion of Honour 298

Lime Juice 28, 88, 95, 156, 158, 215, 217, 268, 295

Liverpool 166, 170, 172, 180, 188–189, 279, 290, 303

London Gazette 34, 37, 53, 70, 223, 278, 297–299

Luscombe, Dr Edward Thornhill 28, 44, 329

Luxations 224, 234, 245, 251–252, 258

Lyons, Admiral Sir Edmund 120, 137, 151, 157, 276, 323

Maclean, Professor William Campbell 304, 323, 330

Macleod, Dr George Husband Baird 219–220, 296, 331

MacMunn, General Sir George 37, 81, 84, 96, 131, 334

McDonald, Professor Lynn 30–31, 89, 107, 128, 215, 219, 253, 265–267, 273, 277, 290, 334

Malaria 22–23, 212, 214, 230

Malta ii, 24, 47, 73, 82, 94–95, 98, 100, 124–127, 139, 164–165, 167–171, 173–174, 202, 212, 227, 323

Marines 84, 157, 300

Marmora, General Alfonso Ferrero de al 209

Martineau, Harriet 36, 97, 136, 229, 246, 290–291, 331

Maxwell, Peter Benson (Hospitals Commissioner) xviii, 18, 52, 55, 61, 80–81, 85, 96, 103, 131, 261–262, 264–265, 267, 288, 294, 321, 324, 330

Mayall, John Jabez Mayall. xii, 307–308
McGrigor, Sir James 29–30, 55, 219, 262, 286, 323, 325, 336
McMurdo, Colonel William Montague Scott (Director General, Land Transport Corps) 67, 148, 150, 324
McNeill, Sir John (Supplies Commissioner) 79, 267–268, 324
Medical and Surgical History viii, 23, 31, 33, 35, 37, 41–42, 44, 46, 48–49, 51–52, 54, 56, 59, 74–75, 77, 98, 100, 104, 106–107, 109, 111–113, 117, 119–120, 122, 127, 130, 133, 143, 152, 155, 158–160, 179–180, 185, 187, 190, 192, 194, 196–198, 200, 202–204, 207, 209–215, 218–220, 222, 224–228, 231, 233, 235–238, 242–245, 251–252, 255–259, 266, 274, 281–282, 295, 328
Medical Board 22, 127
Medical Department iii, vi, xiv, 23, 29, 35, 39, 41, 55, 65, 68, 70–72, 74–75, 88, 90, 98, 105, 108, 111, 123, 136, 144, 149, 152, 168, 189, 213, 217, 254, 261, 270, 282, 284–286, 322–323, 325–326, 328–329, 333, 338
Medical Officers iii, 28–29, 46, 52, 55–57, 60, 67–73, 76, 78, 90, 94, 110, 114, 120, 122–123, 125–127, 138–139, 141–142, 148–149, 151–155, 157–158, 161–162, 165–166, 170–171, 173–174, 183, 187–188, 191, 203–205, 209, 217, 220, 246, 269, 274–275, 277, 280–282, 284–286, 289–291, 294, 297–299, 302, 315, 319, 327, 331
  Regimental 55, 115, 282
  Senior 58, 71, 148, 274, 278, 298
  Staff 55, 57, 77
Medical equipment/supplies/stores iv, 68, 77, 138, 152, 156, 161, 165, 293
Medical Staff Corps (MSC) iii, xiv, 29, 43, 62, 64–65, 72, 133, 139, 187, 194, 300, 338
Medical Times and Gazette 38, 69–71, 73, 101, 106–107, 117, 123, 129, 170, 176, 178, 182–184, 187, 189, 202, 204, 206–207, 211, 263, 281, 285, 289, 297–298, 316, 331
Medicines/Medical comforts 59, 77, 115, 124, 138, 140, 151–152, 167–168, 177, 268, 286
Mediterranean Fleet 24, 323

Mediterranean Sea and Region iv, 124, 214, 328
Medway, River 179–180, 183
Military Authorities 23, 30, 49, 55, 65–66, 69, 76, 95, 100,114, 128, 135–136, 139–140, 142, 155, 167, 169, 176, 192, 230, 271, 277, 289, 320
Military Secretary (Crimea) 50, 57, 67, 81, 87, 128–129, 132, 148, 161, 163, 215, 278, 280
Military Secretary (Horse Guards) 60, 66, 97–98, 126, 134–135, 148, 166, 168–169, 176, 178–180, 186, 187–188, 217, 297
Military Surgeons iii, 27–28, 56, 67, 71, 73, 78, 298, 302
Military Undersecretary (War Officer) 63, 70, 108, 125–127, 133, 164, 166–167, 189, 191, 204, 282, 324
Milroy, Dr Gavin (Sanitary Commissioner) 38, 218, 219, 220, 269, 323–324, 331
Mitra, Sidda Mohana 30, 66, 74,108, 137–138, 150, 202, 268, 281, 330
Monastery Hospital 36, 98–99, 120, 130, 222, 236
Monro, Dr Donald 28, 329
Mules 52, 90, 92, 116, 123, 129, 133, 140, 145, 147–150, 154

Napoleon Bonaparte/Napoleonic Wars 24, 28, 39, 44–45, 79, 230, 260
Napoleon III/Emperor of France 39, 174, 260, 300
Naval Authorities 95, 120, 125, 137, 157, 163,
Naval Brigade 121, 203
Naval Hospitals 34, 121, 188
Naval Medical Department 189, 213, 254
Netley Hospital 60, 182, 191
Newcastle, , Henry Pelham Clinton, 5th Duke of 26, 30, 44, 49, 57, 60, 63, 67, 73–74, 80, 82, 85, 95, 98, 100, 105, 108, 111–112, 127–128, 131, 135, 160, 26530, 44, 49, 57, 60, 63, 67, 73–74, 80, 82, 95, 100, 105, 108, 111–112, 127–128, 131, 135, 26530, 44, 49, 57, 60, 63, 67, 73–74, 80, 82, 95, 100, 105, 108, 111–112, 127–128, 131, 135, 160, 26530, 44, 49, 57, 60, 63, 67, 73–74, 80, 82, 95, 100, 105, 108, 111–112, 127–128, 131, 135, 265–267, 301, 304, 317, 324, 327

Nightingale, Florence ii, xv, xvii–xx, 29–32, 36–37, 52, 76, 89–90, 107, 128–131,149, –150, 215, 219–220, 230, 247, 250, 253–254, 262, 265–267, 271–273, 277, 287–288, 290, 295, 307, 313–314, 316, 320, 322, 324–325, 331–336
Nosocomial (hospital acquired) infections v, 195, 218–219, 228, 247

Omer Pasha 47
Ordnance x, xiv, 33, 42–43, 81, 86, 92, 94, 145, 180, 186, 190, 209, 212, 256, 293, 299, 328
Osborne, Hon. the Revd Sidney Godolphin 73, 159–160, 263, 265, 288, 324, 331
Ottoman Empire 24, 38, 307, 332, 335, 339

Palmerston, Henry John Temple, Viscount 26, 46, 69, 81, 165, 182, 205, 269–270, 283, 301, 307, 324, 327
Panmure, Fox Maule, 2nd Baron xix, 19, 25–26, 30, 36, 46–47, 50, 53, 57–58, 64, 67, 71–73, 82, 85, 94, 103–104, 106–112, 120, 125–128, 133, 142, 148, 157, 164–165, 182, 186–187, 204, 209, 223, 230, 267, 269–271, 274–275, 279–280, 285, 289–290, 297, 301, 311–312, 316, 318–320, 323–324, 328–329
Parkes, Dr. Edmund Alexander 74, 104, 111, 113, 324, 331
Paulet, , Major General Lord William 62–63, 67, 101, 103–107, 109, 111, 124–125, 127–129, 149–152, 160, 162, 165, 267, 270–271, 275, 317, 324–325
Peninsular War 30, 97, 231
Pirogov, Nikolai 39–40, 335, 337
Plymouth xii, 95, 165, 171–172, 174–177, 179–180, 187–189, 257
Pneumonia 195, 222, 229, 247
Port Admiral 80, 120, 157, 262, 275–6, 322–3
Portsea xi, 173, 184–185, 188
Portsmouth vii, xi–xii, 95, 164–166, 169, 171–180, 183–190, 192, 257
Pack animals 66, 82, 85, 92–93, 96, 293
Précis of Letters 35, 37, 54, 56, 58–60, 62–67, 70, 72, 74, 94, 97, 100–101, 104, 106–111, 114, 119, 123–129, 133–135, 137, 143, 145, 148, 157, 162, 164–169, 171–173, 176, 178–180, 184–190, 202, 274, 282
Principal Medical Officer (PMO) xiv, 65, 67, 204

Balaklava 62, 140–141, 152, 154, 160, 162, 172, 275
Chatham/Fort Pitt 171, 179–180, 183
Corfu 125
Devonport 172, 187–188
Of Divisions 66, 68, 72, 91, 114, 122, 140–141, 144–145, 148–149, 153, 282–283, 322
Liverpool 188
Malta/Gozo 124–126
Plymouth 164–165
Portsmouth 165–166, 169, 171, 173, 176, 178–180, 184, 187–188
Scutari 60, 62–63, 67, 69, 100–101, 104–106, 114, 125, 129, 137, 151, 160, 163, 169, 190, 215, 219, 262, 271, 323
Pringle, Sir John 28–29, 316, 329, 338
Prophylaxis 23, 203–204, 217
Punishment 53, 195–197, 223–225, 251–252, 337
Purveyors/Purveyor's Department 59, 64–65, 76, 100, 125, 142, 151, 173, 177, 187, 209, 261, 266

Quartermaster General (QMG) xiv, 45, 49, 63, 66–67, 73, 78–79, 82, 84, 88, 90–92, 94, 98, 100, 104–105, 108–110, 116, 119–120, 125, 127, 129, 136–140, 142–145, 147–148, 150–154, 157, 163, 169–170, 172, 179, 185–190, 268, 276–280, 291, 306, 318–319, 322
Queen's Regulations 46, 67–68, 89, 152, 162, 168, 277–278, 332
Quinine 204, 214, 268

Raglan, Field Marshal Fitzroy James Henry Somerset, 1st Baron 25, 30, 38, 49, 52, 57–58, 60, 63, 67, 69, 72–74, 78, 80–83, 85, 87–88, 92, 95, 98, 100–101, 103–105, 107, 111, 114–115, 125, 128–129, 131–133, 135, 137–138, 140–142, 144, 148–152, 155, 161–162, 165, 168, 170, 202, 210, 226, 235, 262, 265–267, 270, 275, 277–279, 294, 301, 307, 315, 317–319, 323–325, 333, 335, 337
Railway x, 24, 43, 81, 83–84, 86, 96, 122, 133, 150, 163, 176, 179, 233, 260, 267, 293, 321, 333
Rawlinson, Mr Robert (Sanitary Commissioner) 269, 279, 324
Recruitment/Recruits iii, 44–47, 49–51, 53,

Index 347

60–61, 64–65, 72–73, 85, 98, 105, 120, 132, 157, 220, 291
Regimental and Divisional Hospitals iii, iv, vii, xi–xii, 35, 62, 75–76, 93, 97–98, 115, 119, 121, 123–124, 131, 150, 163, 192, 200, 233, 235–236, 247–250
Renkioi iv, x, 36, 73–75, 77–78, 93, 98, 100, 104–105, 107–108, 111–113, 155–156, 192, 236–237, 322, 324, 331, 335, 338
Repatriation iv–v, 164, 191, 255–258
Respiratory diseases 31, 107, 196, 222, 226–228, 259
Rhodes 100, 128
Roads 49, 79–84, 86, 95–96, 133, 140, 142, 145, 149, 153–154, 160, 163, 267, 317, 319
Roebuck, John i36, 261, 325
Romaine, Deputy Judge Advocate General William Govett 45, 149, 223, 325, 330
Royal Army Medical Corps (RAMC) Archive xiv, xvii, 30, 34, 37, 46, 50, 52, 56–58, 60, 62, 64–65, 69–70, 74, 78, 89–90, 92, 98, 100–101, 103–105, 108–111, 114–116, 119–120, 124–125, 127–129, 135, 137–138, 140, 143–145, 147–155, 161–163, 168, 190, 202, 206–207, 215, 217, 233, 239–241, 254, 270, 272, 275, 278, 282–283, 293–294, 318, 338
Royal Artillery (R.A)/Artillery viii, x, xiv, 25–26, 33, 35, 37, 41–42, 45, 47, 53, 55–56, 66, 78–79, 84, 87, 102, 133, 141, 144, 180, 186, 209, 226, 242–243, 245
Royal Commission/Royal Commission Report vi, 28, 30, 34, 37, 60, 62–64, 68, 72, 74, 90–91, 97–98, 101, 108, 110, 113–114, 119–120, 122, 125, 127–129, 133, 138, 140–141, 143–145, 149, 151, 164–167, 170, 179, 187, 191, 215, 217, 261, 271–273, 276–278, 280–282, 286–287, 289, 292, 322–323, 325, 327
Royal Dock Yards 95
Royal Engineers (RE)/Engineers xiv, 25–26, 32, 35, 41, 45, 53, 78, 83, 86, 113, 122, 131, 171, 177, 242, 253, 263, 272–273, 311, 322, 330
Royal Navy/Navy iv, 24, 37, 49, 81, 86, 95, 114, 135–137, 139, 157, 165, 167, 180, 191,206, 210, 212–213, 301, 313, 327,337
HMS *Albion* 311
HMS *Arethusa* 100, 125, 171
HMS *Belleisle* 135

HMS Bellerophron 171
HMS *Britannia* 166, 172, 187–188
HMS *Caledonia* 187–188
HMS *Centaur* 176,
HMS *Cressy* 175
HMS *Diamond* 121
HNS *Firebrand* 176
HMS *Highflyer* 171
HMS *Leander* 120, 157
HMS *Malacca* 171, 177
HMS *Neptune* 170, 176–178, 184–185
HMS *Resolute* 176
HMS *Retribution* xi, 173, 175, 184
HMS *Sanspareil* 83
HMS *Simoom* 162
HMS *Transit* 186
HMS *Urgent* 341
HMS *Valorous* 162
HMS *Vulcan* 155, 164
HMS *Wasp* 120, 157, 161
Royal Patriotic Fund vi, 300–301, 328, 332
Royal Sappers and Miners (RS&M) viii, xiv, 25–26, 33, 41–42, 180, 184, 186, 209, 242–243, 245
Russell, William Howard 69, 81–82, 86, 119, 129, 138–139, 150–152, 154, 223, 275, 294, 303–304, 313, 325, 330, 333
Russia and the Russians iii, 21–27, 34–36, 38–40, 69–7, 87, 94, 101, 129, 148, 206, 228, 230, 242, 246, 249, 272, 293, 302, 304, 313, 325, 328, 330–333, 337
Russian Government 39, 94
Russian Medical Department/Services/Hospital 39 306, 328, 338

Sailing ships/transports/vessels 81, 156–158, 165, 167, 190–191, 328
Sanitary Commission/Commissioners vi, xix, 17–19, 27, 36, 103, 129, 155, 160, 205, 213, 230, 250, 253, 262, 267, 269–276, 278–282, 284–285, 287–290, 296, 316, 320–321, 323–325, 328, 331, 338
Sardinian Army/Sardinians 22. 25, 38, 71, 83, 112, 209
Sayer, Captain Frederic v, 25–26, 32, 41–42, 47–48, 159, 233, 242–243, 278, 325, 332
Scurvy v, xi–xii, 28, 31, 79, 88, 95, 107, 194, 196–197, 215–218, 220, 228, 247–248, 256, 268, 282–283, 295–296, 315, 336

Scutari iv–vii, x–xii, xviii–xix, 30, 34, 36–37, 39, 59–63, 65–67, 69, 73, 75, 89, 93, 98, 100–112, 114–116, 119, 121, 125, 128–131, 137, 139, 141, 149–153, 155–156, 159–160, 162–165, 169–170, 172, 174, 177, 187, 190, 192, 208–209, 215, 218–220, 228, 230, 247, 249–250, 253–254, 256–258, 261–263, 265–267, 270–271, 273–274, 280, 283, 287–288, 290, 294, 301, 306, 310–313, 316–317, 323–325, 327, 330–331, 337

Sea of Marmora 128–129, 171

Seacole, Mary xviii, 76, 308, 335

Secretary at War (Sidney Herbert) 170, 299

Secretary for War (Duke of Newcastle and Lord Panmure) 58, 98, 291, 299

  Deputy Undersecretary for War (Benjamin Hawes) xiv 62, 64, 90, 110, 313, 323

  Undersecretary for War (Frederick Peel, MP) xiv 60, 170, 324

Select Committee on Sebastopol/Roebuck Committee vi, ix, xviii, 36–37, 45–46, 59, 61, 63, 72, 79, 83, 87–88, 103, 132–133, 135, 145, 150–151, 160, 192, 254, 261, 263–267, 288, 294, 324 326

Select Committee on the Army Medical Department vi, 71, 75, 111, 261, 285–286, 326

Sevastopol/Sebastopol viii, x–xii, xvii–xviii, 19, 21, 25–26, 39, 40–42, 50, 53, 56, 74, 76, 84, 113, 115, 123–124, 139, 143, 146–148, 156, 158, 192, 195, 200, 207–208, 212–213, 220, 223, 225, 228, 232, 238–241, 247, 250, 253, 263, 273, 277–279, 281, 290, 294, 296, 298, 300, 306, 308–309, 316, 318, 321, 325–326, 334–335

Shaftsbury, Anthony Ashley Cooper, 7th Earl of xix, 275, 280, 333

Shepherd, John 22–23, 28–29, 36–38, 60, 66–67, 69, 73, 75, 78, 90, 93, 104, 121–123, 132–133, 141–142, 155, 163, 191, 200, 213, 217–218, 220, 222, 225, 233, 235, 237, 261, 273–274, 278, 294–296, 335, 338

Sillery, Major Charles 101, 103, 262, 325

Simpson, General Sir James 25, 50, 53–54, 67, 84, 127, 148, 154, 274, 279–281, 319, 325

Simpson, William 154, 281, 305, 329

Sinope 24, 100, 129, 337

Smith, Dr Sir Andrew iii, xi, 23, 30, 37, 54–56, 58–67, 70–75, 94–95, 97, 100–101, 103–104, 106–111, 114, 116, 119, 123–129, 132–138, 143, 145, 147–148, 151, 153, 157, 161–162, 164–173, 176, 178–180, 183–192, 202, 204, 207, 212, 215, 217, 219, 226, 262, 267–268, 274, 278, 282, 288, 293,295, 319–320, 322–325, 334

Smyrna iv, x, 36, 47, 73–75, 77–78, 98, 100–101, 105–111, 116, 128, 155–156, 165, 167–168, 192, 215, 236–237, 325, 327–329

Snow, Dr John 28, 205, 212–213, 318, 331

Soap 187, 282–283

Sore throat 195, 197, 224, 251–252

South African War vii, 22–23

Southampton x, 93, 171, 174–175, 177, 191

Soyer, Alexis 89–90, 330, 332–333

Spence, DIGH Thomas (Hospital Commissioner) 157, 261–262, 325

Spithead 171–172, 174–176

Staff surgeons x, 56–57, 60, 68, 105–106, 113, 123, 126, 160, 162, 168, 170, 175–176, 183, 274, 276, 296, 298–299

Stafford, Mr Augustus 71, 73, 261, 265, 285, 288, 325

Steam-powered ships/steamers/steam xi, 24, 81, 92, 109, 135, 137, 139, 151, 156, 158–159, 163, 165, 167, 169, 171–172, 174, 176, 261, 291, 276, 293, 303, 328, 341

Stretchers/Bearers 133, 140–141, 147, 155, 160, 173, 233, 262

Stores 43, 62, 68, 77, 81, 84–88, 94–95, 115, 120, 126, 138, 152, 155, 160–161, 165, 317, 327

Storks, Major General Henry Knight 74, 104–109, 112, 187, 325

Stoicism iii, 51–52, 55

Stratford Canning, Viscount Stratford de Redcliffe 26, 52, 87, 101, 103, 105–106, 128, 162, 167–168, 262, 267, 312–313, 317, 325, 330

Strood 170, 179, 183

Supplies, non-medical 22, 25, 36, 49, 81–85, 91, 95–96, 116, 121, 132, 143, 145, 151, 154, 177, 210, 217–218, 267–268, 283, 288, 293, 296, 298, 315, 317, 324–325, 327, 330

Index 349

Supplies Commission/Commissioners vi, 36–37, 66, 79, 82, 91–93, 116, 121 132, 143. 145, 154, 217–218, 267–268, 283, 324, 325, 327
Surgeons/Doctors, Civilian vi, 37, 71–72, 77–78, 109, 210. 285–286, 298
 Aitken, Dr William 322
 Bryce, Dr Charles 39, 113, 129, 215, 302, 329
 Lyons, Dr Robert D 50, 74, 322-3
 Macleod Dr George Baird 219
 Meyer, Dr John 74, 108, 110
 Wells, Dr Spencer 107, 116–117, 122, 263
Surgeons, Military (Regimental and Staff) iii, x, 27–29, 55–58, 60–62, 67–73, 75, 78, 87, 91, 105, 115, 121, 123, 127, 136, 149, 151, 160–162, 175, 183, 188, 198, 202, 210, 225, 235, 244–245, 279, 283, 286, 293, 295, 298–299, 302
 Alexander, Staff Surgeon Thomas 68, 90, 322
 Armstrong, Staff Surgeon 126
 Baxter, Staff Surgeon Francis Hastings 168
 Bostock, John Ashton (Scots Fusilier Guards) 145, 329 (letters)
 Brady, Assistant Staff Surgeon Thomas Clarke 299
 Cattell, Assistant Surgeon William (5th Dragoons) 206–207, 225
 Cowan, Assistant Surgeon James McHattie (55th Regiment) 123
 Cumming, IGH Alexander (sometime Hospital Commissioner) 63, 89, 100–101, 103–104, 106–107, 109, 125, 128–129, 190, 261, 267, 271, 323
 Dartnell, Staff Surgeon George Russell 182–183, 336
 Dumbreck, DIGH David 23, 113–114, 139, 141, 151–153, 215, 265–266, 294, 298, 323
 Fair, Acting Assistant Staff Surgeon, George 299
 Gibb, Acting Assistant Surgeon Spencer Boyd (1st Dragoons) 178
 Gibbons, Assistant Surgeon John (44th Regiment) 299
 Gibson, DIGH James Brown 126–127, 298
 Greig, Assistant Staff Surgeon David 94–95, 149, 329 (letters edited by Hill)
 Hale, Assistant Surgeon Thomas Egerton (7th Regiment) 71, 297
 Jeeves, Assistant Surgeon William Young (38th Regiment) 299
 Lawson, Assistant Staff Surgeon George 91, 133. 329 (letters edited by Bonham-Cater and Lawson)
 Lawson, DIGH Robert 91, 107, 152–153, 162, 323
 Linton, DIGH William 23, 114, 202, 298
 Longmore, Surgeon Thomas (19th Regiment) 32, 301–302, 331
 Ludlow, Assistant Staff Surgeon Henry Harvey 274
 Macartney, Surgeon, (77th Regiment) 282 (though not named)
 MacKinnon, Assistant Surgeon William (42nd Regiment) 296
 Menzies, DIGH Duncan 67, 69, 98, 137, 160, 262, 265, 324
 Mitchell, Staff Surgeon John 23
 Moorhead, Staff Surgeon Thomas 106
 Mouat, Surgeon James (6th Dragoons) 71, 284–285, 289, 297, 299
 O'Callaghan Acting Assistant Staff Surgeon Charles 299
 Odell, Staff Surgeon William 174
 Rutherford, Staff Surgeon William 296
 Sandwith, Acting IGH Humphrey 299
 Saunders, Staff Surgeon George 170
 Scott, Assistant Surgeon John James (57th Regiment) 274
 Sylvester, Assistant Surgeon Henry Thomas (23rd Regiment) 71, 297, 299
 Taylor, Assistant Staff Surgeon Arthur Henry 153
 Taylor, Staff Surgeon George 90
 Teevan, Staff Surgeon Thomas 176
 Watt, Surgeon William Godfrey (23rd Regiment) 245 (though not named), 283
 Williams, Assistant Surgeon John Ignatius Purcell (Rifle Brigade) 144
 Wilson, Assistant Surgeon Robert (7th Hussars) 70 (though not named)
 Wrench, Assistant Surgeon Edward Mason (34th Regiment) 226, 274, 306
Surgeons, Naval 103, 160–161, 202, 206, 211, 298
 Deas, IGH&F David 254, 298

Sutherland, Dr John (Sanitary Commissioner) 124, 205, 211, 253, 267, 269, 271, 273, 276, 279–281, 283–285, 289, 325, 327, 331–332
Sweetman, John 29, 38, 43, 64, 79–80, 85, 87, 96, 299–300, 335, 338

Tchernaya, Battle of xii, 25, 148, 309
Telegraph 24, 108, 164–165, 174, 293
Tents 49, 82, 93–94, 98, 115–116, 121–122, 126, 154, 203, 218, 220, 226–227, 277, 279–280, 282–283, 320
The Times 30, 34, 37, 46, 53, 65–66, 69, 81, 86, 89, 116, 119, 126–127, 131, 133, 135, 137–139, 141, 150–155, 160–161, 164–167, 169–174, 176–178, 180, 182–190, 202, 209–210, 218–219, 223, 227, 263, 265–267, 274–275, 280, 283–284, 294, 301, 304, 307, 312–314, 317, 325, 333
Transport ships and tugs 37, 81, 103, 108–109, 114, 134–137, 155, 158–159, 162–164, 167–168, 170, 175–176, 191, 227, 276, 328
  Adelaide 106, 171, 190
  Alma 170–171
  Alster, 82
  Andes 137–138
  Arabia 170, 174, 177–178, 186
  Argo 171
  Assistance 167
  Australian 109, 120, 151, 157, 176, 185
  Avon 136, 152, 162, 174, 178, 184–185, 202, 323
  Black Prince 176
  Blake 100
  Bombay 101, 103, 114, 137
  Brandon 89, 104, 106–107, 109–110, 151, 158, 186, 332
  Cambria 137–138, 170, 189
  Camperdown 176
  Candia 97, 171, 173, 177, 184
  Canterbury 186
  Cape of Good Hope 171
  Chapman 186, 190
  Charity 167
  City of Norwich 185
  Clifton 158
  Colombo 136, 160–161
  Columba 171
  Comet, 176
  Confreance 176
  Conrad 175
  Cornwall 137, 175, 186
  Culloden 183
  Cumberland 171
  Croesus 170, 185
  Dragon 171
  Drobak 171–172
  Duke of Cornwall 185
  Dunbar 125, 136, 139, 155, 171, 174, 183
  Earl of Mulgrave 126
  Echo 176
  Emeu 100, 104, 106, 168–169, 176
  Europa 227, 336
  Euxine 170
  Germania 171, 175
  Gibraltar 171–172, 176
  Golden Fleece 164, 171, 185
  Great Britain 170, 322
  Great Tasmania 165–167, 170–171
  Hansa 185
  Harbinger 164, 171, 174, 178
  Himalaya xi, 162, 169, 171–177, 184–185
  Hope 171
  Hydaspes 170, 185
  Imperador 107, 123, 158
  Imperatriz 170
  Indiana 185, 190
  Jason x, 102
  John Masterman 138–139
  Julia 170, 190
  Jura 100, 125
  Kangaroo 104, 136, 139, 155
  Lady Eglington 169
  Lancashire 176
  Libertas 164, 168, 176, 183
  Lord Raglan 170
  Magicienne 171
  Mangerton 164
  Mauritius 173, 178, 184, 186
  Medina 162
  Medway 106, 174
  Melbourne 104, 106, 109, 151, 158, 185
  Mercia 114, 137
  Monachy 137
  Niagara 164, 170, 185
  Orient 120, 157
  Orinoco 164, 170, 178, 184
  Ottawa 109, 120, 157
  Oudine 190
  Perseverance 171

Index   351

Palmyra 164
Poietiers 120, 123, 157
Prince 88, 91, 126, 261, 325, 327
Prompt 167
Pygmy 176
Ripon 100, 170–171, 175
Robert Lowe 104, 120, 157, 170
Rockliffe 185, 190
Saldanha 165–167
Severn 107, 109–110, 120, 123, 151, 157–158, 171–172
Shearwater 171
Simla 171
Sprightly 176
St Hilda 120, 157
Sultana 124, 170, 178, 183
Sydney 107, 109, 151
Talavera 124, 171, 177, 186
Teignmouth 137
Thames 165, 171–172
Tonning 164
Trent 100, 136, 161–162
Tynemouth 53, 106, 186, 190
Victoria 174, 176
War Cloud 176
White Falcon x, 93
Wm Jackson 120, 157
Trenches/Trench warfare xi, 22, 25–26, 46, 49, 52, 55, 61, 83, 123, 134, 149, 207–208, 210, 217, 226, 239, 240, 242, 246, 264, 277, 281, 290, 306, 308, 317, 319
Tuberculosis/Phthisis 179, 185, 193–194, 222, 229, 256–257
Tulloch, Colonel Alexander Murray (Supplies Commissioner) vii, 32–33, 66, 79, 132, 267–268, 325–328, 331
Turks and Turkey iv–v, viii–ix, xi, xiii, xviii–xix, 22–25, 27, 29, 35–36, 41, 55, 59–60, 71, 77, 81, 84, 97–101, 103–106, 109, 120, 129, 131, 136, 139, 155, 157, 163–165, 167–168, 179, 189–190, 199, 208, 210, 215, 223, 230, 235–236, 246–247, 249–250, 256–257, 262, 269, 271, 293, 298, 324–325, 327–329, 331–332, 337–338
Turkish Army 38, 47, 211, 213, 329

Turkish Contingent 37, 47, 212
Typhoid 214, 230, 260, 316
Typhus 197, 213–215, 220, 229–230, 247, 260

Ulcers 195–197, 224, 251–252, 256–257, 282

Varna 36, 60, 92, 98, 113–115, 130, 138, 155, 231
Venereal disease (VD) 195–197, 220, 224, 228 251–252
Victor Emmanuel II, King of Sardinia 299, 328
Victoria, Queen/'the Queen' 27, 44–45, 177, 182, 191, 307, 312–313, 317, 329–330, 335
Victoria Cross (VC) vi, xiv, 71, 78, 285, 292, 297–298, 337
Vienna 82, 92, 126

Walcheren expedition 21–22, 333
War Department 43, 74, 79, 94, 159, 165, 331
War Office xiv, 34, 57, 59, 71, 90, 96, 111, 131–132, 164, 176, 190, 299, 324
Ward, Sir Henry 318
Wardmasters 60–63, 65, 125–126
Water 23, 27–28, 31, 112, 120, 123–124, 129, 153, 203–207, 212–213, 217, 225, 253, 262–263, 270, 277–278, 283–284, 290, 293, 295, 318, 321, 328, 337
Wellington, Duke of 30, 69, 79
Westmorland, John Fane, 11th Earl of 30, 82, 92, 126
Wetherall, Major General Sir George (see also Adjutant General (AG), Horse Guards) 45, 65, 84, 316, 325
Wheeled transport 82–83, 93, 95, 133, 145, 178 231, 367, 317
Carriages 66, 145, 148, 317
Wives 172, 184
Women 75, 103, 139, 164, 169–170, 176–177, 179, 185–186
Wood, for fuel 84, 92, 94, 283, 286
Woolwich 172, 178, 180, 186, 190

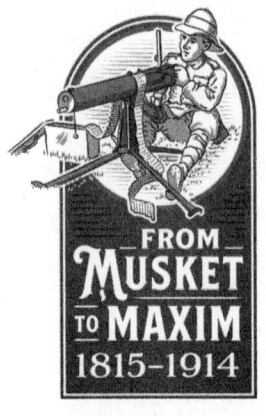

The period 1815-1914 is sometimes called the long century of peace. It was in reality very far from that. It was a century of civil wars, popular uprisings, and struggles for Independence. An era of colonial expansion, wars of Empire, and colonial campaigning, much of which was unconventional in nature. It was also an age of major conventional wars, in Europe that would see the Crimea campaign and the wars of German unification. Such conflicts, along with the American Civil War, foreshadowed the total war of the 20th century.

It was also a period of great technological advancement, which in time impacted the military and warfare in general. Steam power, electricity, the telegraph, the radio, the railway, all became tools of war. The century was one of dramatic change. Tactics altered, sometimes slowly, to meet the challenges of the new technology. The dramatic change in the technology of war in this period is reflected in the new title of this series: From Musket to Maxim.

The new title better reflects the fact that the series covers all nations and all conflict of the period between 1815-1914. Already the series has commissioned books that deal with matters outside the British experience. This is something that the series will endeavour to do more of in the future. At the same time there still remains an important place for the study of the British military during this period. It is one of fascination, with campaigns that capture the imagination, in which Britain although the world's predominant power, continues to field a relatively small army.

The aim of the series is to throw the spotlight on the conflicts of that century, which can often get overlooked, sandwiched as they are between two major conflicts, the French/Revolutionary/Napoleonic Wars and the First World War. The series will produced a variety of books and styles. Some will look simply at campaigns or battles. Others will concentrate on particular aspects of a war or campaign. There will also be books that look at wider concepts of warfare during this era. It is the intention that this series will present a platform for historians to present their work on an important but often overlooked century of warfare.

Submissions

The publishers would be pleased to receive submissions for this series. Please contact series editor Dr Christopher Brice via email (chrismbrice@yahoo.com), or in writing to Helion & Company Limited, Unit 8, Amherst Business Centre, Budbrooke Road, Warwick, Warwickshire, CV34 5WE.

BOOKS IN THIS SERIES:

1. *The Battle of Majuba Hill The Transvaal Campaign 1880-1881* John Laband (ISBN 978-1-911512-38-7)*

2. *For Queen and Company Vignettes of the Irish Soldier in the Indian Mutiny* David Truesdale (ISBN 978-1-911512-79-0)*

* Denotes books are paperback 248mm × 180mm, other books are hardback.